THIRD EDITION

NURSING RESEARCH

PRINCIPLES, PROCESS AND ISSUES

KADER PARAHOO

palgrave
macmillan

First edition 1997
Second edition 2006

Third edition published 2014 by
PALGRAVE MACMILLAN

Palgrave Macmillan in the UK is an imprint of Macmillan Publishers Limited, registered in England, company number 785998, of Houndmills, Basingstoke, Hampshire RG21 6XS.

Palgrave Macmillan in the US is a division of St Martin's Press LLC, 175 Fifth Avenue, New York, NY 10010.

Palgrave Macmillan is the global academic imprint of the above companies and has companies and representatives throughout the world.

Palgrave® and Macmillan® are registered trademarks in the United States, the United Kingdom, Europe and other countries.

ISBN: 978–1–137–28126–5

This book is printed on paper suitable for recycling and made from fully managed and sustained forest sources. Logging, pulping and manufacturing processes are expected to conform to the environmental regulations of the country of origin.

A catalogue record for this book is available from the British Library.

A catalog record for this book is available from the Library of Congress.

Typeset by Aardvark Editorial Limited, Metfield, Suffolk.

Printed in China

To Roisin, Yasmin and Ciaran for keeping my feet on the ground,
and to Eilis for her love and friendship.

Contents

List of Research Examples

List of Figures and Tables

Figures

Tables

Preface to the Third Edition

By the time this third edition is in print, this book will have reached its 18th birthday. That it has endured so long is a testimony to the fact that the core principles of research tend to remain the same even while the research process and issues can change. New ways to conduct and disseminate research are constantly being developed. And, of course, change is necessary for progress.

The increasing recognition that qualitative approaches can make a valuable contribution towards understanding people's experience of interventions in randomised controlled trials is particularly welcome. Researchers worldwide are beginning to be more open to the use of multiple methods in the same study. One of the strengths of this book from the first edition onwards has been the integration of quantitative and qualitative approaches in all its chapters.

Advances in the field of information technology and the increasing accessibility of the internet and all that it can offer have opened up new arenas where research can be learnt, conducted and disseminated. This gives rise to new practical, ethical, methodological and financial implications. No doubt discussions of these issues will fill the pages of journals for years to come.

This edition takes into account these new trends while retaining its focus on the core principles of research. Feedback from readers of the previous edition indicated a thirst for more knowledge of qualitative approaches. To this end, three new chapters (on phenomenology, grounded theory and ethnography) have been added to provide readers with a good grasp of these approaches and of their potential use in addressing nursing and health issues. The rest of the book has been updated, particularly in terms of the research examples.

In writing this third edition, the main consideration has been to keep what is good and enhance it by taking current research issues into account. The result is an updated text that can continue to help readers acquire the necessary skills to read, understand, critically appraise and use research.

Acknowledgements

The authors and publishers would like to thank John Wiley and Sons for permission to reproduce Fig. 8.1, originally from Carter H, MacLeod R, Brander P and McPherson K (2004) Living with a terminal illness: patients' priorities. *Journal of Advanced Nursing*, 45, 6:611–20 © 2004 Blackwell Publishing Ltd; Table 19.1, originally Table 2 (p. 331) from Ussher J M, Perz J and Gilbert E (2013) Information needs associated with changes to sexual well-being after breast cancer. *Journal of Advanced Nursing*, 69, 2:327–37 © 2013 Blackwell Publishing Ltd; Fig 19.1, orignally from Röndahl G, Innala S and Carlsson M (2004) Nurses' attitudes towards lesbians and gay men. *Journal of Advanced Nursing*, 47, 4:386–92 © 2004 Blackwell Publishing Ltd; and Fig. 19.2, originally from Gudmundsdottir E, Delaney C, Thoroddsen A and Karlsson T (2004) Translation and validation of the nursing outcomes classification labels and definitions for acute care nursing in Iceland. *Journal of Advanced Nursing*, 46, 3:292–302 © 2004 Blackwell Publishing Ltd. Figures and tables all reproduced with kind permission from John Wiley and Sons Ltd.

Introduction

Nursing research, globally, has a relatively short history dating back to the 1950s, and one of uneven development. The USA, Western Europe, Canada and a handful of countries such as Australia, Hong Kong and Taiwan among others have experienced meaningful growth in terms of the status of nursing research, funding and publication. Of these countries, none rivals the USA, with its establishment of the National Institute of Nursing Research in 1993, supported by significant funding. In many Middle Eastern, Asian, African and Eastern European countries, nurses are still struggling to build a viable and sustainable research base in nursing.

There is no doubt that one of the preconditions for the development of nursing research is the integration of nursing education into tertiary-level education. There is a direct link between degree-level nurse education and the growth in nursing research. This is understandable given that a nursing degree programme, like other degree programmes, involves basic training in research. The provision of doctoral-level education is also crucial in developing research capacity. The availability of research funding (from governments, businesses and voluntary organisations) is also important. Underpinning the rationale for investing in and supporting nursing research is the recognition that nurses need knowledge and skills as well as compassion in order to provide timely, safe, humane and effective intervention. Commenting on the UK government's announcement that nursing would become an all-degree profession in England by 2013, Bernhauser (2010), explains the rationale for the change:

> Over the next 15 years and even beyond, nurses will meet challenges relating to changes in demography, disease patterns, lifestyle, public expectations and information technology. We will see the greatest demands in healthcare met by nursing or other therapy care. There will also be a growing need for healthcare professionals with advanced practice skills and they will need to develop these from a graduate knowledge base.

Early nursing research focused on nurses' roles, nurses' characteristics and nurse-related issues, as well as on nurse education. There was, however, a recognition that research should focus more on what nurses do. This led to a widening of the scope of nursing research to include a focus on clients (their healthcare needs, experience and perceptions), nursing interventions, the provision of nursing care, nursing concepts and theories and research methodologies. Both quantitative and qualitative approaches featured in the research strategies used by nurse researchers.

A number of 'new' developments are likely to influence nursing research in the future. These are the impact of research on the economy and on people's lives, the increasing importance of multidisciplinary research, the use of information technology for research, and the growth in the use of mixed methods in nursing and health studies.

The emphasis on research impact requires researchers to focus more on the outcome or 'product' of their research and their engagement with users. Researchers will have to demonstrate the difference that their findings make to people's health, to healthcare organisations and to the economy in general. Working closely with users and involving them meaningfully in research can ensure that nursing research is relevant to their needs. While this already happens to some extent, it is likely that it will be the norm in the future. Users, aided and abetted by information technology, are becoming more knowledgeable, skilful and engaged in meeting and articulating their information needs.

Researching health is not the exclusive domain of nurses. Multidisciplinary research is increasingly becoming the norm. This is a positive and welcome trend. Equally important is the need for research capacity development in nursing to continue in order that nurse researchers can be, more and more, part of multidisciplinary and multiprofessional research teams.

Information technology is rapidly changing our behaviour and the world we live in. The opportunities to harness it to serve our research objectives are only now becoming clear. Online data collection through Skype, blogs, Facebook and web-based questionnaires are only a start in what could be a revolution in the way we do research. There is no limit to where this may take us. What is certain, though, is that research will become more global. We need to prepare ourselves to be at the forefront of the use of this technology and to rise to the challenge that this will bring.

The quantitative–qualitative debate is defunct. It has been replaced by discussions of how to use different methods in the same study, and the methodological and epistemological implications that mixing entails. Nursing deals with concepts such as the 'body', 'mind', 'rationality', 'emotions', 'rigour' and 'creativity', among a host of others. Nursing is the perfect arena for the eclectic use of research methodologies. Our focus on patient experience has found its way into the stronghold of quantitative research – the randomised controlled trial (RCT). The UK Medical Research Council (2008) now recognises that both the intervention and the patient's experience of it are legitimate outcomes in RCTs. Qualitative methods are an essential part of such research.

These new developments and trends are likely to lead to a new breed of nurse researcher and to an increasing scrutiny on research outcomes. For research to impact positively on health and well-being, nurse researchers will have to pay more heed to the utility of their findings for users and ways in which knowledge transfer can become real. Nurses in clinical practice, too, will play their part in shaping the future of nursing research. They have to justify what they do with sound evidence. They will also need more training in how to critically read and implement research in their practice. New skills for accessing databases and for research appraisals will feature more in nursing curricula.

The role of nurses in research

To understand the role of nurses in research, one has to refer to what 'nursing' itself is. According to the International Council of Nurses (2010):

> Nursing encompasses autonomous and collaborative care of individuals of all ages, families, groups and communities, sick or well and in all settings. Nursing includes the promotion of health, prevention of illness, and the care of ill, disabled and dying people. Advocacy, promotion of a safe environment, research, participation in shaping health policy and in patient and health systems management, and education are also key nursing roles.

There is significant scope and potential for research to inform all these areas of policy, practice and education. The extent to which this is achieved depends on how nurses perceive their role in research. This is likely to vary according to the levels at which they practise. First-level (qualified) nurses are expected to be able to search for and evaluate the relevant evidence to inform their decisions and actions. By questioning their practice, they should be able to identify problems and issues that require research investigation. Nurses need to understand the ethical implications of research and of the different methodologies in order to be in a better position to protect patients from potential harm when participating in research and to safe-guard patients' rights. To do this, they must first acquire the necessary skills and knowledge to be able to read research critically.

One of the competencies for entry to the register of the Nursing and Midwifery Council (2010) in the UK, in relation to research, is that:

> All nurses must appreciate the value of evidence in practice, be able to understand and appraise research, apply relevant theory and research findings to their work, and iden-tify areas for further investigation.

This book is written mainly for those who have little or no prior knowledge of research. It is intended to equip them with a comprehensive understanding of the concepts and principles of nursing research so that they can begin to read research critically. Postgraduate students will also find sections of the book useful. Of neces-sity, this book provides an introduction to the principles, process and issues in nursing research, as it is intended for beginners. The challenge in writing this book is to explain research in a way that attracts the interest of those who want or need to gain a basic understanding of research. No doubt readers will want to know more. For this, there are whole books written on, for example, interviewing, randomised controlled trials or grounded theory.

Book structure and content

This book opens with a discussion of the relationship between research and practice. It puts research in the context of other ways of knowing, such as intuition, tradition and experience, as well as the potential contribution of research towards enhancing practice and to the development of nursing as a profession.

There are four distinct parts to this book:

- The philosophical foundations of research (Chapters 2–5)
- The research process and research designs (Chapters 6–15)
- Methods of data collection and analysis (Chapters 16–19)
- Evaluating research studies and evidence-based practice (Chapters 20 and 21).

An understanding of the relationship between knowledge and science and the different research paradigms helps readers to put research knowledge into perspective (in relation to other belief systems). Chapter 2 explains how research has become a dominant form of knowledge production, and how our perception of reality or 'truth', and the means of studying it, can influence our choice of approaches and methods.

What constitutes nursing research and research evidence is itself problematic. There are different perspectives on research, on how it should be carried out and on its actual and potential benefits. The growing trend in mixed methods studies has given rise to new discussions about the merits and limitations of combining qualitative and quantitative methods in the same study. This book deals with many of the issues raised in this new debate. The potential contribution of both approaches is compared and contrasted, and the benefits and drawbacks of mixing them are explored. The strengths and weaknesses of a range of methodologies, in particular research methods, are also discussed. These issues are dealt with in Chapters 3–5.

The rest of the chapters follow closely the stages of the research process. Chapter 6 gives an insight into the process of different types of research as well as the main ethical implications of conducting research with humans. These issues are further raised at relevant points in the book. Chapters 7 and 8 explore the meaning and processes of literature reviews and the relationship between theory and research in quantitative and qualitative studies, while Chapter 9 deals with the formulation of questions and operational definitions.

Although a range of research designs is discussed in Chapter 10, experimental and quasi-experimental designs are given a separate and lengthy treatment in Chapter 11. Those conducting RCTs have generated a wide range of research jargon. This is explained and illustrated with examples from actual research studies. The strengths and weaknesses of the RCT, as well as its appropriateness for the study of nursing phenomena, are also considered.

Three of the most popular qualitative approaches in nursing research (phenomenology, grounded theory and ethnography) are given a chapter each (Chapters 12, 13 and 14). Readers are introduced to the different versions of each approach and to their main features. The research process in each approach is outlined, and their strengths and limitations are discussed. Their potential contribution to nursing knowledge is also explored.

Samples, sampling techniques and data collection methods are described and discussed in Chapters 15–18, while Chapter 19 is designed to help readers make sense of research findings. This book is about understanding and reading research. The penultimate chapter explores ways in which readers can evaluate research studies.

Finally, the last chapter takes a critical look at the concept of evidence-based practice and its relevance to nursing. The book ends with the topic with which it began – the relationship between research and practice. This chapter outlines the process of evidence-based practice and takes a critical look at its relevance for nursing practice. It is a reminder of the *raison d'etre* (reason for being) of nursing research.

There are three strands that run through most of the chapters:

- the integration of quantitative and qualitative concepts;
- ethical issues;
- research critique.

Although there are separate chapters on each of these topics, they are also explored in other chapters as well. For example, while Chapter 6 deals with general ethical principles, the ethical implications of interviewing are also discussed in the chapter on interviews. In this way, readers are able to put ethical principles into the context of interviewing.

One of the main features of the book is the use of examples to explain abstract concepts. In these Research Examples, the relevant parts of the articles are described or quoted, and are followed by comments designed to illustrate concepts or issues raised in the text. Therefore they should be treated as part of the text.

Finally, in an attempt to avoid the clumsy and inelegant form 'she/he', the female gender is used in this book to refer to researchers. The flipping of a coin was the 'scientific' strategy used to select the pronoun. It is, of course, acknowledged that researchers are both men and women.

To conclude, this book is not designed to teach readers how to do research but to help them to acquire a thorough and comprehensive understanding of research principles, concepts, processes and issues in order to be able to read research critically. The view taken here is that both qualitative and quantitative approaches have a contribution to make towards advancing knowledge. Research is put in the context of other ways of knowing. Throughout this book, both the potential benefits of research and the danger of blind faith in research findings are emphasised.

References

Bernhauser S (2010) Moving to an all graduate profession is a necessity. Retrieved from http://www.nursingtimes.net/moving-to-an-all-graduate-profession-is-a-necessity/5015335.article (accessed 19 November 2013).

International Council of Nurses (2010) Definition of nursing. Retrieved from http://www.icn.ch/about-icn/icn-definition-of-nursing/ (accessed 18 November 2013).

Medical Research Council (2008) *Developing and Evaluating Complex Interventions: New Guidance* (London: MRC).

Nursing and Midwifery Council (2010) Competencies for entry to the register – adult nursing. Retrieved from http://standards.nmc-uk.org/PreRegNursing/statutory/competencies/Pages/Competencies.aspx (accessed 18 November 2013).

Research and Nursing Practice

Opening thought ▶ Research without practice is like building castles in the air.
Practice without research is building castles on slippery grounds.

Introduction

This introductory chapter will examine the sources of knowledge for practice and the meaning of, and rationale for, nursing research. The role of nurses in research and the relationship between research and practice will also be explored.

Sources of knowledge for nursing practice

Much has been written about the variety of sources of knowledge from which practitioners draw. Of these, the main ones are tradition, intuition, experience and research.

Traditional knowledge

The bulk of our knowledge has been accumulated over centuries and passed down to us through literature, art, music, oral history and other such media. Traditional nursing knowledge is learnt mainly from books and journals, by word of mouth and by observing the practice of others.

Much traditional practice takes the form of rituals. For example, a traditional fasting rule for patients admitted for elective surgery is nil by mouth from midnight for a morning theatre procedure, or a light breakfast for an afternoon one (Rycroft-Malone et al., 2012). Yet there is robust evidence to show that 'it is safe for healthy adult patients undergoing elective surgery to have clear water and clear fluids up to two hours before the induction of anaesthesia and food up to six hours prior to induction' (Rycroft-Malone et al., 2012). While fasting times are generally prescribed by doctors, there are many rituals in nursing practice, such as routine blood pressure monitoring, set feeding times or putting all patients to bed at the same time, regardless of whether they want to go to sleep or not.

Jefford et al. (2009) explain that routinely performing a vaginal examination during birth to check for the nuchal cord is a ritual that started in the late seventeenth century when all aspects of birth were 'medicalised through fear'. According to them, 'when the midwife avoids routine invasive checking for the cord and instead makes individual clinical decisions for each particular woman and baby, this may be a marker of her willingness to practice as an autonomous decision maker and not just a follower of ritual'.

Traditions are important not only in passing down knowledge, but also in giving groups in society a sense of identity, belonging and pride. Through socialisation, we learn the culture of those who have gone before us. Similarly, traditional nursing knowledge and practice are learnt by novice nurses through the process of socialisation in educational institutions and clinical areas. Much of this traditional knowledge and many ritual practices are the outcomes of sound reasoning. Today's new knowledge and practices will likewise eventually become traditional. The term 'traditional' is sometimes used in a negative sense, meaning backward, outdated or unprogressive. Knowledge in itself is harmless; it is the use people make of it that can be harmful or beneficial. It should neither be rejected too quickly nor clung to rigidly, if we are to benefit from the experiences of our predecessors and continue to make progress.

Debating 'the pros and cons' of routines, Barton (2011) explains that a routine can 'be desirable, bringing comfort, certainty and quality to life, or constraining, monotonous and ineffective'. Semple (2011), on the other hand, sees 'rituals as characterised by mechanistic repetitious actions that lack thought and detract from individualised care'. However, he concedes that some routines may have a role in healthcare. No one denies that routines can provide some structure to one's practice, without which there could be confusion and misunderstanding. Guidelines and checklists can, to some extent, if used insensitively, lead to routine practice.

Intuition

Intuition by its very nature is not easy to define. It is a form of knowing and behaving that is not apparently based on rational reasoning. The use of intuition in nursing is only now beginning to attract nurse researchers' interest, so not much is known about 'how' nurses come to know there is something 'wrong' or whether they have a 'sixth' sense that tells them what to do. According to Kenny (1994), nurses use empathetic intuition in their daily practice:

> This type of intuitive thinking often occurs within the context of a nursing situation, and feeling, rather than conscious thinking, seems to predominate. Nurses know that there is something wrong but cannot explain what it is.

Intuition involves the use of all human senses such as touch, smell, hearing, sight and even taste, as well as previous experience (in the form of tacit knowledge) to assess, and react to, a situation. It happens in ways which seem to be beyond comprehension. McCutcheon and Pincombe (2001) studied nurses' understanding of intuition and their perceptions of their use of intuition, and assessed the impact of intuition on nursing practice. They found that intuition is the result of a complex interaction between a number of factors including knowledge, experience, expertise, personality and environment.

Greenhalgh (2011), who believes that intuition has a place in medical practice, explains that:

> Intuition is not unscientific. It is a highly creative process, fundamental to hypothesis generation in science. The experienced practitioner should generate and follow clinical hunches as well as (not instead of) applying the deductive principles of evidence-based medicine.

Experience and reflective practice

Nurses and midwives base their practice on their own experience and on the experience of others. Experience is a useful way of learning. There is a wealth of untapped knowledge embedded in the practice and 'know-how' of expert nurse clinicians (Benner, 1984). It is also reckoned that what we learn by experience is more enduring than what we are taught. However, our experience in itself is rather narrow. For example, in treating depression, a nurse may use one or two approaches. While the experience obtained is invaluable, she will be unfamiliar with other treatments and may either be reluctant to try them or may reject them out of hand.

We also learn a lot from the people we care for, as they have a wealth of experience with the conditions we are trying to grapple with. Livesley (2004), in her paper on 'How a personal account contributes to nurse knowledge', argues that story-telling is an important tool for nurses seeking to explore and discover the meanings of their own personal and professional experience and the experiences of those with whom they work.

There is also a degree of trial and error when learning by experience. While this may be inevitable in a few cases, there is, by and large, a risk of reinventing the wheel and a greater risk of unsafe practice. Experience is therefore an important source of nursing knowledge, but relying solely on it and overstating its importance can be detrimental to nursing practice.

A number of studies have shown that experiential knowledge and information gained by consulting colleagues are the main sources that nurses draw upon when making clinical decisions (Gerrish and Clayton, 2004; Pravikoff et al., 2005; Thompson et al., 2005). In a recent study in Ireland, Yadav and Fealy (2012) found that 'psychiatric nurses in Ireland get most of their knowledge from their everyday experiences of nursing patients and from fellow practitioners, but few seem to get knowledge to guide their practice from sources such as published professional and research journals'.

We all engage in reflection in our daily lives. This type of informal, ad hoc reflection can be deliberate or may happen spontaneously. Reflective practice, on the other hand, is a formal reflection on our actions. Although there is no consensus of what reflective practice is, it is a term that can simply mean 'adopting a thinking approach to practice' (Finlay, 2008). The degree of formality and the models, theories or frameworks that practitioners can use to guide their reflection vary between individuals and professions. Critical reflection is generally believed to be 'a process by which practitioners can better understand themselves in order to build on existing strengths and take appropriate future action' (Somerville and Keeling, 2004).

Reflective practice requires practitioners to think though the process of decision-making that leads to particular actions. The two types of reflective practice that are generally referred to are 'reflection-on-action' and 'reflection-in-action' (Schön, 1987). The former is a retrospective 'analysis' of an action that has already taken place, while the latter involves reflecting while the action is taking place. Now and then, we must stop and consider what we do, why and how we do it and to what effect, otherwise we will turn what we do into thoughtless routines. For progress to take place, we must ask if we are doing the right things and if there are alternative ways to make things better. According to Rolfe (2001), in order to become 'knowledge generators', practitioners can use reflective practice 'to uncover the rich store of experiential knowledge that lies buried within their own practice'.

Reflective practice has its own limitations. It assumes that the practitioner is capable of reflecting in a meaningful way on his or her decisions leading to a particular action, despite the acknowledgement that the rationale for action can be intuitive and difficult to verbalise. It is also believed that we can examine our prejudices, which may underpin our practice. Yet people are generally reluctant to admit their prejudices, many of which they may not be conscious of. The process of group reflection can be a daunting and threatening experience with ethical and political implications. The use of diaries and journals for reflective purposes has been criticised by Mackintosh (1998) as giving rise to issues of confidentiality. Problems and poor practice, when identified, have to be addressed; otherwise this can lead to frustration, low morale and ethical dilemmas.

Reflection as a concept to learn about our actions and about ourselves has much to commend it. Despite its problems and limitations, it should not be rejected, nor should it be the only strategy for developing practice. It must be recognised that all methods of generating knowledge have limitations, and that closing our minds to other methods can be unproductive and often dangerous.

Reflective practice has the potential to raise questions that can thereafter be explored by other means, including research. In Paget's (2001) study of practitioners' views of how reflective practice has influenced their clinical practice, some of the respondents reported that reflective practice encouraged the use of research findings in their practice. Elliott (2004) describes how the use of the 'critical incident technique' (which involves reflection on a particular incident to find out what worked or did not) led to a literature review and the identification of a researchable topic in intensive care.

Research

Research, in contrast to tradition, intuition and reflective practice, is a systematic way of knowing and lays bare its methods for all to see. Researchers collect and analyse data systematically and rigorously, and this process is described to others by means of oral and/or written presentations. Research findings by themselves are not solutions to problems. They provide new insight into phenomena or add to, confirm or reject what is already known. Decisions still have to be taken about whether the findings should be used (or not used), and how.

One may argue that, by using common sense, nurses can take the right decisions. However, they still need relevant and valid information in order to do so. What may seem simple and straightforward is not necessarily so. For example, in some cultures babies suffering from diarrhoea are not given fluids because it is believed that this will aggravate the situation. To the parents, it makes sense that in order to stop the baby from passing 'watery' faeces, they must stop the administration of fluids. In doing this, the baby is put at risk of dying from dehydration.

One of the important factors in decision-making is the availability of relevant and up-to-date information. Traditional knowledge, although an important source of information, needs to be updated. What was relevant a decade ago may not be so now. Research has the potential to provide up-to-date information that may facilitate decision-making. The perception of research data as superior to other forms of knowledge is not purely a matter of personal preference, but is dependent on the quality of the research itself. Traditional knowledge may have suited a world in which 'authority' was not questioned, people did what they were told and things were right because someone 'important' said so. However, we now live in an age when most clients are no longer the passive recipients of services, and those who hold the purse strings require business plans for the allocation and use of funds. The need to justify one's practice is greater now than it has ever been.

Using more than one source of knowledge

By separating the sources of knowledge for the sake of explanation, the impression may be given that practitioners use one source to the exclusion of others. In practice, nurses and other practitioners use a combination of these, consciously and unconsciously, depending on what their interventions consist of. Referring to the lack of consensus about what kind of knowledge is at work in the actions of social workers, Nygren and Blom (2001) ask:

> What is the role of theoretical knowledge in the moment of action, when a child is separated from its parents, when a dialogue is opened with a drug abuser, or when the client is told how much money she or he will get? To what extent is it a question of personal talent, creativity or charisma that is crucial to what will happen? Is knowledge applied in a prescriptive or instrumental way, or does it take the shape of a 'mass' or a matrix of knowledge – a more or less conscious background against which social workers reflect their sensory impressions.

Benner et al. (2008) point to the relationship between experiential learning and scientific investigations:

Often experience and knowledge, confirmed by experimentation, are treated as oppo-
sitions, as either–or choice. However, in practice it is readily acknowledged that experiential knowledge fuels scientific investigations, and scientific investigations fuels
further experiential learning. Experiential learning from particular clinical cases can help
the clinician recognize future similar cases and fuel new scientific questions and study.

It must be acknowledged, however, that there can be potential conflict when knowledge drawn from various sources is different and contradictory.

The meaning of nursing research

'Nursing research' is a broad term for all research into nursing practice and issues.
It aims to provide insights into, and an understanding of, nursing practice and its
effects on patients and their families and on the use of resources. Other areas of
nursing research include the education and training of nurses, the organisation and
delivery of services, the conditions in which nurses work, their influence on the
work environment and the effects of work on the nurses themselves.

Definitions of nursing research are difficult to find mainly because of the lack of
consensus in the definition of nursing and because nurses' roles are constantly
evolving and expanding in order to meet new demands. The definition of nursing
research is often implicit in the goals of nursing organisations. According to the
National Institute of Nursing Research (NINR; 2013), one can define nursing
research simply as research that supports and develops the work that nurses do in
order 'to promote and improve the health of individuals, families, communities and
populations'. Nursing research develops knowledge to:

- build the scientific foundation of clinical practice;
- prevent disease and disability;
- manage and eliminate symptoms caused by illness;
- enhance end-of-life and palliative care.

Healthcare is delivered not by nurses alone, but by multiprofessional teams whose
aim is to provide the best possible care for patients and their families. It follows, then,
that multidisciplinary research should be an approach of choice. Yet there are boundaries around the areas that each professional group deals with, and although these
areas can overlap, health professionals generally are aware of what constitutes their
domain of practice. There are aspects of care that are entirely or mostly delivered by
nurses, and it is legitimate that nurses seek to develop their practice with the use of
research. Both multidisciplinary and unidisciplinary research are important, and one
should not be developed at the expense of the other.

One can ask whether nursing research should be carried out only by nurses. In
theory, it may not seem important that research is 'produced by members of the
professions to whose practice it is directly or indirectly relevant' (Higher Education
Funding Council for England [HEFCE], 2001). In practice, it would be odd if

members of these professions did not engage in researching their practice. Clinically relevant questions can be developed mainly by clinicians themselves.

Clinicians are also well placed to decide on priority areas for research. According to the Department of Health (2000), there are 'two principal dimensions to influencing the research and development agenda: ensuring that important areas of research about nursing receive appropriate priority; and ensuring that general priority setting benefits from a nursing perspective'. The HEFCE (2001) explains that because it 'recognised the importance of maintaining healthy links between research, practice and teaching, it would be concerned if entire sub-fields became dominated by researchers from outside the professions'.

Nursing research uses designs and methods taken mainly from the natural and the social sciences, since nursing is concerned with the physical, psychological, social, environmental and spiritual aspects of patients and their carers. In return, nursing also provides fertile grounds for testing the theories and methods of these sciences. Nursing research is eclectic (that is, it uses a variety of methods and approaches) and sometimes modifies these methods to suit its own ends. In doing so, nursing research further develops these approaches and methods, and often gives them particular 'slants' or interpretations more suited to the context and the reality of nursing practice. Thus, nursing research makes a unique contribution to the development of approaches and methods for the study of its core issues.

The rationale for nursing research

Nurses are the largest professional group among healthcare workers worldwide. How such a workforce fulfils the health service agenda and what use they make of the sizeable budget they consume should be of concern to those responsible for the health of the population, to nurses and to society itself. Nurses are the health professionals who have most person-to-person contact with patients. They carry out thousands of interventions with patients and their carers, and their decisions and actions affect the lives of whole populations. It makes sense, therefore, that nursing practice should be based on sound evidence. As the UK Clinical Research Collaboration (2006), observes:

> Nurses play a pivotal role within the NHS (National Health Service), providing front line services and support to patients, and they can make a unique contribution to health research. In particular, they can bring distinctive patient-focused insights to the kind of research which offers greatest benefits to patient care, and to the practical methodological issues which need to be addressed for research to produce relevant outcomes.

If what nurses do is important, it needs to be done well. To ensure that nursing practice is efficient and effective from the perspectives of both patients and nurses, it has to be questioned and, where necessary, improved. Research is one of the main tools available to question practice and seek answers. Aristotle differentiated between two types of knowledge: 'know-how' and 'know-why' (Laudan, 1996). Put simply, 'know-how' is the knowledge that the craftsman possesses, for example when a shipbuilder knows that wood, when properly sealed, floats (Laudan, 1996). 'Know-why' would require him to know the principle by which wood floats over water (buoyancy). 'Know-why' knowledge is mainly generated by research, both basic and applied. Basic research involves answering general questions such as, for example, why, and in which circumstances, do people conform? This type of knowledge can be used to understand why patients conform. Applied research focuses on a specific question in an area of practice: for example, why do patients with diabetes comply (or not) with professional advice?

'Know-how' knowledge is necessary but not enough for progress. This type of knowledge involves learning by 'trial and error', which can be costly and time-consuming. If practitioners are reasonably satisfied with their work, it could lead to a tendency to leave things as they are, thus maintaining the status quo. 'Know-why' knowledge, on the other hand, can be divorced from practice. This is why this type of knowledge needs to be generated in collaboration with practitioners, otherwise it could remain in its 'ivory towers'. Together, 'know-how' and 'know-why' knowledge are necessary for the enhancement of nursing practice.

Nurses are at the front line in the battle for better healthcare. They have first-hand experience of working directly with the public, and as such they are aware of the needs of their clients. They can act as advocates for patients, and nurses' full potential for advocacy can be realised if they support their arguments with research evidence.

Another reason for using research to generate knowledge for nursing practice is to contribute towards the development of nursing as a profession. One of the hallmarks of a profession is the possession of a body of knowledge based on research. The accumulation of knowledge on different aspects of nursing constitutes a 'body of knowledge' that nurses and others can draw upon and contribute to. This body of knowledge is the sum total of nursing knowledge (theories, research findings, experience and so forth) contained mainly in books, journals, reports, theses and other audiovisual forms. The progress made in the creation of nursing's body of knowledge can be gauged by the availability of books on different aspects of nursing and the number of nursing journals currently on the market compared with the early 1970s, when the number of books on nursing in the UK probably amounted to only a handful. The creation of a body of knowledge distinct to nursing is an important step in establishing nursing as a profession. Nursing relies heavily on knowledge from other disciplines, such as biology, chemistry, sociology, philosophy and psychology. While nursing will continue to draw upon, and contribute to, knowledge from these other disciplines, it is imperative that it continues to create a body of knowledge to inform its own practice.

The status of nursing as a profession will be enhanced when other professions recognise that nursing is not just common sense but is based on knowledge derived from research and organised in the form of concepts and theories. The creation of a body of knowledge is the means by which parity with other professions can be achieved, and research is the process by which this knowledge can be developed and validated. Below is an editorial that appeared in the *New York Medical Journal* in 1914 (quoted in Messer, 1914):

> Nursing is not, strictly speaking, a profession. A profession implies professed attainments in special knowledge as distinguished from mere skill (Century Dictionary); nursing is an honorable calling, nothing further, implying proficiency in certain more or less mechanical duties; it is not primarily designed to contribute to the sum of human knowledge or the advancement of science. The great and principal duty of a nurse is to make a patient comfortable in bed, something not always attained by the most bookish of nurses. Any intelligent, not necessarily educated woman can, in a short time, acquire the skill to carry out with implicit obedience the physician's directions. The graduate of the unregistered hospital or sanitarium or of the short term school, or any woman who reads conscientiously a course of instruction in nursing and practises assiduously at home what she learns, is fully competent to undertake any ordinary case of illness. Where special skill is required, as in a major surgical case, a laparotomy for example, we admit that hospital training is, if not indispensable, at least highly desirable, and for such cases the hospital-trained nurse might exclusively reserve her services at a wage higher than the ordinary. Nursing is an honorable, a remunerative, a noble calling, but efforts to exalt it into a profession or to rank it with the higher branches of learning and culture are the apotheosis of the absurd.

This was written at the beginning of the twentieth century. While there is no doubt that the status of nursing as a profession has been raised considerably in many countries since then, there is still a view among some members of the public, politicians and nurses themselves that nursing does not require its practitioners to be trained at degree level. In response to this, uninformed perception, Watson (2011) defends the need for an all-graduate profession in the UK:

> In reality, nursing is a complex subject reflecting the complexity of the job. Biology, psychology, medicine, pharmacology and – to the horror of many – sociology all contribute to the unique mixture that is nursing. Clearly, nurses need to know how the body works in sickness and in health, and how it responds to treatment. Nurses – like doctors – need to be able to contextualise their work, thus the sociology. Nurses need to understand why children with chronic illnesses living on sink estates have different health-education needs than the children of middle-class parents. Are they stupid? Don't they care? Or do they simply face competing pressures and have fewer role models? The more you know, the less judgemental you will be. The less judgemental care is, the greater its effect.

Research is an integral and important part of nursing degree curricula. It has a central role in contributing to safe and efficient practice based on evidence. It is unacceptable that, in the twenty-first century, nurses have to justify why they need to be properly trained for them to deliver the quality of care that their clients deserve.

The role of nurses in research

As explained above, nurses have an important role in creating a body of knowledge and using it to inform their practice. This is what is meant by nursing being a research-based profession (Briggs, 1972). Yet it is not always clear to nurses what exactly they are expected to do. With competing demands on their time and the need to acquire a range of skills, they may wonder whether they are expected to be researchers as well as nurses. This perception may be based on the fact that research is relatively new to nursing.

Nurses' primary duty is to give the best possible care to patients. This involves creating and maintaining a safe, caring environment and using interventions that, to the best of their knowledge, are the most appropriate and effective in bringing about the desired effects. To do this, they should question the knowledge and rationale on which they base their practice and seek to develop new ways to improve what they do. The answers to some of these questions can be obtained in various ways, including research. An important step in integrating research and practice is for nurses to be research-minded.

To be research-minded involves an attitude and an ability to ask questions of one's practice that can be answered through the process of research. While the next step involves finding the answers to those questions, it does not mean that all practitioners are expected to carry out research studies. The answers may already be available in the form of published research. In this case, a literature search and review would be undertaken. In cases where there is no research, the role of nurses is to identify and work with those who have research experience and who are in a position to carry out a new study. To complete the process, the findings of the literature review or the research study should be critically appraised and, where appropriate, they should be disseminated and implemented.

Nurses' role in research extends beyond asking questions, and seeking and implementing evidence. It includes protecting patients' rights by ensuring that patients are fully informed of the implications of participating in research, that informed consent is sought, that no pressure is exerted – directly or indirectly – on them to participate, and that their right to withdraw at any time is respected. This advocacy role applies throughout the duration of the project and beyond (see Chapter 6 for more discussion of these issues).

The methods and skills used by researchers can also be of use to nurses and midwives in their daily practice. These health professionals and others consistently collect and analyse data in the assessment of patients and in the evaluation of outcomes. The skills of interviewing and observing in clinical practice can be sharpened though learning some of the research method skills. Hayes (2002) explains how her research experience prior to starting nurse training was useful to her as a nurse:

> My research background has helped me develop an enquiring mind and the ability to see the broader picture. It helps me question my practice and its impact on patients. The skills I developed while working as a researcher are relevant to everyday practice

on the wards. For example, they give me the confidence to tackle new information and communicate with people. Interview skills help me to sensitively obtain information for patient assessments and analytical skills help me develop care plans.

Although it is rare that a student nurse would have research experience before undertaking nurse training, this example shows how learning research skills can benefit practice.

Maximising the potential contribution of research to practice requires knowledge of what research means, its strengths and limitations, knowledge of the research process (including the main research designs) and an appreciation of the ethical and political implications of research. Knowledge of the resources available to support research is often very important. The skills required include the ability to identify aspects of practice that would benefit from research, to formulate research questions, and to differentiate between questions that can be answered by research and those which can be answered by other means such as audit and reflection on practice (or by a combination of these).

Another fundamental skill for research-based practice is the ability to search and critically appraise research studies. Information technology has greatly facilitated access to research and other literature. To fully reap the benefits, nurses need the skills to search, obtain and critically read appropriate and relevant literature. Critical appraisal skills are likely to be more useful to most nurses than the skills to carry out research. Finally, the skills to implement findings and to manage and evaluate change are crucial if research is to have any impact on practice.

How nurses should acquire these fundamental skills remains a subject for discussion. Anecdotal evidence in the UK suggests that this has been interpreted differently by different institutions, with the result that some courses require students to carry out a literature review on a topic related to practice, while others expect students to formulate a research proposal or even carry out a small-scale project. The consensus in the nursing profession seems to be that qualified nurses should be able to read and use research critically and have a sense of the need for research to underpin their practice. The task of conducting research should rest with those who have acquired further education and training, especially in research methodology.

The role of nurses in research-based practice, as described above, applies to all nurses, since they should all identify researchable questions and seek and implement evidence. However, depending on the nature of their jobs, positions or responsibilities, some nurses may put more emphasis on certain aspects of these roles than others. For example, nurse managers may have more of a leadership role in encouraging and facilitating others to enhance their practice through research and by supporting them with the necessary resources. Nurses play a pivotal role within the National Health Service (NHS), providing front-line services and support to patients, and they can make a unique contribution to health research. In particular, they can bring distinctive patient-focused insights to the kind of research that offers greatest benefits to patient care, and to the practical and methodological issues that need to be addressed for research to produce relevant outcomes.

It is important in any profession that some of its members focus their attention on research. In the UK, Briggs (1972) proposed that the 'active pursuit of serious research must be limited to a minority within the nursing profession'. To carry out in-depth research, nurses need a degree of knowledge and skills that is not usually attainable in basic training. The research training of undergraduate nurses varies in the UK, as explained earlier. Anecdotal evidence, as well as a perusal of the nursing literature, shows that more and more staff nurses in the UK conduct research, often in collaboration with members of multidisciplinary teams and academics. Practising nurses are frequently asked to collect data for other researchers, be they nurse researchers, doctors, psychologists or others. Their clinical nursing experience can be valuable to the research enterprise. Nurses are also in a position to identify problems that need investigation through research.

On the other hand, the researcher can also bring her detached perspective to bear on the problem being researched. This is illustrated by the following example. A researcher was called upon to help to improve care in a ward of older people through research. She had a hunch that constipation might be a problem in this group of patients. The ward sister did not think so until they both examined the notes and found that 11 out of 19 patients were prescribed laxatives, some three times daily. While discussing each patient individually, the ward sister also observed that those who were not prescribed laxatives were also the most confused patients on the ward and would probably not have been able to ask for medication. Without clinical insight, the researcher would have missed this important observation. This highlights the important and unique contribution that nurses can make to the research enterprise in nursing.

The American Nurses Association's (ANA; 2003) position statement on education for participation in nursing research states that, at undergraduate level, 'an attitude of enquiry, as well as an introduction to the research process should be initiated'. Nurses should also learn about how to look for, critique and utilise research in their practice. According to the ANA (2003), the responsibility for the conduct of research begins at master's level, when nurses are prepared to be active members of research teams. At doctoral level, nurses should be able to contribute to knowledge through 'the conduct of research aimed at theory generation or theory testing' (ANA, 2003).

The danger of leaving the conduct of research to a minority of nurses within the profession is that practitioners may not see research as integral to their practice. While there is some evidence from the nursing journals of staff nurses conducting research, it is too much to expect first-level nurses to do so, even though many are very capable of it. Whether they conduct research or not often depends on their research training, their interests and their skills, and on the available resources and opportunities. Although nurses should collaborate with others, they should seek to become full members of the research team. The opportunities to register for a higher degree must also be considered. Nurses have grown in confidence from the early days when they were mostly handmaidens to medical and other researchers, collecting data with little to show for it.

A number of triggers and reasons can make you question your practice. These include:

- when you carry out a task even though you have doubts about whether it is effective, harmful or even necessary, as shown in Research Example 1;
- when you want to know more about something that arouses your curiosity (Research Example 2);
- when you wonder whether there is a better way to care for patients (Research Example 3);
- when you want to introduce a new policy or practice (Research Example 4).

Implementation of fasting guidelines through nursing leadership *Lorch (2007)*

One of the most enduring 'common' practices is the policy of fasting patients for longer periods than necessary before an anaesthetic for surgery. In her role as a specialist nurse coordinator in trauma and orthopaedics, the author was concerned about the 'long periods of starvation of the very young and elderly' on the three wards within the trauma unit. She carried out a 'snapshot study' of 50 patients over the age of 60 with limb fractures. She found that '16 patients were inappropriately starved with the average fasting period of 7–12 hours'. Following this, she embarked on a study on 'the implementation of fasting guidelines through nursing leadership'.

Research example 1

Nasogastric tube feeding – which syringe size produces lower pressure and is safest to use? *Knox and Davie (2009)*

Knox and Davie (2009) explain that 'the impetus for this study was a combination of curiosity about the safety issues relating to feeding via different syringe sizes and the rising cost of syringes for nasogastric feeding'. They questioned the National Patient Safety Agency's recommendation on the size of syringes for use in adults (50 ml) and children (20 ml or 50 ml). To Knox and Davie, it 'seemed illogical, as the use of smaller syringes ought surely to be safer in larger patients'.

Research example 2

An action research project to improve the quality of nursing documentation on an acute medicine unit *Lees (2010)*

The aim of this action research study was to improve nursing documentation and the quality of nursing assessments. The rationale for the study was that, despite regular audits of nursing documentation and assessment (in one foundation trust), nurses continued to experience 'challenges in upholding the established standards'.

Research example 3

Using action research to develop a thoracic support nurse role to enhance quality of care   *Bellman and Corrigan (2010)*

Due to the increasing number of thoracic patients requiring surgery, a senior research development nurse and a consultant cardiac care nurse at a foundation trust decided to explore how the delivery of the existing service could be improved to meet the needs of these patients. As they explain: 'We anticipated that the development of a thoracic support nurse (TSN) role would lead to improved patient care and a potential reduction in length of stay'.

The development of nursing research

It is beyond the scope of this chapter to give a detailed account of the development of nursing research worldwide. The origins of nursing research can be traced back to the time of the Crimean War, when Florence Nightingale collected data on mortality rates in the hospital where she worked. However, it was not until the beginning of the twentieth century in the USA, and in the 1950s in the UK, that nursing research began to develop.

Although the pace and extent of the development of nursing research worldwide vary from country to country, there are remarkable similarities in the way nursing research began and progressed thereafter. This is mainly due to some of the similar issues faced by nurses everywhere, namely the low status of nursing relative to other health professions, the education and training of nurses at the margins of higher education and the lack of resources to carry out research.

In 1985, nursing research in the USA became part of the National Institutes of Health (the US medical research agency and the largest source of funding in the world for health and medical research) despite political opposition at the highest level of government and differences of opinions among nurse leaders about the creation of the National Centre for Nursing Research (NCNR). Since then, nursing research in the US has made a significant contribution to nursing and to society as a whole. Cantelon (2010) explains that:

> since 1986, the NINR (National Institute of Nursing Research) and its predecessor the NCNR, have served as the nucleus for the advancement of nursing science, providing the profession with national leadership on the federal level and financial support for research initiatives throughout the country.

Tierney (1997, 2005) offered an insightful analysis of the development of nursing research in some European countries, including the UK. She described the 1960s as the emerging years in which 'lone pioneers' played a great part. The 1970s are credited with the 'beginnings of collective activity', both internationally and nationally, throughout Europe. Tierney (1997) explained that collaboration among pioneer nurse researchers across Europe led to the formation of the Workgroup of

European Nurse Researchers in 1978. The 1980s are described as the period of 'growth of activity and infrastructure', underpinned by the nursing profession's expanding association with universities. Finally, the 1990s was an era in which 'the development of research in nursing in Europe' was steered 'strategically and with a greater sense of political acumen'.

Tierney (1997) also recognised that the advancement of nursing research has occurred more rapidly in countries with strong and stable economies. Not surprisingly, therefore, the development of nursing research in less developed countries has lagged behind. The *International Journal of Nursing Studies* (volume 27, issue 2, 1990) published a series of papers on the development of nursing research in the UK, Norway, Sweden, Denmark, Finland and Canada. In Canada, nursing research has experienced inconsistent growth over the past four decades, although from 1980s onward funding became available from the Medical Research Council of Canada and the National Health Research and Development Program (Jeans et al., 2008). For more information on the development of nursing research in Canada, see Stinson et al. (1990), Kerr (1996) and Pringle (2004). Australia has also experienced positive growth in nursing and health research (see Wilkes et al., 2002; Australian Nursing Federation and Royal College of Nursing, Australia, 2007).

Not much has been written about the development of nursing research outside Europe, Australia and North America. In India, there are positive signs, such as research being part of the basic nursing curriculum, that nursing research is being embraced by the nursing profession, yet the 'research base in nursing is yet to develop' (*The Hindu*, 4 January 2011). In Turkey, where nursing education has been offered at university level since 1955, nursing research has been growing slowly, but not 'sufficient in relation to the development of global nursing research' (Özsoy, 2007). Researchers in countries such as Taiwan, Hong Kong, Thailand and Malaysia, as well as the in Middle East, are increasingly publishing in highly rated journals. In mainland China, nursing research has been growing rapidly in the last 10 years, although this varies between regions (Li at al., 2009). The lack of investment and the low status of nursing are contributory factors for the slow development of nursing research in many of these countries. There are, however, positive signs that progress is being made, such as the increase in the number of research conferences and publications and the provision of doctoral programmes.

There are real benefits of investing in nursing research. For example, in Ireland, the Department of Health and Children (2003) published the first ever *Research Strategy for Nursing and Midwifery in Ireland*. It recognised the 'considerable importance' of research in providing a solid base for nursing and midwifery practice. It also made a number of recommendations including the provision of funding. A review of what the strategy achieved (Department of Health and Children, 2010) reported that 'the capacity of the professions to generate and utilise research has expanded inextricably since the strategy commenced' and that 'champions of research are emerging within the professions and across the sectors both in developing research generation and in its utilisation'. The report also noted 'the concentration of activity on producing research to inform nursing and midwifery practice and enhance the service or care provided to patients and clients'.

Summary

The role of research-based knowledge in decision-making is crucial for effective practice, and the need to have a sound rationale for one's practice has increased over the last decade. It is not incumbent on every nurse to carry out research, but all should be research-minded enough to value the contribution of research to practice, identify problems that can be explored through research, be aware of research findings, collaborate with others in research activities and protect the rights of patients with regard to their involvement in research projects.

While nursing research must be carried out by nurses in order to create a nursing body of knowledge, a multidisciplinary and multiprofessional approach is also required as nurses work with other health professionals and share the same goal.

Nursing research has come of age in some countries, while in others it is still in its infancy. The momentum created by nursing research must be maintained and increased if it is to contribute positively to patient care and achieve the recognition it deserves.

References

American Nurses Association (2003) Education for participation in nursing research. Retrieved from http://nursingworld.org/readroom/position/research/rseducat.htm (accessed 18 April 2003).

Australian Nursing Federation and Royal College of Nursing, Australia (2007) Nursing research: joint position paper. Retrieved from http://www.rcna.org.au/ (accessed 3 October 2013).

Barton D (2011) The pros and cons of routine. *Nursing Management*, **18**, 5:11.

Bellman L and Corrigan P (2010) Using action research to develop a thoracic support nurse role to enhance quality of care. *Nursing Times*, **106**, 22:18–21.

Benner P, Hughes R G and Sutphen M (2008) Clinical reasoning, decision making and action; thinking critically and clinically. In: R G Hughes (ed.) *Patient Safety and Quality: An Evidence-based Handbook for Nurses* (Rockville, MD: Agency for Healthcare Research and Quality).

Benner R (1984) *From Novice to Expert – Excellence and Power in Clinical Nursing Practice* (Menlo Park, CA: Addison-Wesley).

Briggs A (1972) *Report of the Committee on Nursing* (Briggs Report). Cmnd 5115 (London: HMSO).

Cantelon P L (2010) *NINR: Bringing Science to Life* (Bethesda, MD: National Institute of Nursing Research).

Department of Health (2000) *Towards a Strategy for Nursing Research and Development – Proposals for Action* (London: DoH).

Department of Health and Children (2003) *Research Strategy for Nursing and Midwifery in Ireland* (Dublin: DoHC).

Department of Health and Children (2010) *Research Strategy for Nursing and Midwifery in Ireland 2003–2008 – Review of Attainments* (Dublin: DoHC).

Elliott M (2004) Reflective thinking turning a critical incident into a topic for research. *Professional Nurse*, **19**, 5:281–3.

Finlay L (2008) Reflecting on 'reflective practice'. Open University Practice-based Professional Learning Centre. Retrieved from http://www.open.ac.uk/cetl-workspace/cetlcontent/documents/4bf2b48887459.pdf (accessed 18 December 2013).

Gerrish K and Clayton J (2004) Promoting evidence-based practice: an organizational approach. *Journal of Nursing Management*, **12**:114–23.

Greenhalgh T (2011) Intuition and evidence – uneasy bedfellows. *British Journal of General Practice*, **52**:395–400.

Hayes L (2002) Research provides valuable skills that can be applied to everyday practice on the wards. *Nursing Standard*, **17**, 8:24.

Higher Education Funding Council for England (2001) *Research in Nursing and Allied Health Professions* (Bristol: HEFCE).

Jeans M E et al. (2008) Nursing research in Canada: a status report. Ottawa, Ontario: Canadian Health Services Research Foundation. Retrieved from http://www.cfhi-fcass.ca/Migrated/PDF/ NursingResCapFinalReport_ENG_Finalb.pdf (accessed 3 October 2013).

Jefford E, Fahy K and Suudin D (2009) Routine vaginal examination in order to check for the nuchal cord: a medical procedure becomes a midwifery ritual. *British Journal of Midwifery*, **17**, 4:248–51.

Kenny C (1994) Nursing intuition: can it be researched? *British Journal of Nursing*, **3**, 22:1191–5.

Kerr J (1996) The financing of nursing research in Canada. In: J Kerr and J MacPhail, *Canadian Nursing Issues and Perspectives* (Toronto: Mosby).

Knox T and Davie J (2009) Nasogastric tube feeding – which syringe size produces lower pressure and is safest to use? *Nursing Times*, **105**, 27:24–6.

Laudan L (1996) *Beyond Positivism and Relativism: Theory, Method and Evidence* (Oxford: Westview Press).

Lees L (2010) An action research project to improve the quality of nursing documentation on an acute medicine unit. *Nursing Times*, **106**:37 (early online publication).

Li M, Wei L, Liu H and Tang L (2009) Integrative review of international nursing research in Mainland China. *International Nursing Review*, **56**, 1: 28–33.

Livesley J (2004) How a personal account contributes to nurse knowledge: Rachel's story. *Professional Nurse*, **19**, 5:293–5.

Lorch A (2007) Implementation of fasting guidelines through nursing leadership. NursingTimes.net, **103**, 18:30–1.

Mackintosh C (1998) Reflection: a flawed strategy for the nursing profession. *Nurse Education Today*, **18**:553–7.

McCutcheon H H I and Pincombe J (2001) Intuition: an important tool in the practice of nursing. *Journal of Advanced Nursing*, **35**, 5:342–8.

Messer M A (1914) Is nursing a profession? *American Journal of Nursing*, **15**, 2:122–4.

National Institute of Nursing Research (2013) Nursing research. Retrieved from http//www.ninr.nih.gov/ (accessed 20 July 2013).

Nygren L and Blom B (2001) Analysis of short reflective narratives: a method for the study of knowledge in social workers' actions. *Qualitative Research*, **1**, 3:369–84.

Özsoy S A (2007) The struggle to develop nursing research in Turkey. *International Nursing Review*, **54**:243–8.

Paget T (2001) Reflective practice and clinical outcomes: practitioners' views on how reflective practice has influenced their clinical practice. *Journal of Clinical Nursing*, **10**:204–14.

Pravikoff D S, Tanner A B and Pierce S T (2005) Readiness of U.S. nurses for evidence-based practice. *American Journal of Nursing*, **105**, 9:40–51.

Pringle D (2004) The realities of Canadian nursing research. In: M McIntyre, E Thomlinson and C MacDonald (eds) *Realities of Canadian Nursing: Professional, Practice and Power Issues*, 2nd edn (Philadelphia: Lippincott, Williams & Wilkins).

Rolfe G (2001) *Knowledge and Practice* (London: Distance Learning Centre, South Bank University).

Rycroft-Malone J, Seer K, Crichton N et al. (2012) A pragmatic cluster randomised trial evaluating three implementation interventions. *Implementation Science*, **7**: 80.

Schön D A (1987) *Educating the Reflective Practitioner* (San Francisco: Jossey-Bass).

Stinson S, Lamb M A and Thibaudeau M F (1990) Nursing research: the Canadian scene. *International Journal of Nursing Studies*, **27**, 2:105–22.

Semple M (2011) The pros and cons of routine. *Nursing Management*, **18**, 5:11.

Somerville D and Keeling J (2004) A practical approach to promote reflective practice within nursing. *Nursing Times*, **100**, 12:42–5.

Thompson C, McCaughan D, Cullum N, Sheldon T and Raynor P (2005) Barriers to evidence-based practice in primary care nursing: why viewing decision-making as context is helpful. *Journal of Advanced Nursing*, **52**, 4:432–44.

Tierney A J (1997) Organization report: the development of nursing research in Europe. *European Nurse*, **2**, 2:73–84.

Tierney A (2005) Nursing research: progress and challenges. Retrieved from http//www.dbfk.de/download/Tierney-2005-09-11.pdf (accessed 23 July 2013).

UK Clinical Research Collaboration (2006) *Developing the Best Research Professionals. Report of the UKCRC Subcommittee for Nurses in Clinical Research (Workforce)* (London: UKCRCR).

Watson R (2011) We need the IV Leaguers. Retrieved from http://www.timeshighereducation.co.uk/416935.article (accessed 1 November 2013).

Wilkes L, Borbasi S, Hawes C, Stewart M and May D (2002) Measuring the outputs of nursing research and development in Australia: the researchers. *Australian Journal of Advanced Nursing*, **19**, 4:15–20.

Yadav B L and Fealy G M (2012) Irish psychiatric nurses self-reported sources of knowledge for practice. *Journal of Psychiatric and Mental Health Nursing*, **19**:40–6.

Knowledge, Science and Research

Opening thought   Knowledge and human power are synonymous.
                                                          Francis Bacon

Introduction

Science has evolved as a dominant and legitimate mode of knowledge production in modern societies, and research plays an important part in the scientific enterprise. This chapter examines the relationships between knowledge, science and research. While there is agreement on the distinction between the supernatural, metaphysical and scientific belief systems, there is no consensus on a common definition of science. The traditional scientific method used in the natural sciences and alternative qualitative approaches are outlined and discussed in this chapter. It will be argued that they can both contribute to the understanding of social, health and nursing phenomena, and that it is the research question that determines the design and method of a study.

The need for knowledge

Humans have always had a need for knowledge. Our prehistoric ancestors had to 'know' their environment in order to survive: know what food to eat and how and where to get it. Knowledge brings with it a degree of power. Sheer force and numbers have sometimes not been enough to win battles; those with a superior knowledge of weapons, the battlefield and tactics have often had the advantage. Authority and status are bestowed on people who possess knowledge. Those who appear on our television screens to display their knowledge on particular issues are referred to as 'experts'. Professionals are highly regarded because they possess a body of knowledge in their particular disciplines. Although some knowledge is to satisfy our curiosity, most of us need to 'know' in order to make decisions in our daily lives.

We have come a long way since humans felt at the mercy of the environment. As Sigerist wrote in 1943 in his classic book, *Civilisation and Disease*:

We have created the means of lighting up the darkness and can heat our dwellings to the temperature of summer in the middle of winter. We have learned to produce food in the quantity and quality desired, sometimes even in complete disregard of the seasons.

Since then, humans have invented the nuclear bomb and the microchip, and sent people to the moon. We seek knowledge to change not only our environment, but also ourselves. Behaviour therapy and genetic engineering are but some of the products of this quest for knowledge, which began with our ancestors' need to know how to adapt to their environment in order to survive. In 1927, Freud wrote that the 'principal task of civilisation, its actual raison d'être, is to defend us against nature'.

The knowledge we have acquired seems to have put nature at our mercy. Indeed, a mark of modern civilisation is how nature is protected by, and from, humans.

Belief systems

Knowing what happens only partly satisfies the thirst for knowledge; humans also need to know why things happen. For example, knowing how day follows night, that the tide comes in and goes out or that someone has abdominal pain is not enough. We need to know why these things happen. The first two phenomena can be explained by the movement of the planets, and the last could be food poisoning. However, the same phenomena would have been explained differently in the tenth century BC, in the Middle Ages or during the Renaissance. In the history of humans, different belief systems have provided the frameworks within which phenomena can be interpreted. Adam (2009) explains the meaning of belief:

> A belief is a system of thought that is comprised of the information we have accumulated and stored in our brains. Collectively this provides a worldview and mechanism by which we interpret new information and assess how our experience in the world should be managed. What is important to understand is that such a belief does not have any intrinsic validity beyond the fact that it is the way in which data has been organized within our brains and it appears to provide us, individually, with a model against which we interpret the world around us.

Three belief systems that have been dominant in the West are the mythical or theological, the metaphysical and the scientific.

Mythical or theological beliefs

In primitive times, people predominantly believed that supernatural objects or beings had power over their lives. Thus, gods, spirits, planets, mountains, rivers and trees were thought to possess magical powers, and everything that happened was determined by them. According to Sigerist (1943), 'primitive man found himself in a magical world, surrounded by a hostile nature whose every manifestation was invested with mysterious forces'.

Later, organised religions emerged and provided the framework for people to make sense of themselves and the world in which they lived. Judaism, Christianity and Islam seemed to have put some order into the mythical world by providing the notion of one supernatural being, God, instead of a number of gods or spirits, but they kept some of the elements of pre-religious times (Sigerist, 1943).

Metaphysical beliefs

When people began to question and doubt the power of the supernatural and relied more on their own observation of the world around them, they began to put more faith in nature, which did not appear to be as threatening as they had previously thought. Endo and Nakamura (1995) explain that the Ayurvedic theory of the three *doshas* (wind, bile and phlegm), the Buddhist theory of the four elements (earth, wind, bile and phlegm) and the Greek theory of the four humours (blood, yellow bile, black bile and phlegm) were put forward as explanations for why people became ill and what they should do to keep healthy (that is, by keeping a balance between these elements). While the Greek theory of the four humours has long been rejected, the tridosha theory underpins the current practice of Ayurvedic medicine that is prevalent on the Indian subcontinent.

Scientific beliefs

Metaphysical thoughts had elements of science and influenced earlier scientific theories, but they were limited because most of their explanations were based on speculation. The beginnings of modern Western science are generally traced to the sixteenth century, a time in which Europe experienced profound social changes and a resurgence of great thinkers and philosophers (Polgar and Thomas, 1991). The next stage in the evolution of human thought was to put some of these theories to the test. We began to rely more on what we could observe in order to explain phenomena. However, casual observations were not enough: there was a need to observe systematically and rigorously so that the explanations offered could be verified by others. Experiments became the medium through which scientific knowledge was created, and this area of activity became known as research. Galileo was the first person to carry out systematic observations of the movement of the planets. These observations supported the claim by Copernicus that the earth was not flat and that it moved around the sun. Copernicus had arrived at his theory by mathematical calculations.

The scientific age is characterised by the belief that nature can be controlled, that phenomena can be prevented and predicted. Epidemics were no longer thought to be a punishment for human transgressions of religious laws but were seen to be caused by the spread of infections. Therefore, by preventing the spread, the disease could be contained. In laboratory experiments, the infectious organisms could be identified, and the ways in which they were transmitted could be observed.

Belief systems and knowledge

The world is made up of more belief systems than can be described here. However, the three systems described above are believed to have dominated Western thought. Although they are presented here in chronological order, different belief systems have also coexisted throughout history. Scientists and philosophers worked and lived amidst primitive societies, and spiritual, religious and scientific beliefs coexist to this day. A recent survey published by THEOS (a religion and society think tank in the UK) reported that over three-quarters (77 per cent) of all adults and three-fifths (61 per cent) of non-religious people believe that 'there are things in life that we simply cannot explain through science or any other means' (THEOS, 2013). Almost 60 per cent believe in the existence of some kind of spiritual being, 30 per cent in God 'as a universal life force', 30 per cent in spirits, 25 per cent in angels, and 12 per cent in 'a higher spiritual being that can't be called God'.

People are also eclectic in their beliefs. This means that they can borrow elements from different belief systems in order to make sense of their world. For example, some people who believe that AIDS is caused by a virus may believe at the same time that it is also a punishment for what they perceive as 'sin'. According to McLaughlin and Braun (1998):

> Native Americans (also) place great value on family and spiritual beliefs. They believe that a state of health exists when a person lives in total harmony with nature. Illness is viewed not as an alteration in a person's physiological state, but as an imbalance between the ill person and natural or supernatural forces. Native Americans may use a medicine man or woman, known as a shaman.

Many would also consult a doctor trained in modern medicine as well.

By contrasting these three belief systems – the mythical, the metaphysical and the scientific – a number of issues can be raised. First, each system seems to have evolved from the failure of the dominant system at the time to satisfy the curiosity of human beings, science being the latest attempt to explain natural phenomena.

Second, they each have their own interpretation of the same phenomena. For example, in the mythical age, disease was explained by spirit possession or punishment from God or other supernatural beings. Metaphysical philosophers thought that the balance between the sick person and nature was disturbed, while science attempts to identify the causal agents by means of blood tests, X-rays and other scanning devices.

Third, their sources of knowledge differ. In the mythical or theological age, knowledge was thought to be acquired through divination, revelations or dreams. Knowledge was invested in witch-doctors, healers, prophets and religious leaders. Metaphysical knowledge was obtained through speculation, inspiration and no doubt as the result of some forms of limited observation. Scientific knowledge, on the other hand, is derived mainly from research.

Finally, each of these systems has rules for what should or should not be questioned or studied. The knowledge of spiritual healers or religious leaders was not to be questioned. There was a mystique concerning where this knowledge came from and how it was passed down. By and large, religions were concerned with souls and forbade the study of the human body.

The metaphysical age, which can be thought of as a transition between the other two periods, opened the way for people to question everything. Philosophers speculated on the soul as well as the body. Science, on the other hand, dictates that only what can be observed can be studied: the body, not the soul, is now the central focus of study.

Science and knowledge

The term science is derived from the Latin word *scientia*, meaning knowledge. However, it is difficult to find one definition of science that is acceptable to all. The Science Council (2013) defines science as 'the pursuit and application of knowledge and understanding of the natural and social world following a systematic methodology based on evidence'. This definition would be acceptable to most people, but the notion of science as searching for universal laws to explain and predict human behaviour would be challenged by many who do not believe that the scientific methods used in the natural sciences can be readily applied to the study of humans.

The aim of science is to produce a body of knowledge that can enhance our understanding of phenomena, and, where possible, to predict, prevent, maintain or change them. For example, the theory of gravity was conceived or developed by Newton and built upon by other scientists. Through an understanding of such phenomena as gravity and speed, it was possible, later on, to fly an aeroplane without it falling from the sky. Thus, by understanding gravity, it was possible to control it. The question is, can the methods used in the natural sciences produce the kind of theories or laws that can explain, predict and control human behaviour? This will be addressed further on in this chapter.

Science and research

Scientists construct knowledge through the process of induction and deduction. Induction means that, after a large number of observations have been made, it is possible to draw conclusions or theorise about particular phenomena. A theory, simply defined, is an explanation of why certain phenomena happen (see Chapter 8). The inductive method consists of description, classification, correlation, causation and prediction. The scientific study of plants (botany), for example, initially necessitated a description of the different types of plant species. The next inevitable step was to classify these, according to whether they were trees, flowers or grass, or whether they were edible or poisonous, for example. Through observation, it was possible to discover that the same plants grew better in certain conditions.

After a large number of observations, scientists were able to theorise that some plant species thrived better with adequate light and water. They found that there was a correlation between light, water and growth (of certain plants). To understand whether there was a causal relationship, experiments were carried out. Scientists were able thereafter to predict the conditions under which plants would thrive or wither. According to Bronowski (1960), 'science puts order in our experience'. Without descriptions, classifications and theories, we would be exposed to a mass of information about plants that we would find difficult to make sense of. Wilson (1989) reminds us that:

> in the natural sciences vast amounts of time and energy were – quite rightly – consumed in their early stages by way of simply observing and classifying and describing phenomena (think of zoology, for example): only much later, and with great difficulty, could scientists move toward anything like a theory.

One of the most used classifications is the periodic table of chemical elements developed by the nineteenth-century Russian chemist and inventor, Dmitri Mendeleev.

Other scientists, however, formulate a theory or a hypothesis (a mini-theory) and then collect data in order to support or reject it. This approach to knowledge acquisition is called deduction. For example, if the proposed theory is that heat causes iron to expand, experiments will be carried out to put it to the test. This theory will be supported as long as no one shows, in one or more experiments, that heat does not cause iron to expand. If this happens, the theory is falsified, and a new theory may emerge. The testing process has been termed 'falsification' by Popper (1969). According to him, theories formulated by researchers must be 'put to the test' by the scientific community. As Chalmers (1980) explains:

> When a hypothesis that has successfully withstood a wide range of rigorous tests is eventually falsified, a new problem, hopefully far removed from the original solved problem, has emerged. This new problem calls for the invention of new hypotheses, followed by renewed criticism and testing. And so the process continues indefinitely. It can never be said of a theory that it is true, however well it has withstood rigorous tests, but it can hopefully be said that a current theory is superior to its predecessors in the sense that it is able to withstand tests that falsified those predecessors.

There is normally some form of generalisation from observations prior to the formulation of a theory. For example, casual observations made during the Napoleonic wars showed that injured servicemen left unattended for days were found to have higher survival rates if their wounds had been infested by maggots (*Sunday Times*, 1995). These observations, however unscientific, led to the hypothesis that maggots help wound healing. This could then be tested in laboratory-type experiments.

What is research?

In our daily lives, we use deductive and inductive approaches in gathering information, drawing conclusions or having a 'hunch' about something, and we look for evidence to support our beliefs. For example, you may find that some patients always look drowsy after taking a certain medication. You may conclude (after finding that this has happened a number of times) that there is a connection between the drug and drowsiness. You have, therefore, used the inductive approach to collect this information. On the other hand, you may have a hypothesis or hunch that a particular form of treatment is ineffective. Subsequently, having found out that a number of patients who were given this treatment did not get better, you may conclude that your hypothesis is right. You have, therefore, used a deductive approach.

The 'scientific' research process or the 'scientific method' consists mainly of formulating questions or hypotheses, collecting data using research methods such as observations, interviews or questionnaires, and analysing data. You may be right in thinking that this is what we do all the time. We always have questions to which we seek answers; we either observe or talk to others in order to gather our information, and we process this information and come to some conclusions. There are, however, crucial differences in the way in which non-researchers and researchers find out about phenomena.

Researchers are rigorous and systematic in their approach. Suppose, for example, that a researcher is studying the 'effects of authoritarian management on the job satisfaction of nurses'. A literature review will be carried out to help her to arrive at definitions of 'authoritarian management' and 'job satisfaction' that are acceptable to others. It must be clear that what is being measured or observed is actually job satisfaction and not another concept. If, for example, the researcher observes nurses' interaction on the wards rather than asking them questions about their level of satisfaction, the data collected would not be valid because interactions in themselves do not tell us whether or not nurses are satisfied with their jobs. A method is valid when it measures what it sets out to measure.

The people from whom data are eventually collected must represent the population referred to in the research question. In the above example, the researcher is studying the job satisfaction of 'nurses'. Therefore she must draw a sample who will be representative of nurses, be objective in her choice and avoid selecting her friends or only those who volunteer to take part; she must be rigorous and systematic in her selection of respondents. If the sample is biased, the data will not be reliable because the answers may not reflect the views of those who did not have a chance to be selected. Similarly, if some nurses in the sample understand the questions differently from others, or have not all been asked the same questions, the answers may not be reliable. Reliability refers to the consistency of a particular method in measuring or observing the same phenomena.

Once the data have been collected, the researcher will analyse them systematically. She cannot reject answers that do not reflect her views. Thus, the difference between lay people finding answers to questions in their daily lives and a researcher studying a particular phenomenon is that the latter is rigorous and systematic in her approach. She must not let her prejudice influence the decisions and actions she takes. She must describe in detail all the steps taken in order for others to follow what she has done and to verify her findings, if they so wish, by replicating the study. Replication refers to the process of repeating the same study in the same or similar settings using the same methods with the same or equivalent samples.

Research can be defined as the study of phenomena by the rigorous and systematic collection and analysis of data. Research is a private enterprise made public for the purpose of exposing it to the scrutiny of others, to allow for replication, verification or falsification. Some researchers may not, however, believe that research has to be systematic. For example, they may not ask the same questions to all respondents, or use large random samples, and may not subject their data to systematic statistical analysis. They may use a flexible approach which they believe allows them to get closer to the essence of phenomena. One can still argue that they develop their own 'systems' of collecting and analysing data but that their systems are more flexible (see Chapter 4).

Science and non-science

So far, we have distinguished science from other forms of beliefs such as the supernatural and the metaphysical. But where do other forms of knowledge production that do not use the traditional scientific method fit in? According to Wolpert (1993), for a subject to qualify as science it needs at least to satisfy a number of criteria:

> the phenomena it deals with should be capable of confirmation by independent observers; its ideas should be self-consistent; the explanations it offers should be capable of being linked to other branches of science; a small number of laws or mechanisms should be able to explain a wide variety of apparently more complex phenomena; and ideally, it should be quantitative and its theories expressible by mathematics.

Wolpert goes on to question whether the social sciences can match the 'methods of the "hard" sciences – from physics to biology'. He concludes that, because of the complexity of the subject matter in the social sciences, it is difficult to disentangle causal relationships.

Laudan (1996), on the other hand, quotes Aristotle, who stated that 'science is distinguished from opinion and superstition by the certainty of its principles'. One can ask whether it is feasible and realistic to formulate laws and theories that can predict human behaviour and social phenomena with the same certainty with which phenomena in the natural sciences can be described and predicted. Laudan believes that the 'quest for a specifically scientific form of knowledge, or for a demarcation criterion between science and non-science, has been an unqualified failure'. He adds:

> There is apparently no epistemic feature or set of such features which all and only the 'sciences' exhibit. Our aim should be, rather, to distinguish reliable and well tested claims to knowledge from bogus ones.

Laudan challenges 'traditional' scientists and social scientists to devise their own methods and criteria for testing their claims (knowledge). Whether one accepts (non-supernatural, non-metaphysical) knowledge as 'scientific' depends on the particular paradigms one believes in.

Paradigms

The term 'paradigm' was coined by Kuhn (1970). A paradigm can loosely be described as a school of thought with a set of beliefs. Smith (1991) describes paradigms as:

> different scientific communities [who] share specific constellations of beliefs, values, and techniques for deciding which questions are interesting, how one should break down an interesting question into solvable parts, and how to interpret the relationships of those parts to the answers.

From this description, it seems that paradigms influence:

- the nature of phenomena (for example, whether they have an autonomous existence or depend on our interpretations);
- the way they can be studied (for example, whether the researcher should adopt a 'detached' stance or interact with participants);
- the designs and methods that are the most appropriate to answer the research questions, taking the above into account.

In any era, one paradigm is likely to be dominant. When this paradigm, also called normal science, is no longer effective and influential in addressing topical research problems, a crisis occurs (Kuhn, 1970). According to Kuhn, a 'scientific revolution' takes place in which the dominant paradigm is replaced by a new science, which in turn becomes normal and dominant until it is in turn challenged and replaced, and so the process continues.

Positivism

One paradigm that has influenced much research in the health and social sciences is positivism, a movement that evolved as a critique of the supernatural and metaphysical interpretations of phenomena in the early nineteenth century. The name 'positivism' derives from the emphasis on the positive sciences – that is, on tested and systematised experience rather than on undisciplined speculation (Kaplan, 1968). Developments in the natural sciences, especially physics and chemistry, led early sociologists (in the mid-eighteenth century) to the belief that the methods of these sciences could be applied to the study of human behaviour. As Ayer (1969) explains:

It was the belief of positivists [that] the empire of science was to be extended to every facet of man's nature; to the workings of men's minds as well as their bodies and to their social as well as their individual behaviour; law, custom, morality, religious faith and practice, political institutions, economic processes, language, art, indeed every form of human activity and mode of social organisation were to be explained in scientific terms; and not only explained but transfigured.

Positivists believe in the unity of science. This means that the scientific method used in the natural sciences should equally be appropriate for the study of social phenomena (for example, suicide, life satisfaction or social solidarity). Equally, they believe that it is possible to deduce universal laws to explain human and social phenomena in the same way as there are laws in physics, chemistry or biology. This is known as reductionism, which, in this case, means reducing complex phenomena (for example, why people commit suicide) to simple laws. These laws are expected to predict with precision the probability of an event or phenomenon happening. The higher the degree of certainty, the more 'scientific' the knowledge on which the prediction is based. Positivists believe that such laws can be uncovered for social phenomena as well.

Throughout history, mathematics was thought by philosophers to be the science potentially able to explain and predict human actions. Bertrand Russell (1971) pointed out that positivists regarded mathematics as the pattern to which other knowledge ought to approximate, and thought that pure mathematics, or a not dissimilar type of reasoning, could give knowledge of the actual world. Many phenomena or events in the physical world can be explained by mathematical formulae. Mathematical calculations played a central role in sending men to the moon and bringing them back. Some physicists hope to discover a formula that explains how the world came into existence. Alchemists, the precursors of chemistry scientists, were preoccupied for centuries with finding a formula for mixing substances to produce gold or to develop a potion for eternal life. Taken to the extreme, positivists in the social sciences would aspire to develop mathematical formulae to explain human phenomena. For example, an editorial in the (British) *Daily Mail* newspaper (8 August 2003) made the following comments on the work of Professor James Murray of the University of Washington, who formulated equations to predict whether a couple would stick together or divorce:

Wondering whether your fiancée is really the girl for you? Then wonder no longer. Simply sit her down, talk to her for 15 minutes about a subject on which you disagree, and then work out the following equation: $w(t + 1) = a + r1*w(t) + ihw[h(t)]$. If you are a woman, wondering whether the man you fancy is really Mr. Right, then you should adopt the same procedure, but apply a slightly different equation: $h(t + 1) = b + r2*h(t) + iwh[w(t)]$. The higher values you arrive at for $w(t + 1)$ and $h(t + 1)$ the better advised you will be to dump your intended and find someone else.

This formula claims it can predict with 94 per cent accuracy whether a couple will stick together or divorce.

While this example may seem to portray an extreme form of the use of mathematics to understand human phenomena, Smith (1996) points out that, from its very beginning, the Royal Statistical Society in the UK has sought to promote informed quantitative reasoning as 'the dominant modality in public debate, as well as in decision-making processes of government, business and individuals'. Politicians cite statistics 'ad nauseum' to support their arguments.

Positivists take a 'realist' view of social phenomena: that the world has an existence independent of our perception of it, and that there is an objective way of knowing what it is. They believe in the separation between researchers and their object of enquiry. If we take a social phenomenon such as the war in Vietnam, positivists believe that it actually happened whether or not we are conscious of it (independent of what we think). Only one true version of it exists, and it is the task of historians to find this version. They can do so provided they take an 'objective' stance.

Another important characteristic of positivism is empiricism, according to which only what can be observed by the human senses can be called facts. Positivists also believe in the notion of cause and effect (determinism) and look for explanations in empirical data. They adopt the hypothetico-deductive approach of physics and chemistry. This means that hypotheses or theories are put to the test by the deductive process during the course of experiments.

Postpositivism

Positivist beliefs, in their original forms, lasted from the middle of the nineteenth century to the beginning of the twentieth century. The founding fathers – Auguste Comte and Herbert Spencer and their followers such as Emile Durkheim – through their fascination with the progress made in physics and chemistry, had what has been described as a 'naïve faith' in the ability and appropriateness of the scientific method to study social phenomena. This position came under criticism, which led to a number of adjustments and revisions. There are different versions of these adaptations; however, the main beliefs described below represent what is called 'postpositivism'.

There was a realisation that the idea of 'reality' independent of the experience of people was thought to be 'naïve'. Using the above example of Vietnam, postpositivists might say that there are so many different ways to look at what happened that it is not possible to give one true account of it. Instead, postpositivists believe that it is possible to get as close as possible to (an approximation of) the 'truth'. This position became known as 'critical realism'. The positivist notion that social phenomena can be observed in a detached way has been questioned. Observation is believed to be influenced by the researcher's frame of mind, and by social and cultural conditioning (Corbetta, 2003). According to postpositivists, these influences or biases can be avoided by devising strategies to make tools more objective.

Postpositivists seem to have abandoned the quest for universal laws to explain social phenomena. They realise that it is not possible to predict a social event with the same degree of certainty that natural scientists can with physical events. For example, if research shows that divorce affects the mental health of children involved, one cannot state with certainty that this will happen to every child whose parents go through a divorce. Postpositivists are more realistic and acknowledge the 'probable' nature of predictions in social science. The search for 'causes' and 'effects' in the study of human and social behaviour has, to a great extent, been replaced by efforts to establish 'correlations' (relationships) between variables. Postpositivist researchers still aim to produce generalisable findings, but they are more cautious about how this can be done. It must also be pointed out that the nature of all knowledge is probabilistic. Even though natural scientists can predict physical events, there is still a degree of uncertainty.

The positivist notion of empiricism, whereby only what can be observed by the human senses (sight, hearing, touch, taste and smell) can be called social facts, would exclude the study of such concepts as anxiety, well-being or life satisfaction. Postpositivists accept that these phenomena may not be observable but can be studied by means of self-reports (provided that tools to measure these concepts are valid and reliable).

Despite these adjustments, the legacy of positivism still persists. 'Naïve realism' has been replaced by 'critical realism', but the belief in the existence of 'one truth' is still there, although it is acknowledged that it cannot be accessed easily. Corbetta (2003) explains that, despite these changes, postpositivism has retained much of the original characteristics of positivism:

> The new positivism redefines the initial presuppositions and the objectives of social research; but the empirical approach, though much amended and reinterpreted, still utilizes the original observational language, which was founded on the cornerstone of operationalisation, quantification and generalisation ... The operational procedures, the ways of collecting data, the measurement operations and the statistical analyses have not fundamentally changed. Conclusions are more cautious, but the (quantitative) techniques utilized in reaching them are still the same.

As can be seen from the above, postpositivistic research adopts the scientific process whereby research questions (or hypotheses) are formulated in advance, the key terms are operationalised (defined), the methods of data collection are selected prior to data collection and the analysis of data is mainly quantitative. Some qualitative methods can be included in the study and made to fit in this process. The designs of postpositivistic research are mainly surveys and experiments.

Interpretivism

Postpositivistic reaction to the limitations of positivism in its original form is to devise strategies to overcome them while keeping the positivistic principles. Interpretivists, on the other hand, reject these principles, as will be shown below.

Interpretivism has been put forward as an alternative to positivism. It is 'the belief that the social world is actively constructed by human beings' and that 'we are continuously involved in making sense of' or interpreting, our social environments (Milburn et al., 1995). Interpretivists share the philosophical belief that human behaviour can only be understood when the context in which it takes place and the thinking processes that give rise to it are studied. This approach also recognises that researchers have preconceptions that must be either 'bracketed' (that is, prevented from influencing the research process) or discussed in relation to their implications for the data.

Interpretivists focus on subjective experience, perception and language in order to understand intention and motivation that can explain behaviour. For example, when a man loses his job, he may be depressed. It does not mean that he will be depressed each time he loses his job, nor can we say that everyone who loses their job becomes depressed. Therefore, not only does the same person not necessarily react in the same way every time he is under the same pressure, but different people may also react differently when subjected to the same pressure. Apart from the loss of a job itself, there may be other factors, such as whether or not the man liked his job, that may precipitate or prevent the depression.

Humans can also be affected by the fact that they are being studied, and their actions cannot be understood without access to the thinking processes of the person. We do not always mean what we say, nor do we always say what we mean, even when we are not lying or drunk. Sometimes we do not know if and why we behave the way we do. Therefore empirical observations only skim the surface of the behaviour being studied. The intentions and motivations of the person need to be examined if we are to make sense of a behaviour. Ayer (1969) pointedly asks:

> May it not be that there is something about the material on which these sciences have to work, something about the nature of men, which makes it impossible to generalize about them in any way comparable to that which has made the success of the natural sciences?

In order to study subjective perceptions and experiences, interpretivists know that they cannot behave as detached observers. Instead, through interactions, they can get an insight into how and why people behave the way they do. Such interactions cannot be pre-planned and structured, as interactions between humans are not predictable in terms of process and outcome. Therefore the methods used by interpretivists are interactive and flexible. The types of data collected are mainly in the forms of conversations and narratives. These are not normally analysed statistically. The findings have limited generalisation value and are not expected to lead to universal laws. Interpretivists believe that their findings are context related, although they may have significance beyond the setting where the study is carried out.

It is possible for interpretivists to share the notion of 'critical realism' with post-positivists. This means that they see their (interprevist) methods and approaches as capable of producing findings that represent reality as closely as possible. However, not all interpretivists share these beliefs. Constructivists, for example, put forward the idea of 'multiple realities'. They do not believe that there is one reality, but that there are different perceptions of what the reality is. According to them, knowledge is constructed or co-created through interactions with others and with the environment. Such ideas sit uncomfortably with those who want to uncover the 'truth'.

However, if we take the view that social phenomena and human behaviour are complex, dynamic and changeable, that participants and researchers bring their own prejudices to the research process and that the tools we use can reveal different aspects of the same phenomenon, it is not difficult to understand why research does not always provide unequivocal and uncontestable results.

Different perceptions of the same phenomenon are uncomfortable but can lead to reflection and negotiation. For example, if users and professionals view a particular service differently, or different users have different perceptions of the same service, this could lead to discussions of why this is so. In practice, it is likely that the perceptions that are given more credibility are the ones that the users of the findings find more acceptable and that serve the purpose for which the study was carried out. Different historian researchers would produce different accounts of the Vietnam War, and these accounts will be accepted or rejected according to how they match the perceptions of different groups in society. Multiple realities can also be heuristic (have a learning function) in that people would be made aware how others view the same phenomenon.

There are various strands of constructivism, including social, physical and radical. For more understanding of interpretivism and constructivism and how they are used in research studies, see Brandon and All (2010), Scotland (2012), Hall et al. (2013) and Galanek (2013).

Modernism and postmodernism

Beliefs about the nature of physical and social realities are not only of relevance to the fields of science and research. They also reach and influence people's thoughts in different aspects of society including the arts, the humanities and politics. What is known as 'modernism' is a set of ideas that emerged during the enlightenment period (in the eighteenth century) as a reaction to earlier supernatural and metaphysical belief systems. Rational thinking began to take hold, and people put faith in the ability of science to improve their lives. Knowledge based on science and rationality was seen as a liberating force. Scientific knowledge was supposed to increase as scientists built upon previous knowledge. The aim was to produce theories that could explain everything in the world.

By the end of the 1950s, intellectuals began to challenge some of these ideas for what they saw as the modernists' failure to improve the circumstances of people worldwide and the limitations of their scientific ideas and methods in producing meaningful findings. This new movement, called 'postmodernism' (which has a number of strands), rejected the notion of 'truth' or 'reality' as objective, and rationalism as the only way to think. It questioned how knowledge was created and for whose benefit.

Postmodernists support the notion that knowledge is socially constructed or co-created. Interpretation and meanings have a central place in knowledge production. According to Bouffard (2001), postmodernists 'repudiate' universal laws and believe that the attempt to produce meta-narratives (grand theories) 'is misguided and should be replaced by smaller narratives that are local, contextual, and time-bound'.

There is by no means a consensus among the proponents of the different strands on what constitutes postmodernism. This brief outline hardly does justice to the ideas on which these two movements are based. For fuller discussions of modernism and postmodernism, readers are directed to the works of Toulmin (1990), Lyotard (1992), Fox (1993), Cahoone (1996) and Rolfe (2001).

Qualitative research

The terms 'interpretivism' and 'qualitative research' are sometimes used interchangeably in the literature (Williams, 2000). 'Qualitative research' is a broad umbrella covering a number of approaches which subscribe to the notion that phenomena can realistically be understood by studying the meaning that people give to them and the context in which they happen. It rejects the idea that researchers can remain detached (objective) and replaces it instead by interactive, flexible and inductive methods capable of gaining access to people's experiences and perceptions.

Beyond this, the different strands of qualitative research vary in many ways, including their focus, their process and the type of data that they produce. They draw upon different theories and conceptual frameworks from a wide range of disciplines including philosophy, sociology, anthropology, psychology and semiotics. Atkinson (1995) argues that there is too much diversity in the qualitative approach for it to constitute a paradigm. This will be further discussed in the chapter on qualitative research.

Summary

In this chapter, we have looked briefly at the need of humans for knowledge, and we have examined the relationship between knowledge, science and research. We have seen that each of the three main belief systems not only interprets phenomena differently, but also has its own ways of 'knowing'. Science is the latest attempt to produce and organise knowledge, and research plays an important part in generating and testing theories, which remain the ultimate goal of scientific endeavours.

There is, however, no consensus on what research is and how it should be carried out. The two main paradigms in social, health and nursing research (positivism and interpretivism) have their own assumptions of how phenomena should be studied and of what constitutes scientific knowledge.

The nature of science and knowledge is such that no one school of thought can have a monopoly on the definition and the production of knowledge, although the dominant or favoured paradigm tends to influence what is researched and how. Dzurec and Abraham (1993) sum up succinctly the relationship between knowledge and research:

All research is an effort to fulfil cognitive needs, to perceive, and to know. These needs emerge from curiosity about the world as expressed in a desire to understand it and from an incessant attempt to gain a sense of mastery over self and world. Consequently, if differences among researchers exist, it is not because they aspire to different ends, but because they have operationalized their methods for reaching those ends differently.

References

Adam G (2009) Belief, knowledge, and truth. Retrieved from http://www.science20.com/gerhard_adam/belief_knowledge_and_truth (accessed 15 September 2013).

Atkinson P (1995) Some perils of paradigms. *Qualitative Health Research*, **5**, 1:117–24.

Ayer A J (1969) *Metaphysics and Common Sense*, 2nd edn (London: Macmillan).

Bouffard M (2001) The scientific method, modernism and postmodernism revisited: a reaction to Shephard (1999). *Adapted Physical Activity Quarterly*, **18**:221–4.

Brandon A F and All A C (2010) Constructivism theory analysis and application to curricula. *Nursing Education Perspectives*, **31**, 2:89–92.

Bronowski J (1960) *The Commonsense of Science* (Harmondsworth: Pelican).

Cahoone L (ed.) (1996) *From Modernism to Postmodernism: An Anthology* (Malden, MA: Blackwell).

Chalmers A F (1980) *What Is This Thing Called Science?*, 2nd edn (Buckingham: Open University Press).

Corbetta P (2003) *Social Research: Theory, Methods and Techniques* (London: Sage).

Daily Mail (2003) The right formula. Editorial, 8 August 2003.

Dzurec L C and Abraham I L (1993) The nature of inquiry: linking quantitative and qualitative research. *Advances in Nursing Science*, **16**, 1:73–9.

Endo J and Nakamura T (1995) Comparative studies of the tridosha theory in Ayurveda and the theory of the four deranged elements in Buddhist medicine. [Japanese]. *Kagakushi Kenkyu*, **34**, 193:1–9.

Fox N J (1993) *Postmodernism, Sociology and Health* (Buckingham: Open University).

Freud S (1927) *The Future of an Illusion* (London: Hogarth Press).

Galanek J D (2013) The cultural construction of mental illness in prison: a perfect storm of pathology. *Culture, Medicine and Psychiatry*, **3**, 1:195–225.

Hall H, Griffiths D and McKenna L (2013) From Darwin to constructivism: the evolution of grounded theory. *Nurse Researcher*, **20**, 3:17–21.

Kaplan A (1968) Positivism. In: D L Sills (ed.) *International Encyclopedia of the Social Sciences* (New York: Macmillan/Free Press).

Kuhn T (1970) *The Structure of Scientific Revolutions*, 2nd edn (Chicago: University of Chicago Press).

Laudan K (1996) *Beyond Positivism and Relativism: Theory, Method and Evidence* (Oxford: Westview Press).

Lyotard J F (1992) *The Postmodern Explained to Children* (London: Turnaround).

McLaughlin L and Braun K (1998) Asian and Pacific Islander cultural values: considerations for health care decision-making. *Health and Social Work*, **23**, 2:116–26.

Milburn K, Fraser E, Secker J and Pavis S (1995) Combining methods in health promotion research: some considerations about appropriate use. *Health Education Journal*, **54**:347–56.

Polgar S and Thomas S A (1991) *Introduction to Research in the Health Sciences*, 2nd edn (Melbourne: Churchill Livingstone).

Popper K R (1969) *Conjectures and Refutations* (London: Routledge & Kegan Paul).

Rolfe G (2001) Postmodernism for healthcare workers in 13 easy steps. *Nurse Education Today*, **21**:38–47.

Russell B (1971) *Logic and Knowledge: Essays 1901–1950*, 5th edn (London: George Allen & Unwin).

Science Council (2013) What is science? Retrieved from http://www.sciencecouncil.org/definition (accessed 16 September 2013).

Scotland J (2012) Exploring the philosophical underpinnings of research: relating ontology and epistemology to the methodology and methods of the scientific, interpretive, and critical research paradigms. *English Language Teaching*, **5**, 9:9–16.

Sigerist H E (1943) *Civilisation and Disease* (Chicago: University of Chicago Press).

Smith A F (1996) Mad cows and ecstasy: chance and choice in an evidence-based society. *Journal of the Royal Statistical Society*, **159**, 3:367–83.

Smith H W (1991) *Strategies of Social Research*, 3rd edn (St Louis: Holt, Rinehart & Winston).

Sunday Times (1995) Hospitals use maggots to heal infected wounds. 21 January, pp. 1, 20.

THEOS (2013) The spirit of things unseen: belief in post-religious Britain. Retrieved from http://www.theosthinktank.co.uk/files/files/Reports/Spirit%20of%20Things%20-%20Digital%20(update).pdf (accessed 25 October 2013).

Toulmin S (1990) *Cosmopolis: The Hidden Agenda of Modernity* (Chicago: University of Chicago Press).

Williams M (2000) Interpretivism and generalisations. *Sociology*, **34**, 2:209–24.

Wilson J (1989) Conceptual and empirical truth; some notes for researchers. *Educational Research*, **31**, 3:176–80.

Wolpert L (1993) *The Unnatural Nature of Science* (London: Faber & Faber).

3

Quantitative Research

Measure what is measurable, and make measurable what is not so.
Gallileo Gallilei

Introduction

Positivism and postpositivism rely on measurable and quantifiable approaches to the study of phenomena. In this chapter, we will continue to explore the type of knowledge and evidence that the quantitative approach produces.

Quantitative research has a long tradition in nursing, dating back to the time of Florence Nightingale, who collected statistical data to establish the causes of mortality during the Crimean War. For many researchers, it produces 'hard', scientific knowledge, the highest form of evidence, vital for evidence-based practice. It is caricatured and vilified by others who reject it as a viable approach in nursing research. In this chapter, the characteristics usually associated with quantitative research, its usefulness in advancing nursing knowledge and the criticisms levelled at it, will be outlined and discussed.

What is quantitative research?

It is important from the outset to differentiate between the quantitative approach and quantitative methods. In this context, the terms 'research', 'approach' and 'tradition' will be used interchangeably to designate a particular paradigm. An approach is the whole design, including the researcher's assumptions, the process of enquiry, the type of data collected and the meaning of the findings. The quantitative approach comes from a philosophical paradigm that views human phenomena as being amenable to objective study, in particular to measurement. It has its roots in positivism, although most recent studies reflect a postpositivistic stance. According to Hammersley (1993), 'there are probably few social researchers today who would call themselves positivists, but the influence of positivism persists'.

The process of quantitative research mirrors that of the traditional scientific method used in the natural sciences. It consists of stating, in advance, the research questions or hypotheses, operationalising the concepts (see Chapter 9) and devising or selecting, in advance, the methods of data collection and analysis. Finally, the findings are presented in numerical and/or statistical language.

The quantitative approach to research involves the use of data collection methods such as questionnaires, structured observations, structured interviews and a number of other measuring tools. On the other hand, in-depth interviews and unstructured observations are normally associated with qualitative research. Researchers have to choose methods that are appropriate for answering their research questions. Methods of data collection such as the questionnaire or the interview do not belong exclusively to particular paradigms; however, selecting them is not a neutral, value-free or haphazard exercise. Instead, the choice reflects, consciously or unconsciously, the particular beliefs and values of the researcher in relation to the phenomenon she investigates. For example, an attitude scale is devised and used, based on the belief that attitudes can be measured. As Hughes (1980) claims:

> No technique or method of investigation … is self-validating: its effectiveness, its very status as a research instrument making the world tractable to investigation, is dependent, ultimately, on philosophical justification. Whether they may be treated as such or not, research methods cannot be divorced from theory; as research tools they operate only within a given set of assumptions about the nature of society, the nature of man, the relationship between the two and how they may be known.

Distinguishing between quantitative and qualitative research (whatever the merits of the exercise) is problematic. The popular notion that quantitative research deals with quantity and numbers, and qualitative research deals with quality and description, is too simplistic and unhelpful. Differentiating between these two approaches on the basis of data collection methods or sampling procedures alone can be misleading. The essential difference between quantitative and qualitative approaches lies in their philosophical assumptions, which are inferred but not always stated. These assumptions in turn guide the data collection and analysis process. According to Blumer (1969), the kinds of question asked and the kinds of problem posed determine the subsequent lines of enquiry, and 'the means used to get data depend on the nature of the data to be sought'.

The main purpose of quantitative research is to measure concepts or variables (for example, attitudes) objectively and to examine, by numerical and statistical procedures, the relationship between them (for example, attitudes and occupation). Blumer (1969) describes a quantitative researcher as 'someone who casts study in terms of quantifiable variables, who seeks to establish relations between such variables by use of sophisticated statistical and mathematical techniques, and who guides such study by elegant logical models conforming to special canons of the "research design"'.

Quantitative research has been described as being reductionist, deterministic and deductive. Its findings are expected to be replicable and generalisable. Each of these characteristics is discussed below.

The role of measurement in quantitative research

Measurement has been defined as 'the process of assigning numbers to objects to represent the kind and/or amount of attributes or characteristics possessed by those objects' (Waltz et al., 2010). Measurement occupies a central position in the traditional scientific method. Quantitative researchers, therefore, try to achieve scientific status in their studies by aiming to measure the concepts and variables they deal with, as objectively and as accurately as possible. Objective knowledge, in the natural sciences, is the highest form of knowledge. For quantitative researchers, objective, valid and reliable measurements remain the goal, although, in practice, this is not always possible.

It has been argued that qualitative researchers also use measurement in their studies. For example, such terms as 'most' or 'a few' (respondents) indicate 'quantity', although actual numbers are sometimes used. There is no reason, of course, why numbers cannot be used in qualitative research, as they are part and parcel of the language of communication and understanding. Sandelowski (2001) explains that while numbers generally have a less prominent place in qualitative research, they are, nevertheless, useful – for example in showing how samples are selected, in identifying patterns and themes and in generating hypotheses. Similarly, 'words' are equally important to quantitative researchers. It is sometimes believed that the latter deal with numbers and do not understand that words can convey different meanings. The care and attention that is required in choosing the appropriate words and phrases for questionnaires and scales is evidence of the importance of words to quantitative researchers.

Numbers are used not only to describe the distribution of certain characteristics in a population, but also to determine relationships between them. Most data in quantitative research are collected or converted in the form of numbers. These numerical data are analysed mathematically and/or statistically to produce answers to the researchers' questions. Although statistical findings can be interpreted in different ways, the figures tend to speak for themselves.

Objective and subjective measurements

Measurement in quantitative research can be objective or subjective, although in practice researchers may use a combination of both. Objective measurements are those which can be empirically observed, recorded and verified. Examples of objective measures include blood sugar levels, temperature readings or weight loss. The degree of error and bias in these measures is low (although instruments can be faulty and human errors can happen). Thus, measuring the weight of person with a scale is high on objectivity because neither the researcher nor the person being measured can influence (alter) the outcome. This exercise can be repeated by the same or other researchers and the results should be the same. This type of measure is therefore verifiable and replicable.

Objectivity in the quantitative approach means that researchers 'stand outside' the phenomena they study. The ways in which data are collected and analysed are expected to be free from bias on the part of the researcher and the participants in the study. The whole process of quantitative research should reflect objectivity. For example, in measuring the level of satisfaction with district nurses' services, the researcher hands out, or posts, questionnaires to the participants. The researcher will try to be as little involved with the participants as possible. In effect, it is the tool that does the measurement and not the researcher (although later on we will discuss how the values and beliefs of researchers may influence the development of questionnaires or other measuring instruments). Objectivity is also shown by selecting samples through random techniques (see Chapter 15) and by analysing data using statistical tests that will show the same results no matter who performs them.

Quantitative researchers also engage in the study of human concepts that are often not amenable to objective measurement. For example, attitudes, pain, spirituality and fatigue are experiences or beliefs that can only be conveyed by the participants themselves. The task of quantitative researchers is to construct scales (or use existing ones) that can best capture these concepts. Typically, researchers select and offer a number of responses (in the form of statements) that participants are asked to rate or indicate their agreement or disagreement with.

An example of a subjective rating scale is the 'Epworth Sleepiness Scale' (Johns, 1991). As Smyth (2012) describes:

> The Epworth Sleepiness Scale (ESS) is an effective instrument used to measure average daytime sleepiness. The ESS differentiates between average sleepiness and excessive daytime sleepiness that requires intervention. The client self-rates on how likely it is that he/she would doze in eight different situations. Scoring of the answers is 0–3, with 0 being 'would never doze' and 3 being 'high chance of dozing'. A sum of 10 or more from the eight individual scores reflects above normal daytime sleepiness and need for further evaluation.

Subjective measurements, therefore, are essentially responses by participants to structured questions or scales. Alternatively, a researcher could use a similar scale or checklist (see Chapter 16) to record when patients fall asleep and in what type of situation.

Subjective measures can be crude or rigorous. An example of a crude way to measure quality of life is by asking respondents to indicate if their quality of life is either 'high', 'medium' or 'low'. On the other hand, researchers can go to great lengths to develop tools by carrying out interviews with people, reviewing the literature and consulting experts on the topic. These tools are then subjected to validity and reliability tests before they are used in projects (see Chapter 16 for how this can be done). In time, other researchers will comment on the strengths and limitations of these instruments, thereby contributing further to their validity and reliability. Once developed, a tool represents the phenomenon it seeks to measure. For example, the self-esteem scale represents a definition of self-esteem. This is not to say that everyone agrees with this definition; those who will read and appraise the study have to decide whether they accept it or not.

Quantitative research is often described as being reductionist. To measure non-observable, subjective psychosocial concepts, researchers resort to measurement by proxy. For example, a complex concept such as self-esteem is reduced to 10 statements. This reductionist approach is commonly used in measuring physical concepts such as density, gravity or speed. The latter, for example, is measured by the time it takes for an object to travel from A to B. Time itself is measured by the movements of the 'hands' on a clock. As explained in Chapter 2, reductionism also means reducing complex phenomena to universal laws.

Objective measures are considered to be more valid and reliable than subjective measures, as the latter depend on self-reports. Researchers often measure an outcome such as 'smoking cessation' or 'abstinence' by asking respondents if they have stopped smoking. These self-reports may not provide accurate evidence and are not as reliable as the urinary cotinine test or the measurement of breath carbon monoxide. As pointed out earlier, some subjective measures are crude and others are robust, depending on how they are constructed and validated. Whether or not they are accepted as evidence depends on what else is available and how these measures are rated by the research community. In theory, valid, reliable, replicable and objective measures remain the ideal that quantitative researchers aim for. In practice, this is not always possible. Therefore they use measures they believe are appropriate in the circumstances.

Types of quantitative data

Quantitative researchers collect a range of numerical data in their attempt to answer their research questions. Typically, they use such terms as level, extent, frequency, number, amount, prevalence, incidence, trends, patterns and relationships. At their most basic, quantitative data are collected to classify, group and describe the attributes and behaviour of populations, and activities within organisations. These attributes or variables can be classified as physical (for example, height, weight and gender), physiological (for example, blood sugar level, urinary pH and cortisol levels), psychological (such as anxiety, attitudes and dependency levels), social (occupation, education, social support) or behavioural (smoking status, self-care activities). Some of these attributes fall within more than one of these areas. For example, nutritional status is, at the very least, a physiological as well as a physical attribute. Data on activities, events, patterns or trends include, for example, hospital attendance rates, attrition rates, number of visits and skill mix.

Studying relationships between concepts by the use of measurements and statistical tests is another characteristic of the quantitative approach. Researchers are interested in how variables or concepts are related. For example, a researcher may want to know if social support for carers is associated with their quality of life. Thus, both 'social support' and 'quality of life' can be measured, and their relationship can be tested statistically. For the findings of this study to have any influence on policy and practice, the researcher would have to show that these concepts (social support and quality of life) were adequately measured, that appropriate statistical tests were carried out and that the relationship between the two concepts was statistically significant (see Chapter 19).

Randomised controlled trials (see Chapter 11) rely on quantitative measures in order to determine whether interventions have the desired effects, although qualitative methods can also be used to explore some issues related to the intervention or the outcomes. This type of approach is often termed 'deterministic' as it studies 'cause' and 'effect'. For example, Hawkes et al. (2013) carried out a randomised controlled trial to evaluate the 'effects of a telephone-delivered multiple health behavior change intervention on health and behavioral outcomes in survivors of colorectal cancer'. A number of tools were used to measure primary outcomes such as physical activity (the Godin Leisure-time Exercise Questionnaire), health-related quality of life (the Health-related Quality of Life Short Form-36) and cancer-related fatigue (the Functional Assessment of Chronic Illness Therapy Fatigue Scale). Secondary outcomes including body mass index, diet, alcohol intake and smoking were measured at baseline and at 6 and 12 months thereafter. Data analysis included a range of measures and statistical tests (Hawkes et al., 2013).

These examples show that quantitative research can provide data to describe the distribution of characteristics or attributes in populations, to measure variables and concepts, to explore correlations between them as well as to determine cause-and-effect relationships. The same study can often collect data to perform all these functions, as in a study by Cook et al. (2013) that evaluated the effects of an educational intervention on the knowledge, confidence and practice of nursing staff in the care of children with mild traumatic brain injury (Research Example 5).

Research example 5

A quantitative study

Effect of an educational intervention on nursing staff knowledge, confidence, and practice in the care of children with mild traumatic brain injury *Cook et al. (2013)*

The authors tested the effects of an educational intervention for mild traumatic brain injury on nurses' knowledge, confidence and perceived change in practice. This was a single-group study with pre- and post-test measurements.

'Knowledge' was measured by a multiple-choice questionnaire. 'Confidence' and 'change in practice' were measured by self-report Likert scale statements.

Comments
1 In this study, the data collection tools were developed by the researchers prior to the study. They were administered in the same way to all nurses in the study. The questionnaires were also structured. Therefore the tools were predetermined, standardised and structured. The three variables (knowledge, confidence and change in practice) were also quantified (scored). Statistical analyses were carried out.

2 'Knowledge' was objectively measured, while 'confidence' and 'change in practice' were subjectively measured (that is, by means of self-reports). It is important to note that self-reports can be quantified.

Quantitative approach as deductive

Quantitative research has also been described as 'deductive' – an approach that typically tests researchers' ideas or hypotheses. Quantitative studies that are correlational and deterministic can be described as using a deductive approach since researchers test whether variables are correlated or whether one variable causes a change in another. For example, in a study on 'the interplay between sleep and mood in predicting academic functioning, physical health and psychological health', Wong et al. (2013) set out to test the relationships between sleep behaviours and these variables. This type of research is deductive as it was the researchers who selected these variables ('sleep behaviours' and 'academic functioning', 'physical and psychological health') and decided to find whether a relationship exists between them. Similarly, when Doyle et al. (2011) carried out an experiment to 'evaluate the impact of a communication skills course for nurses on how to handle difficult communication situations in their daily work', they were testing their idea that there may be a relationship between the course and the 'self-efficacy' and 'performance' of nurses in these situations.

Some quantitative studies can also be exploratory. Lewis et al. (2001) wanted to know which factors were related to tobacco use by adolescents. They included the following variables in their questionnaire: age, gender, ethnicity, self-esteem, physical activity, parental smoking and socioeconomic factors. An analysis of data may reveal relationships between those variables and smoking that the researchers did not anticipate. This may lead to the formulation of new questions for study. Therefore one can say that some quantitative studies can generate new hypotheses and can, in this sense, be described as inductive. However, the deductive approach seems to dominate in quantitative studies as it is the researchers who select, in advance, which variables they want to investigate.

Finally, quantitative research is described as producing findings that are generalisable to the setting where samples are drawn or to similar settings. The selection of representative samples by random and objective methods is expected to achieve this aim. In practice, it is not always possible to do this, so researchers also resort to non-random sample selection methods (see Chapter 15). However, a study is no less quantitative if a random, representative sample is not used.

Data collection and analysis

Questionnaires, observation schedules and other measuring tools – such as scales to measure knowledge, skills and competence – and instruments to measure physiological and biomedical indicators, comprise the main methods of data collection in quantitative research. What is common with these methods is that they are all *predetermined*, *structured* and *standardised*. A questionnaire is a predetermined tool (planned in advance) and constructed prior to the commencement of data collection (see Chapter 16). Ideally, it cannot be altered when data are collected, as it would mean that some participants may be asked different questions. In quantitative research, the selection or development of tools such as questionnaires is perhaps the most difficult task for researchers. An analogy to illustrate the importance of this aspect of quantitative research is the skill and precision involved in developing a scale to measure a person's weight. Constructing the scale involves testing and checking whether it can indeed measure weight and whether it can do so consistently. If the scale is well developed, valid and reliable, taking the measurements and analysing the findings are relatively simple tasks.

'Structure' in a questionnaire refers to the way in which the questions and answers are formulated so that respondents can 'tick' or 'circle' their preferred response. The more structured the questionnaire, the less respondents have to write their answers in their own words. An example of a basic structure in a questionnaire is when respondents are asked their age. They may be offered the following responses:

Under 18   ☐
18–25   ☐
26–45   ☐

Scales, such as those measuring attitudes, often offer respondents a choice between 'strongly agree', 'agree', 'neither agree nor disagree', 'disagree' and 'strongly disagree' to select in response to a number of items or statements. The purpose of structure, in quantitative research, is to contribute to the standardisation of responses to facilitate the completion of questionnaires and data analysis. For example, the units (or aspects) of social support are specified in the form of a number of items. The respondents' task is to indicate on scale of 1 to 6 the degree with which they are satisfied or not satisfied with the items. All the respondents are given the same scale and the same instructions. Quantitative researchers collect data in the same way with all respondents in the study. Not only should the questionnaires be the same, but the circumstances in which they are administered should more or less be the same as well. For example, asking some patients to rate their satisfaction with nursing care while still in hospital and giving the same questionnaire to those who have been discharged home may give different results.

As explained earlier, values and numbers are central to the measurement of phenomena in quantitative research. The choice of techniques of data analysis goes hand in hand with the selection or development of data collection methods. Quantitative researchers carry out, wherever possible and appropriate, statistical tests to establish, among other things, the probability of certain phenomena occurring. For example, if the job satisfaction scores of male nurses are higher than those of female nurses, a statistical test may be performed to find out if these scores have been obtained by chance and, if so, what the chances of this happening are. Chapter 19 explains further the analysis of quantitative data.

The value of quantitative research to nursing

As we shall see in the next two chapters, quantitative research is not the only approach that can provide knowledge on which to base practice. Those who prefer, support, fund or do quantitative research believe that it provides hard and objective facts. However, there are those, like Schutz (1962), who maintain that:

> Strictly speaking, there are no such things as facts, pure and simple ... They are, therefore, always interpreted facts ... This does not mean that, in daily life or science, we are unable to grasp the reality of the world. It just means that we grasp merely certain aspects of it, namely those which are relevant to us for carrying on our business of living ...

Therefore the type of data we collect depends on what we need to know. It is the 'business' of nurses to know whether their patients get better. There are a number of indicators such as symptom relief, self-reports from patients or other signs to show whether they get better or not with the care they receive. Quantitative researchers would say that with rigorously designed tools, we should be able to 'grasp the reality' (in this case, measure the indicators of symptom relief and/or other improvements in patients) that they are interested in.

Quantitative research is primarily concerned with measurement and, according to Waltz et al. (2010), measurement is central to everything that nurses do. The large number of tools that have been developed to measure physical, physiological, psychosocial and other concepts and phenomena of interest to nurses is a testimony to the value and importance of quantitative research to nursing. Many of these tools developed for research purposes are also used in clinical contexts to assess patients and to evaluate the care they receive.

Quantitative research provides data for many of the questions that arise out of nursing practice. It is useful in providing the means to measure such concepts as attitudes, anxiety, job satisfaction, critical thinking, empowerment, nursing care, quality of life and many others. Quantitative approaches have been used in needs assessment, in measuring competence, knowledge, attitudes and beliefs, in the evaluation of interventions and in providing data on the organisation, delivery and use of services. Quantitative data are particularly useful in identifying trends and patterns, especially where large populations are involved, and for comparative purposes.

Needs assessment of patients and nurses is a preliminary but essential step in the delivery of care. An example of a quantitative study that focused on the needs of patients is that of Schofield et al. (2012) who used a short version of the Needs Assessment for Advanced Cancer Patients scale with a sample of patients with advanced incurable cancer. There are a number of studies that have assessed the competence, knowledge, skills and attitudes of practitioners (see, for example, Plant and Coombes, 2003; Kao et al., 2013). Other studies have explored, quantitatively, the roles and activities of nurses. For example, Baldwin et al. (2013) explored the role and functions of clinical nurse consultants.

The evaluation of interventions has attracted increasing attention since the introduction of evidence-based practice policies, although nurses have always been concerned about the effects of their practice on patients. Studies on the evaluation of interventions have recently proliferated. An example of such a study is by Hatchett et al. (2013), who evaluated a 'social-cognitive theory-based email' intervention designed to influence the physical activity of survivors of breast cancer.

Ideas for studies on intervention can come from nurses themselves, from research studies and from the literature. For example, McKinney and Melby (2002), after reviewing the literature on 'relocation stress in critical care', concluded that there was a need for 'more research on interventions that aim to reduce anxiety following transfer, such as structured teaching programmes and family conferences'.

Interventions designed to improve nurses' competence or skills have also been studied by means of quantitative research. Such data can be useful in informing the development of effective educational programmes. Adamsen et al. (2003) studied the effects of a 1-year basic research methodology course on clinical nurses' own research activity and the commitment to research in general. There are numerous studies on the effects of courses, workshops and study days on nurses' knowledge, skills, attitudes, competence and other behaviour.

Quantitative data are useful to policy-makers for informing their decisions regarding service provision and delivery. This type of evidence can be used to justify expenditure or support claims for funding to support one service rather than another. Quantitative research can also provide a 'quick and ready' overview of the type and level of services provided. The survey method, with large samples, can provide valuable data within a short period of time, at relatively low costs. Surveys are also successful in 'feeling the pulse' of public opinion. They are not meant to study a phenomenon in any great depth. The Oxford Dictionary defines 'survey' as a 'general view, casting of eyes or mind over something'. Thus, surveys provide a glimpse of, rather than a window into, human behaviour or practice.

This type of data is sometimes all that managers or policy-makers need in order to find out what is happening. McDonnell et al. (2003) carried out a survey of all acute hospitals in England that performed adult inpatient surgery, 'in order to provide an accurate picture of the current level' of acute pain team (APT) provision. They also explored associations between 'the presence of an APT and a number of organisational and clinical initiatives associated with clinical excellence in the management of postoperative pain' (McDonnell et al., 2003).

Quantitative research has a long tradition in nursing, and the current emphasis on evidence-based practice has, to some extent, given it a new impetus.

Criticisms and limitations of the quantitative approach

Supporters of the quantitative approach have described it as the 'highest form of attaining knowledge that human beings have devised'. Those who reject quantitative research point to the limitations of empirical observations in understanding human phenomena. For example, when concentrating on the manifestation of behaviour, it is possible only to study what is observable. Therefore only a partial glimpse of the phenomenon is revealed. By reducing complex phenomena such as stress, anxiety or hope to what can be observed, it is not possible to have a meaningful understanding of what it means to be stressed, anxious or hopeful. Even those defending empiricism admit to the differences between physical and human phenomena and the difficulties in measuring the latter, but they still believe that measurement is possible, as Norbeck's (1987) comments show:

> The inanimate objects in the physical world can be measured, melted down, fractioned and recomposed in predictable and repeatable ways. In contrast, human behaviour is difficult to measure, multideterminant and highly variable. But such difficulties do not necessarily imply that human behaviour defies objective observation.

What appears as objectivity does in fact reflect the values and beliefs of researchers. Based on her own research experience, Burch (1999) wrote a paper in which she argued that 'standardised assessment instruments ignore the social dimensions of interviewing, decontextuative scores and contain implicitly individualistic biomedical ideology of health'. As she explains:

> It is naive to assume that people's 'real' response to a question can be prompted from them by detached interviewing. Many influences operate upon how one decides to answer a question. The 'choice' is not so much between true or false but between the varying aspects of experience and perception which commonly coexist.

Burch (1999) gave many examples of how items on standardised scales can be interpreted differently by participants from what was intended by those who developed them. She concluded that the structured interview (designed to obtain data objectively):

> cannot be assumed to be a neutral data-gathering exercise; scores are not generated in a context-free zone; implicit ideologies of what constitutes good and bad health mean that instruments may tell us more about what society requires of its members than whether interventions are effective for patients.

The view that if researchers do not measure, they are not doing science has given rise to charges of 'scientism' against quantitative researchers. Scientism is the belief that only the scientific method can produce 'hard evidence' worthy to be called science, and that other ways of producing knowledge are inferior. In evidence-based practice, the highest status is given to objective, measurable outcomes. If quantitative data were taken for what they are instead of what they pretend to be, quantitative research would probably not have suffered the barrage of criticism that it has since the 1970s. Data in themselves are not pretentious; it is the claim that they provide 'hard evidence' that elevates the quantitative approach to a level far above others, a position highly contested by its critics.

Summary

In this chapter, the main characteristics of the quantitative approach were outlined and discussed. It was shown that its aim is to produce 'hard evidence' by means of objective and subjective measures. Concepts and variables are measured and, where relevant, the relationships between them are explored with the use of mathematics and statistics. Quantitative studies can be descriptive, correlational and deterministic; they adopt mainly a deductive approach to research. As far as possible, quantitative researchers aim to maintain objectivity throughout the whole process, which models itself on the traditional scientific method used in the natural sciences. It is acknowledged, however, that not all quantitative studies live up to this ideal type. In practice, it is not always possible to measure objectively or to select random samples. Nonetheless, if the aim is to measure, however crudely, and if the scientific method process is used, these studies can claim to be quantitative.

Quantitative research has been instrumental in providing data for over half a century to inform nursing policy, practice and education. It remains a potent research approach to many of the problems, issues and concerns facing nurses and health professionals. It is still the favoured approach for those who provide funding for health research, and it has been provided with a boost by the introduction of evidence-based practice. However, in the last two decades, other approaches have stated their own claims to the production of knowledge for nursing and health practice. We will explore these in the next two chapters.

References

Adamsen L, Larsen K, Bjerregaard L and Madsen J K (2003) Moving forward in a role as a researcher: the effect of a research method course on nurses' research activity. *Journal of Clinical Nursing*, **12**, 3:442–50.

Baldwin R, Duffield C M, Fry M, Roche M, Stasa H and Solman A (2013) The role and functions of clinical nurse consultants, an Australian advanced practice role: a descriptive exploratory cohort study. *International Journal of Nursing Studies*, **50**, 3:326–34.

Blumer H (1969) *Symbolic Interactionism: Perspective and Method* (Englewood Cliffs, NJ: University of California Press).

Burch S (1999) Evaluating health interventions for older people. *Health*, **3**, 2:151–66.

Cook R S, Gillespie G L, Kronk R et al. (2013) Effect of an educational intervention on nursing staff knowledge, confidence, and practice in the care of children with mild traumatic brain injury. *Journal of Neuroscience Nursing*, **45**, 2:108–18.

Doyle D, Copeland H L, Bush D, Stein L and Thompson S (2011) A course for nurses to handle difficult communication situations. A randomized controlled trial of impact on self-efficacy and performance. *Patient Education and Counseling*, **82**, 1:100–9.

Hammersley M (ed.) (1993) *Social Research: Philosophy, Politics and Practice* (London: Sage).

Hatchett A, Hallam J S and Ford M A (2013) Evaluation of a social cognitive theory-based email intervention designed to influence the physical activity of survivors of breast cancer. *PsychoOncology*, **22**, 4:829–36.

Hawkes A L, Chambers S K, Pakenham K I et al. (2013) Effects of a telephone-delivered multiple health behavior change intervention (CanChange) on health and behavioral outcomes in survivors of colorectal cancer: a randomized controlled trial. *Journal of Clinical Oncology*, **31**, 18:2313–21.

Hughes J (1980) *The Philosophy of Social Research* (London: Longman).

Johns M W (1991) A new method for measuring daytime sleepiness: the Epworth sleepiness scale. *Sleep*, **14**: 540–5.

Kao S H, Hsu L L, Hsieh S I and Huang T H (2013) The effects of two educational interventions on knowledge and competence of nurses with regard to conveying gastroscopy-related information to patients. *Journal of Advanced Nursing*, **69**, 4:793–804.

Lewis P C, Harrell J S, Bradley C and Deng S (2001) Cigarette use in adolescents: the cardiovascular health in children and youth study. *Research in Nursing and Health*, **24**:27–37.

McDonnell A, Nicholl J and Read S M (2003) Acute pain teams in England: current provision and their role in postoperative pain management. *Journal of Clinical Nursing*, **12**, 3:387–93.

McKinney A A and Melby V (2002) Relocation stress in critical care: a review of the literature. *Journal of Clinical Nursing*, **11**, 2:149–57.

Norbeck J S (1987) In defence of empiricism. *Image: Journal of Nursing Scholarship*, **19**, 1:28–30.

Plant M and Coombes S (2003) Primary care nurses' attitude to sickness absence: a study. *British Journal of Community Nursing*, **8**, 9:421–7.

Sandelowski M (2001) Real qualitative researchers do not count: the use of numbers in qualitative research. *Research in Nursing and Health*, **24**:230–40.

Schofield P, Gough K, Ugalde A, Dolling L Aranda S and Sanson-Fisher R (2012) Validation of the Needs Assessment for Advanced Lung Cancer Patients (NA-ALCP). *Psychooncology*, **21**, 4:451–5.

Schutz A (1962) *Collected Papers I: The Problem of Social Reality* (The Hague: Martinus Nijhoff).

Smyth C (2012) The Epworth Sleepiness Scale (ESS). *Try This*. Issue 6.2. Retrieved from http://consultgerirn.org/uploads/File/trythis/try_this_6_2.pdf (accessed 17 September 2013).

Waltz C, Strickland O L and Lenz E (2010) *Measurement in Nursing and Health Research*, 4th edn (New York: Springer).

Wong M L, Lau E Y Y, Wan J H Y, Hui C H, Cheung S F and Mok D S Y (2013) The interplay between sleep and mood in predicting academic functioning, physical health and psychological health: a longitudinal study. *Journal of Psychosomatic Research*, **74**, 4: 271–7.

Qualitative Research

Opening thought | All knowledge has its roots in our perceptions.
Leonardo da Vinci

Introduction

The traditional scientific method that relies heavily on measurement is one of a variety of approaches that can be used to answer research questions. In the 1970s, nurse researchers began to realise that many of the core concepts and issues of direct relevance to practitioners and policy-makers could not be adequately addressed by quantitative methods. This led to the adoption of approaches that could potentially provide an in-depth understanding of people's thinking and behaviour. In this chapter, we will examine the purpose of qualitative research, its main characteristics and its potential contribution to nursing knowledge and practice. Four main approaches (ethnography, phenomenology, discourse analysis and grounded theory) will be outlined. Finally, the limitations of qualitative research will be discussed.

What is qualitative research?

Caring for people and promoting or changing behaviour requires an in-depth understanding of concepts such as perception, experience, belief, motivation and intention. Quantitative research, with its adherence to the scientific method and its reliance on measurement, only partially addresses these issues. The frustration with the failure of quantitative researchers to address adequately and meaningfully the core concepts and issues of relevance to those who need them most led to the adoption and development of new research approaches. Simply because some phenomena are not amenable to measurement does not mean that they cannot or should not be studied by other methods. Some researchers began to think that, in order to understand people, one should listen to, and observe, them. Instead of sending out questionnaires, some thought they could learn more by interacting with those they wanted to study. More flexible strategies (than the ones used in quantitative research) to collect and analyse data were also thought to be necessary in order to 'get below the surface'.

What is qualitative research? It is an umbrella term for a number of diverse approaches that seek to understand by means of exploration, human experience, beliefs, perceptions, motivations, intentions and behaviour. They are based on the premise that interpretation is central to the exploration and understanding of social phenomena. Qualitative researchers use interactive, inductive, flexible and reflexive methods of data collection and analysis in order to do this. Their findings are presented in a variety of formats including descriptions, themes, conceptual models or theories.

Main characteristics of qualitative research

What is often called qualitative research is in fact a collection of approaches that share some common characteristics although they have some distinct features as well. Hammersley (1993) explains that 'the time when qualitative research was an apparently unified movement ranged in opposition to quantitative research has largely gone' and that now they are 'free to disagree among themselves'. Some of the differences between qualitative approaches will become clear in the next section.

The essential distinguishing feature of qualitative approaches is exploration as a means to understand the perceptions and actions of participants from their perspectives. It is not uncommon for quantitative researchers to claim that they also explore phenomena (by examining the relationships between variables or the extent to which respondents possess some qualities or characteristics). This type of exploration is quantitative in nature and is achieved by measuring the variables and by examining relationships through statistical tests. Therefore the terms 'explore' and 'exploration' do not by themselves denote whether a study is qualitative or quantitative.

The main features of qualitative exploration are that it is inductive, interactive, holistic and mainly carried out by flexible and reflexive methods of data collection and analysis. The term 'exploration' in qualitative research can best be understood using the analogy of an explorer in a strange land or in uncharted territory. The exploration is undertaken to 'discover' new lands, people or customs and to learn from them. The rationale for the use of exploration in this way is based on assumptions that researchers can only understand perception and behaviour from participants' own perspectives, in their own words and in the context in which they live and work, and that there can be different interpretations of the same phenomenon.

Ultimately, the purpose of exploration is to gain a better understanding of how people think and behave as individuals and as part of a group. For example, health professionals and patients may view the same situation, event or problem differently. This can affect the efficient use of services and expected outcomes. A qualitative study by Yiu et al. (2011), comparing patients' and nurses' perceptions of the information needs of Chinese surgical patients on discharge, reported that nurses did not adequately understand patients' needs regarding information on finance, their illness or condition, psychological support and cultural practices.

Although some people perceive qualitative exploration as conversation or observation without structure and purpose, it is in fact, if properly carried out, a difficult task requiring substantial training and experience. As Blumer (1969) explains:

> It is not a simple matter of just approaching a given area and looking at it. It is a tough job requiring a high order of careful and honest probing, creative yet disciplined imagination, resourcefulness and flexibility in study, pondering over what one is finding, and a constant readiness to test and recast one's views and images of the area.

Inductive approach

Inherent in the quantitative approach is the notion that the researcher knows in advance which variables to study and the answers to her questions. Typically, a set of responses (constructed by researchers) is offered, from which participants are expected to choose those which best fit their views or situations. This deductive approach to research is used to test researchers' ideas or hypotheses. The purpose of qualitative exploration, on the other hand, is to develop concepts, conceptual frameworks and theories from observations, interviews and interpretation of discourses (diaries, letters, biographies, historical documents, and so on). An inductive approach is used, in which the researcher is open to ideas that can emerge out of listening to or observing people, as well as from examining and re-examining her own perspectives on the subject during and after data collection. Blumer (1969) explains that this type of approach is:

> to move toward a clearer understanding of how one's problem is to be posed, to learn what are the appropriate data, to develop ideas of what are significant lines of relation, and to evolve one's conceptual tools in the light of what he is learning about the area of life.

So it is not just listening to people, but a constant reflection on, and analysis of, data from and between participants, and of the researcher's preconceived ideas.

This inductive approach to research is particularly useful when little is known about the topics one wants to study or when existing conceptual definitions or theories are inadequate and do not reflect people's own experience.

Interactive and reflexive process

To avoid bias, quantitative researchers try to study phenomena in a detached way. In qualitative studies, researchers use the interaction between themselves and the participants in order to get closer to the topic under study. The researcher becomes an instrument of data collection. This means that she has to think of questions during the interview or observation, and of other strategies to get as close a glimpse as possible of the perceptions, experiences and behaviour of participants. Using intuition, she can decide when to continue probing, to stop or to steer the interview in other directions. The use of self to facilitate responses and to 'read' the situation is of vital importance.

The tone, hesitation and repetition in participants' responses and the presence of others are all relevant to the researcher who is trying to make sense of what is being said and the context in which it is said. Even silences have meanings (Mazzei, 2003). In order for participants to relate their experience, reveal their personal views or act in front of researchers the way they would normally, a degree of trust is required. Researchers have to use their contact with participants to build this trust and be accepted. A detached or disengaged stance is unlikely to achieve these results. This is succinctly described by Alderson (2001):

> Qualitative research involves being reflexive, which means examining not only what people say and do, but why they might be saying those words and how the interview setting, the questions and themes and the relationship between interviewer and the interviewee might influence how each person reacts, as together they construct and re-construct their conversation.

Holistic exploration

Although a number of variables can be studied in the same research project, quantitative researchers are constrained by the number of variables they can study at any one time. The variables selected for study also reflect what researchers believe are important to focus on. On the other hand, qualitative research allows participants to put their responses in context. For example, if a participant is asked how he is coping with back pain, he has the opportunity of explaining that there are times and circumstances when he can cope or cannot. This may reveal types, conditions and an extent of coping of which the researcher may not have been aware. The participant may also put his coping efforts in the context of his family or work. What is meant here by 'holistic' refers to participants' opportunity to talk about the totality of their experience of a particular phenomenon in their terms and not through the lens of researcher-generated variables.

Researchers also have the opportunity to put participants' responses in context. Participants' experiences can be historically, culturally and socially constructed.

Flexible methods

Qualitative research relies on methods that can allow researchers into the personal, intimate and private world of participants. Flexible, imaginative, creative and varied strategies are used to facilitate this process. These data collection methods include interviews, observations, group discussions and the analysis of video-recordings, letters, diaries and other documents.

In quantitative research, the methods of data collection are selected or constructed in advance. Because they are structured, predetermined and standardised, researchers cannot change the structure or format of the questionnaires, scales or observation schedules. Instead the data are made to fit into these tools. For example, even if a respondent is not too sure whether he should tick 'yes' or 'no', he has to provide an answer.

In qualitative research, data collection methods can be bent and moulded in order to get close to people's perceptions and behaviour. In some ways, qualitative methods resemble everyday conversations and observations, although researchers require considerable training or skills to use them effectively. Researchers often have to be creative and imaginative in order to achieve the understanding they look for. Besser et al. (2012) used semi-structured interviews and drawings to collect data in their study of the perceptions of osteoporosis patients of their illness and treatment. They found that 'drawings elicited more information about the perceived effects of osteoporosis and emotional reactions to the condition'.

The flexible nature of qualitative exploration also applies to the size of the samples and the sampling techniques. Because each interview or observation builds on previous ones, researchers can follow new 'leads' or check emerging ideas. They are not bound by a fixed sample size, decided prior to the study, as is normally the case in quantitative research. Qualitative researchers can decide during the study to interview more participants, often 'hand-picked' because of the particular experience or perspectives they bring to the topic being studied (see Chapter 15). On the other hand, a researcher can decide that no more interviews are necessary when she begins to experience the saturation of data (that is, the same data are being repeated and nothing new is emerging).

The inductive, interactional and holistic goals of qualitative exploration are best achieved by flexible, creative and penetrative methods, as summarised in this extract from Alderson (2001):

> Qualitative interviews and observations can critically address long-held and possibly misleading assumptions: by asking open questions, rephrasing and dwelling on them, and approaching a topic from different angles; by encouraging extended replies during which people may arrive at new insights while they talk; by exploring examples through narrative during which people voluntarily introduce rich examples and incidentally make passing comments that might not occur to them while quickly working through a questionnaire; by examining ambiguities and uncertainties, and reasons for holding stated beliefs; by exploring people's views and experiences through a range of research methods; and by understanding people's responses through the meanings invested in them by the context of their daily lives.

Common approaches in qualitative research

In this section, we will briefly outline common qualitative approaches in nursing research to illustrate their diversity of focus and process and the type of data they normally seek. These approaches are ethnography, phenomenology, discourse analysis and grounded theory. A brief account of studies that make no reference to any of these approaches is also given. There are separate chapters in this book on ethnography (Chapter 14), phenomenology (Chapter 12) and grounded theory (Chapter 13). Discourse analysis is further covered in Chapter 10. Therefore only a brief introduction to these approaches is given here.

Ethnography

Ethnography is an approach that relies on the collection of data in the natural environment. Ethnographers are interested in how the behaviour of individuals is influenced or mediated by the culture in which they live. According to ethnographers, human behaviour can only be understood if studied in the setting in which it occurs. People can influence, and be influenced by, the groups they belong to or are part of. They have shared meanings, perceptions, language, values and norms. By focusing on culture, the ethnographer gains a holistic understanding of their behaviour. It is not about individuals but about how they interact in their groups.

Ethnography means a 'portrait of people'. It seeks to convey a cultural description of groups in society and has its roots in cultural anthropology. It was adopted by early anthropologists such as Malinowski (1922) and Radcliffe-Brown (1964), who went to live in, and study, tribal communities. They immersed themselves in the culture and adopted the manners and habits of the people they studied, as well as taking part in their rituals and customs. Nowadays, ethnographic studies also take place nearer home: in hospitals, schools, prisons, clinics and nursing homes.

In its classical form, the researcher emerges herself in the culture of the group she wants to study, by living and/or working in their midst or spending significant time with them to begin to see the world from their own perspectives. The researcher is the main instrument of data collection, and data are collected from as many sources as possible within ethical and legal boundaries. The main method is participant observation (see Chapter 18), where this is possible and feasible.

Ethnography allows the researcher to study how and why people behave the way they do. Instead of just interviewing them, she can spend time to see for herself and try to put herself in their place. For example, in an accident and emergency department, an ethnographer will experience the busy atmosphere, the noise, the smell, the 'heat', the frustration, the stress and the sense of achievement of the staff and everything as it normally happens. She can see the decisions and actions taken and is able to talk (when appropriate) with practitioners to explore their perspectives. Thus, ethnographers use inductive, flexible and interactive methods to understand the social realities of groups of people.

Phenomenology

Phenomenology, as a research approach, focuses on individuals' interpretation of their experiences and the ways in which they express them. Unlike ethnography, which places a particular emphasis on people's behaviour in relation to their cultural and social environments, phenomenology focuses on describing how the individual experiences phenomena.

Phenomenology as a philosophy (based on the work of philosophers such as Husserl, Heidegger, Merleau-Ponty, Gadamer and others) stresses the notion that only those who experience phenomena are capable of communicating them to the outside world, and that the researcher's empirical observations are limited in understanding people's perceptions. It is concerned with the 'lived experience' of its respondents. As van Manen (1996) explains, phenomenology aims to explore the different ways in which people experience and understand their world and their relations with others and their environment.

The researcher's task is to describe phenomena as experienced and expressed. One of the main features of Husserlian phenomenology is the notion of 'bracketing'. Simply described, it means the 'suspension' of the researcher's preconceptions, prejudices and beliefs so that these do not interfere with or influence her description of the respondent's experience. Heidegger, a student of Husserl, did not believe that getting to know and describing the experience of individuals were enough. Instead, he stressed the importance of knowing how respondents come to experience phenomena in the way they do. Heideggerian phenomenology seeks to find out how individuals' personal history, such as their education and social class, past events in their lives and their psychological make-up, influence the ways in which they experience phenomena. Its focus is not on social structures, as is the case in ethnography, but on the individual's background.

Heidegger believed that it is not possible to carry out 'bracketing'. Instead he put forward the notion of declaring one's (in this case, the researcher's) preconceptions and prejudices regarding the topic under investigation. In this way, it is possible to reflect on them and see how they influence one's interpretation of the participants' responses. Heideggerian phenomenology, far from rejecting or bracketing them, regards such preconceptions as essential to the understanding of how people experience phenomena. There are many different schools of phenomenology, mainly because they come from the work of many philosophers, including Husserl (1970), Heidegger (1962), Gadamer (1990), Merleau-Ponty (1962) and Sartre (1993).

Discourse analysis

Compared with the other two approaches, discourse analysis is a relatively new method in nursing research. Like ethnography and phenomenology, it has a number of strands (and strands within strands). In essence, it is the analysis of discourse. The latter is a term used to describe the systems we use in communicating with others. These include verbal (talk) and non-verbal (which accompany talk) and written materials. Discourse analysis approaches share the belief that language is not neutral in that it just conveys what we mean, but that it plays an active role in creating and changing our identities, our social relations and our world (Phillips and Jorgensen, 2002). How we 'express' ourselves is not a neutral and passive medium. What we say, how we say it, our choice of words, tone and timing are full of values, meanings and intentions. The purpose of discourse analysis is to uncover them and thereby increase our understanding of human behaviour, in particular how, through language and interaction, we shape, and are shaped by, our world. In discourse analysis, what is spoken or written should also be analysed in its social, political and historical context.

The main sources of data are conversations and interactions between participants and/or between participant and interviewer. Written materials in the form of policy documents, case notes, letters and educational programmes have also frequently been the object of discourse analysis. The various strands of discourse analysis draw from a range of philosophical and theoretical perspectives, which lead to particular aims, methods and focus (Phillips and Jorgensen, 2002). Discourse analysts have used frameworks based on the works of Cicourel (1964), Saussure (1960), Laclau and Mouffe (1985) and Foucault (1972) and others. One of the most common strands of discourse analysis is conversation analysis, which according to Corbetta (2003):

> starts from the premise that conversation is one of the most common forms of interaction between individuals, and that, like all forms of interaction, it does not take place haphazardly; rather, it follows a set of unspoken rules and standard patterns, of which the interlocutors themselves are unaware, and which are an integral part of the culture to which they belong.

The purpose of conversational analysis is 'to gain insight into questions about communication, social action and the construction of self; the Other and the world' (Phillips and Jorgensen, 2002). This type of analysis is illustrated in the work of Potter and Wetherell (1987). Conversational analysis uses social psychological concepts. For an example of conversational analysis, see van Nijnatten and Heestermans's (2012) study of 'Communicative empowerment of people with intellectual disability'.

The work of Foucault (1972) has been very influential in the development and direction of discourse analysis. It is particularly used to provide critical frameworks for health and nursing research. According to Traynor (1996), 'Foucaultian analysis aims to unmask power for the use of those who suffer from it and is directed against those who seize power in their name'. This type of analysis has revealed how, through language, we acquire, exercise or lose power. Power relationships as exercised through language are the focus of the Foucaultian approach to discourse analysis in studies on consultation (between patients and professionals), negotiation (between health professions) and decision-making. Discourse analysis is not just about power and dominance. It is also about how we convey and construct meanings in our daily lives through the content and structure of language and the context in which it is used.

Grounded theory

An alternative to the hypothetico-deductive approach of positivism was formulated by Glaser and Strauss (1967), who coined the term 'grounded theory' to mean an inductive approach to research whereby hypotheses and theories emerge out of, or are 'grounded' in, data. Glaser and Strauss believed that existing theories were speculative and did not arise out of observations of behaviour.

Grounded theory itself is not a theory but a description of theories developed from field observations and interviews. The grounded theory approach is useful in explaining social processes and has tremendous potential in increasing our understanding of human behaviour. The purpose of grounded theory is to generate hypotheses and theories, although, as Glaser and Strauss (1967) suggest, once hypotheses or theories have been formulated from observations, they can be tested deductively. Grounded theory, as a research approach, is particularly useful in nursing, an emerging science still seeking to clarify its concepts and develop its own theories. In recent years, there has been a split between Glaser and Strauss. Glaser (1992) believes that Strauss and Corbin's (1990) techniques and procedures 'force' concepts and theories, rather than allowing them to emerge. Other researchers, including Charmaz (2006), Stern (1980) and Keady (1999), have modified and developed their own interpretation of grounded theory and its techniques.

Similarities and differences between approaches

What is common between the qualitative approaches discussed so far is that they are all interpretivist in the broad sense of the term, in that they place emphasis on interpretation (rather than on objective empirical observations). They are interactive because researchers engage in conversations and with texts (for example, in discourse analysis). These approaches collect data from the participants' perspectives and analyse data by taking into account their specific contexts.

These similarities can sometimes lead to 'method slurring' (Baker et al., 1992). Just because the views of individuals are sought does not mean that the study is phenomenological. In the same way, studying individuals in their own environment does not necessarily make it an ethnographic study. Since all four approaches seek to study individuals' experiences and perceptions in the context of their natural environment and at a particular point in time, it is sometimes difficult to differentiate between them. However, if one understands what the focus is for each of these approaches and their particular philosophical and theoretical premises, the differences between them may become clearer.

Ethnography focuses on culture, phenomenology on consciousness, and discourse analysis on language; the aim of grounded theory is the development of theory through induction. However, the target is the same: to understand the actions and reactions of individuals, groups and organisations. Each of these focal points ('culture' for ethnography, 'consciousness' for phenomenology, and 'language' for discourse analysis) provides researchers with a 'window' into the world of their participants. These approaches have their own distinctive methods and procedures that researchers can use or adapt to collect and analyse data. These will be discussed further throughout this book.

Finally, researchers also use two or more qualitative approaches in the same study. Learmonth et al. (2012) used aspects of phenomenology and grounded theory in their study of 'ways in which "community" benefits frail older women's well-being', while Root (2009) went further and used ethnography, discourse analysis, grounded theory and surveys in her study of the 'experiences of body, work, and risk among factory women in Malaysia'. Johnson et al. (2000) argues that this 'pluralistic' approach is 'not only sensible, it is increasingly inevitable', while Morse (1991) believes that such mixing 'violates the assumption of data collection techniques and methods of analysis of all the methods used'. Some of these approaches are difficult to understand singly, let alone when combined in a study. To use more than one would require a good rationale and a thorough knowledge of their philosophical premises and their procedures, and of the implications of mixing them.

Other types of qualitative studies

Questions that are often asked by novice qualitative researchers, in particular undergraduates, are:

● Do I have to use one of these specific approaches (ethnography and so on) as a framework in my study?
● Can I borrow methodological concepts (for example, constant comparison or bracketing) without labelling my study phenomenological or grounded theory?
● Can I develop conceptual or theoretical insight even if I do not use a specific approach?

It is possible to do a study without an explicit mention of a specific approach. In fact, there are a large number of qualitative studies that do not mention any particular approach. On the other hand, there is ample evidence that many researchers who claim to do phenomenological or grounded theory do not in fact show how they use these approaches in their studies. Cooper and Endacott (2007), who reviewed 12 qualitative studies in emergency care, reported that none of them cited a particular research design other than stating that 'they were taking "a qualitative" approach or undertaking an evaluation'.

Addressing the issue of qualitative studies with no explicit approach, Caelli et al. (2003) point out that a number of terms such as 'generic' (Merriam, 1998), 'interpretive description' (Thorne et al., 1997) and 'basic or fundamental qualitative description' (Sandelowski, 2000) have been used to describe these studies. Caelli et al. (2003) describe 'generic' qualitative study as:

those that exhibit some or all of the characteristics of qualitative endeavor but rather than focusing the study through the lens of a known methodology they seek to do one of two things: either they combine several methodologies or approaches, or claim no particular methodological viewpoint at all. Generally, the focus of the study is on understanding an experience or an event.

Sandelowski (2010) revisited her previous paper 'Whatever happened to qualitative description?' (Sandelowski, 2000) and corrected some of the 'several misconceptions' that the paper had generated. Sandelowski (2010) explains clearly that 'qualitative description' is neither her method nor a new method. The term is itself a description of types of study that share some but not all characteristics. She also explains that qualitative descriptive studies involve interpretation and the use of theory even if these are not explicit. As she points out (Sandelowski, 2010):

having no commitment to a theory does not mean not being influenced by theory at all. Every word is a theory; the very way researchers talk about their subject matter reflects their leanings, regardless of whether they present these inclinations as such or even recognize them. For example, even in the absence of any explicit theory of loss or bereavement, to portray miscarriage as a loss is not to define miscarriage, but rather to theorize it.

Thorne et al. (2004) make a distinction between 'interpretive description' and 'traditional qualitative descriptive' approaches. According to them, the former involves more than description: it includes some form of theorising that practitioners can understand and find useful for their practice. According to Thorne et al. (2004), interpretive descriptive studies 'borrow strongly from some aspects of grounded theory, naturalistic inquiry, and ethnography, drawing on values associated with phenomenological approaches inherent in the methods of data collection'.

One of the features of these generic and descriptive studies is that data analysis is quite often at a level that is closer to the data rather than at a deeper, abstract level (Sandelowski, 2010). For Thorne et al. (2004):

> The product of an interpretive description, or the object of the exercise, is a coherent conceptual description that taps thematic patterns and commonalities believed to characterize the phenomenon that is being studied and also accounts for the inevitable individual variations within them. Such descriptions differ in form from those created in qualitative methods whose intent is to generate an entirely original and coherent new truth or metaphor .

An example of a descriptive interpretive study is that of Cooper et al. (2011) in Research Example 6. The findings of this study (Cooper et al., 2011) can be compared with those of Knight et al.'s (2012) study exploring how 'men's conversations about sexual health are constituted by masculine hierarchies'. Knight et al., who used a discourse analysis framework to underpin their study, reported (among other things) that they found:

> situations whereby participants employed a discourse of "manning up" to (i) exert power over others with disregard for potential repercussions and (ii) deploy power to affirm and reify their own hyper-masculine identities, while using their personal (masculine) power to help others (who are subordinate in the social ordering of men).

One can in see, in Knight et al.'s study, a level of interpretation that involves not only describing the participants' behaviour, but also providing an explanation of why they behave in the way they do. Such findings can make a useful contribution to knowledge in theoretical terms. However, they are not in a form that practitioners can readily use in their practice.

The flexible nature of qualitative research allows researchers a degree of freedom to suit their design to the phenomenon that they study. They can use a particular approach (or more than one) to underpin their study. They can borrow methodo-

A qualitative study

A qualitative study exploring the views of users and providers of care of contact-based interventions following self-harm *Cooper et al. (2011)*

The objectives of this study were:

- To obtain user and staff views on treatment following hospital attendance for self-harm in general and contact interventions in particular.
- To gain a further understanding of how such interventions might be of benefit.
- To identify practical issues in the delivery of interventions.

The rationale for the use of a qualitative methodology in this study was:

Qualitative data might help us gain an understanding of the underlying psychological mechanisms and aspects of the design of the interventions that might be of benefit or detriment to patients that a quantitative study could not be expected to elucidate. We wanted to further understand the pragmatic barriers to the implementation of various forms of follow-up contact care by bringing in the perspectives of staff working on the "front line" as a progressive approach to refining treatment'.

The data collection methods were semi-structured interviews and a focus group. The authors conducted thematic analyses. The authors explained that 'data analysis was iterative and used methods of constant comparison with repeated scrutinizing of transcripts to determine the themes emerging from the data'.

The findings were summarised as follows:

Most service users and staff participants identified the period of time directly after discharge as the time of greatest need. A contact-based intervention was viewed by service users as a gesture of caring, which counteracted feelings of loneliness. Delivery by mental health specialists was preferred, initially by phone, but letters were considered helpful later. The intervention should be both genuine in delivery and linked to current services. Potential barriers included means of accessing the service and threats to privacy.

Comments

1 According to Thorne et al. (2004), interpretive description aims to answer questions of relevance to a clinical discipline, such as whether people comprehend their need for our service. In this study, the researchers were interested in obtaining staff's and users' views on the services provided and the type of intervention they would prefer.

2 Constant comparison, a concept in grounded theory (see Chapter 13), was 'borrowed' to analyse the data. However, this study is not described as grounded theory, nor does it use a grounded theory approach.

3 The findings of this study can be directly applied to improve the particular practice that was the focus of this qualitative exploration.

logical concepts from one or more approaches and still not label their study after these approaches. Or they can carry out a study without reference to any approach. However, this flexibility should not be interpreted as 'anything goes'. Labelling one's study is less important than explaining what was done, how it was done and the rationale for, and implications of, the decisions taken. Above all, the study should show evidence of attention to rigour and should be ethically sound.

Qualitative research and nursing

In the early years of the development of nursing research, quantitative approaches were dominant. In the 1970s, researchers began to realise that many of the core concepts and issues of relevance to practitioners and policy-makers could benefit from research approaches capable of providing an in-depth understanding of nursing health phenomena. With the emphasis, in recent years, on users' participation in decision-making in their own care, the need to listen to them and understand their perspectives increased. While questionnaires and scales provide useful data to achieve this objective, qualitative methods are more appropriate for getting to know users' perspectives and experiences.

There is a growing recognition of the value of qualitative research in addressing issues and problems of concern to nurses, midwives and other health professionals such as physiotherapists, occupational therapists, psychologists and doctors, among others. This is evidenced by the increasing number of qualitative studies in their respective journals in the last three decades. A relatively recent trend is the increase in mixed methods studies (see Chapter 5), in particular the use of qualitative approaches for exploring the process of randomised controlled trials. For example, Nelson et al. (2013) carried out a qualitative study as part of a randomised controlled trial comparing a lay-facilitated angina management programme with usual care. They explained that the aim was to explore participants' beliefs, experiences and attitudes to the care they had received during the trial, particularly those who had received the angina management intervention.

Nursing's philosophy is perceived by some (Munhall, 1982; Kirkevold, 2000) as being congruent with qualitative approaches. Apart from being technical, nursing is also patient-centred, holistic and humanistic. Most qualitative approaches share some of these characteristics, which make them suitable for the study of nursing phenomena. Qualitative research, with its focus on the experiences of people, stresses the uniqueness of individuals. In nursing, each patient is a unique individual for whom a specific care plan is developed.

Qualitative researchers collect data from respondents, often in their natural environments, taking into account how cultural, social and other factors influence their experiences and behaviour. Nursing care should ideally be holistic in that the patient and her illness are treated together, rather than the illness being treated separately. The environment in which the patient lives, her partner and her family, should all be taken into account in the planning and delivery of care. The qualitative research focus on experience is also compatible with the person-centred approach to care.

Qualitative approaches value respondents' views and seek to understand the world in which they live. Implicit in some approaches and explicit in others is the notion that respondents have experiences, wishes and rights that must be respected.

Bailey (2001) explains that 'without knowledge of what illness and healthcare mean to people and of how lives are changed, we are left groping or insensitive about what it means to care for people'. As will be shown below, some researchers believe in the empowering potential of research for the participants. Nurses, too, are expected to adopt a humanistic approach to their work, which entails not letting their personal prejudices influence their professional judgement, and respecting and promoting their clients' rights.

Qualitative research is also perceived as contributing more towards ethical healthcare than quantitative research. Alderson (2001), referring to her work on ethical issues relating to the care and treatment of children, points out that 'each case is so individual that research about the elusive processes of children's competent decision-making is understood more clearly through qualitative case studies rather than through standardised questionnaires'. However, it should be noted that quantitative methods also help to ensure that treatments are effective and do no harm, which is at the core of nursing philosophy itself.

Research produces knowledge and has the potential to empower those who carry it out and those who fund it. Some sections of society benefit more than others. Some women in particular feel that research studies by men on women, considering topics chosen mainly by men, do not necessarily serve women's interests and in fact contribute to their domination. Thus, feminist research emerged out of the failure of conventional research to address the issues of relevance and benefit to women. According to Seibold et al. (1994), 'feminist researchers share with critical theorists the need to make a difference through research; that is the desire to bring about social change of oppressive constraints through criticism and social action'. Landman (2006) explains that feminist research 'questions whether mainstream conceptions of objectivity, knowledge and reason proceed from a view of the social world only from the perspective of male or masculine values, interests, emotions and attitudes (i.e. reflect an androcentric perspective)'.

Although the qualitative approach, with its notion of interacting and collaborating with participants, is better suited to feminist research, there are those, like Oakley (1989), who believe that experimental research such as randomised controlled trials can be emancipatory in practice and can be of benefit to those involved in research and to women more generally. For an example of feminist research, see Robinson and VandeVusse (2011). For a review of the trends and contribution of feminist research in nursing, see Im (2010).

Qualitative studies in nursing and health research

In the previous chapter, ways in which quantitative research can enhance policy, practice and education in nursing and other health professions were highlighted. In this section, we will look at examples of the types of problems or concerns of practitioners that can be addressed by qualitative approaches. For the sake of simplification, these studies will be divided into those which:

- explore patients' experience and behaviour;
- explore the experience and behaviour of nurses and other health professionals;
- evaluate interventions and services;
- explore core concepts relevant to nursing and health.

Studies that explore patients' experience and behaviour

Nurses gain their understanding of their patients' experience mainly through direct care and from the literature. Qualitative studies can provide further insight into these experiences. For example, Ekholm et al. (2013) explored, through qualitative interviews, the next of kin experiences of symptoms and distress among patients with colorectal cancer.

To provide efficient, humane and ethical care, nurses need to know why patients behave the way they do, and about the personal and structural factors that influence the way they perceive health, illness and health services. One of the persistent problems in healthcare is the non-compliance of patients with prescribed treatment or the advice of health professionals. Health professionals have their own beliefs and assumptions of why this happens. However, patients themselves have a lot to contribute towards an understanding of this problem. For example, Escamilla Fresnadillo et al. (2008) used focus groups to explore the reasons for non-compliance with therapy in older patients taking multiple medications. They found that the patients' beliefs and lifestyle and the characteristics of the medicine affected their compliance.

Nurses need to know which factors facilitate or hinder their patients or clients in adopting healthy lifestyles or getting better. Tod (2003) explored, by means of interviews, the barriers to pregnant women stopping smoking. The study uncovered a number of factors and barriers, such as the role and meaning of smoking for women with a high caring burden and socioeconomic problems, the influence of family and friends, and their perceptions of the risks of smoking and the nature of the delivery of smoking cessation services (Tod, 2003). These findings have implications for those who provide such services.

Researchers also want to know about the qualities of patients that contribute to positive outcomes. For example, Ablett and Jones (2007) explored 'resilience and well-being in palliative care' with the use of qualitative interviews. The findings allowed them to compare with other similar concepts such as 'hardiness' and 'sense of coherence'. They suggested that their findings have implications for staff training and support.

Qualitative research has also been useful in exploring and assessing patients' knowledge of disease, illness, medication or health services. Dunkley et al. (2009) investigated the knowledge and attitudes of patients and primary care practitioners, in a multiethnic setting, concerning waist circumference measurement (WCM). According to the authors, this study 'adds to our understanding of views on WCM in a multi-ethnic setting, highlighting factors for consideration if WCM is to be facilitated in routine practice'.

Studies that explore the experience and behaviour of nurses and other health professionals

The experience, perceptions, knowledge, attitudes, beliefs and practice of nurses can also influence patients' outcomes. All these aspects have been studied with the use of qualitative research. Wilson et al. (2013), in an ethnographic study of the experiences of novice haemodialysis nurses (HD) and the cannulation of arterio-venous fistulae, identified the interplay between personal and environmental/contextual factors that hindered skill acquisition. They concluded that their findings would 'be helpful in directing future educational, operational, and supportive interventions for novice HD nurses around cannulation skill development'.

Rubarth (2003) described the 'lived experience of nurses who care for newborns with sepsis'. They uncovered many different emotions, reactions and perceptions that they believed could assist nurses to have a better understanding of the role of the nurse and the emotional burden of working in a neonatal intensive care unit.

Nurses' perceptions of the concepts that they deal with on a daily basis have implications for their practice. Thunberg et al. (2001) carried out a grounded theory study of healthcare professionals' understanding of chronic pain. They found that while nurses talked about a biopsychosocial model of care of people with chronic pain, their practice reflected biomedical principles. Thus, qualitative research, using the inductive process, can potentially reveal discrepancies between beliefs and practice.

Studies that evaluate interventions and services

Qualitative research has been used to compare the perceptions of the public with those of practitioners, as there are often wide discrepancies between them. Examples of such studies include Gilmet and Burman's (2003) exploration of 'stroke perceptions of well lay persons and professional care givers' and Yiu et al.'s (2011) study comparing patients' and nurses' perceptions of the information needs of Chinese surgical patients on discharge.

Qualitative approaches can provide data on the effectiveness of tools and interventions that nurses and other health professionals use. For example, Cowley and Houston (2003) examined, by means of interviews and observations, the acceptability and effectiveness of a 'structured health needs assessment tool' from the perspective of health visitors. They found that the tool 'caused anxiety and distress to, particularly, the most vulnerable clients', the 'structured format of the tool appeared to encourage the health visitors to question instead of listen' and 'it did not help to identify all the needs and intruded into normal practice in an insensitive and unhelpful way'. Other researchers have used qualitative research to explore the effectiveness of rapid response teams in a large teaching hospital in the USA (Leach and Mayo, 2013).

Qualitative research can be useful to inform policy as well. For example, Patel et al.'s (2012) study of 'nurses' attitudes and experiences surrounding palliative sedation' was designed to contribute to 'policy and procedural guidelines' regarding palliative sedation in acute care hospitals and hospice programmes.

Studies that explore core concepts relevant to nursing and health

Many of the above examples are of studies that explored the concerns of practitioners, and their findings are often of direct relevance to the population or setting where they have been carried out. However, qualitative research can also contribute to the development of concepts, conceptual frameworks and that which can have wider applications. Kleinman et al. (2013) conducted qualitative research with patients with clinical diagnoses of insomnia and developed 'a conceptual framework and endpoint model' that identifies a hierarchy and interrelationships of potential outcomes in insomnia research.

Blomberg et al. (2008) explored, through the use of focus group interviews, district nurses' care of chronic pain sufferers to create a theoretical model that can explain the variation in district nurses' experiences when caring for these patients. As they explain:

> The result is a theoretical model of district nurses' involvement in pain care. The model: (1) illustrates three main conditions in the care situation that influence district nurses' involvement in pain care and (2) explains the connection between how district nurses actively or passively detect and actively or passively respond to patients with pain problems.

Victorson et al. (2009), from the findings of their qualitative study of the 'experience of dyspnea and functional limitations in chronic obstructive pulmonary disease', developed a 'dyspnea-specific conceptual model in which the most proximal of concepts (dyspnea symptoms) can impair function and are mediated by personal and environmental factors'.

Often, as acknowledged by the researchers themselves, one study can only tentatively develop a conceptual framework or theory. Further research is recommended to build upon these preliminary findings. Combining the results of a number of studies can also contribute towards the development of theories. Kearney (2001) systematically analysed and combined the findings of 13 studies in order to develop a theory of women's experience in violent relationships.

While theories can broaden practitioners' thinking, they can enhance practice directly or indirectly. Morse et al. (1999) describe in detail how theories derived from qualitative research were used to develop the Hope Assessment Guide (Penrod and Morse, 1997) and the Assessment Guide for Bi-polar Disorders (Hutchinson, 1993, 1998). Both guides were implemented and evaluated using qualitative methods in order to modify and strengthen them.

The examples in this section show the relevance and potential contribution of qualitative research to practice, policy, education and theory development. It should, however, be obvious by now that both quantitative and qualitative research can be used to study the same phenomena: views of patients and nurses, barriers to positive health, knowledge, attitudes, effectiveness of intervention and similar issues. The difference, however, is how they study these phenomena. For example, a quantitative researcher may give respondents a list of barriers to a healthy diet and ask them to tick those which apply to them, while a qualitative researcher will explore with them what they think the barriers are without imposing their own views on them. Quantitative researchers study these problems using questionnaires and scales with the purpose of measuring them. Qualitative researchers, on the other hand, explore phenomena by using inductive, flexible and interactive processes.

Criticisms and limitations of qualitative research

The main criticisms of qualitative research are that it is anecdotal and unscientific, and produces findings that are not generalisable. Qualitative research has been described as anecdotal, journalistic, impressionistic and subjective. Green and Britten (1998) point out that there are important differences:

> between anecdotes (stories told for their dramatic or other qualities, without analysis or critical evaluation) and qualitative research. Rigorously conducted qualitative research is based on explicit sampling strategies, systematic analysis of data, and a commitment to examining counter explanations.

All research involves the systematic and rigorous collection and analysis of data, and qualitative research is no exception. All researchers, including qualitative ones, have to demonstrate how they collect and analyse data, justify their decisions and are aware of the strengths, limitations and implications of their selected approach for studying a particular topic or phenomenon.

Qualitative research has been charged with being unscientific in that it does not use methods that have been shown to be valid or reliable (two concepts that are at the heart of quantitative approaches). In particular, it is suggested that researchers get so involved that they cannot be objective. Reliability in quantitative terms is the consistency with which a tool measures what it is supposed to measure. This interpretation of reliability is rejected in qualitative research since it is believed that an interaction between a researcher and a participant (such as in an interview situation) is a unique encounter that happens at a specific point in time and space. Neither the same researcher nor others can reproduce this interaction and the data collected from it. Far from seeing this as a weakness, qualitative researchers point out that it is necessary not to remain detached, otherwise it is not possible to obtain an in-depth understanding of whatever is being studied.

The problem of knowing whether participants tell us what they really think and believe applies to both quantitative and qualitative approaches. The latter involves social interactions of a kind that are conducive to disclosure, in particular if there is a degree of 'cosiness', trust and intimacy. On the other hand, one can argue that intimate, embarrassing and personal details can best be collected by means of questionnaires that can guarantee anonymity.

Qualitative research also allows for questioning, for probing and for clarification of contradictions and inconsistencies in responses, in particular when there is more than one contact with the same participants and where data are collected from a number of sources (as happens in grounded theory and ethnographic research).

In quantitative research, the focus is on producing reliable and valid tools. If a tool is reliable, it is assumed that it will produce reliable findings. While this is usually true of tools measuring physical concepts such as temperature or weight, it is not necessarily so with the measurement of attitudinal or behavioural concepts, since humans can react to tools in a way that temperature cannot do to a thermometer. For example, even if a reliable and valid scale is used to measure research utilisation in clinical practice, one cannot be certain that respondents are giving an accurate account of their practice. It is possible that they consistently give socially desirable answers.

One can conclude that no method or approach has a monopoly on collecting reliable data. It is not a question of whether or not qualitative or quantitative methods are reliable, but rather the degree to which one can assume that they are reliable. This depends on the type of data and the context in which, and the people from whom, the data are collected. Both approaches have devised appropriate and relevant strategies to try to ensure that their findings are reliable.

The concept of validity reflects the accuracy with which the findings reflect the phenomenon being studied. In the final analysis, the findings must be credible to be of any value. Data collection in qualitative research carries with it an in-built process whereby, as the first tentative findings emerge, they are rigorously examined, compared with other participants' responses, viewed within the context of existing knowledge, and confirmed, modified or rejected in further interviews or observations until the researcher is confident that the final findings represent the phenomenon as accurately as possible.

Perhaps the most frequent criticism of qualitative studies is that their findings are not generalisable because small, 'hand-picked', localised, unrepresentative samples are used. Most studies that are carried out well can be of value beyond the sample studied. For example, Bonia et al. (2013) conducted a qualitative exploration of factors associated with mothers' decisions to formula-feed their infants in Newfoundland and Labrador, Canada. They identified themes such as 'the support needed to breastfeed', 'the convenience associated with formula feeding' and 'the embarrassment surrounding breastfeeding in public'. Midwives around the world can compare these findings with their own experiences with women choosing to breastfeed or to use formula feed.

Many qualitative studies are in the form of case studies, the findings of which are often criticised as being applicable only to the case or group being studied. Sandelowski (1997), on the other hand, points out that generalisations can be drawn from and about cases and that 'entire fields of knowledge, such as ethics, law, and several domains in psychology, have been constructed from case generalisations'.

In quantitative research, the findings from large, random, representative samples, are expected to be generalisable to the population from which the samples are drawn. This is appropriate for studies, for example, which seek to know how many people are satisfied with the care they receive or how they score on a 'quality of life' scale. In qualitative research, the aim would be to explore what the concept 'quality of life' means to the participants. For this task, the number of participants is of little relevance. The aim is to find out who can help the researcher to gather as many different perspectives as possible. She has to rely on her knowledge of participants and on the advice of health professionals to explore this concept. A random, representative sample would most likely reveal more of the same. The focus, therefore, is not on generalising to the sample but on developing a concept or theory that represents the phenomenon in its different and varied manifestations.

Qualitative research, like other approaches, has its limitations as well. Since it is believed that one interpretation is as valid as any other, the problem of choosing between them when presented with conflicting ones remains a challenge. Researchers have devised ways such as asking participants if they recognise the researcher's interpretation of what they said, or finding out if other researchers would interpret the data in the same way as the researcher. These strategies are, however, not without their challenges and problems (see Chapter 20).

It is important to note that research paradigms have different philosophical assumptions, rules and norms that researchers follow in order to produce scientific knowledge. It is not helpful to use the rules and criteria of one paradigm to evaluate the process and outcomes of other paradigms. To use an analogy, one cannot use the beliefs of one religion to judge another. Each has its own criteria and rules of what is 'good' or 'bad' and how people should live their lives.

Although the term 'scientific method' is usually associated with quantitative research, other approaches are not less scientific provided they do not explain phenomena in supernatural or metaphysical terms. Alternative approaches to quantitative research recognise that human beings think and act rationally, but that they do not do so all of the time and in all circumstances, and in a mechanical way. They have feelings, emotions, motivations, beliefs, customs and environmental constraints that are difficult for quantitative approaches, with their emphasis on objectivity and measurement, to access in a meaningful way.

Summary

In this chapter, we have discussed the meaning, characteristics and purpose of qualitative research. This is a broad term comprising a number of diverse approaches which share the belief that subjective interpretation is central to the exploration of human and social phenomena. Qualitative researchers use interactive, inductive, flexible and reflexive methods in their studies. Beyond this, some of the main qualitative approaches, such as ethnography, phenomenology, discourse analysis and grounded theory, have their own procedures to collect, analyse, interpret and present data. They are based on theories from such diverse disciplines as philosophy, sociology, psychology or semiotics, or from a combination of these. However, researchers do not necessarily have to use any of these approaches to carry out qualitative studies.

Qualitative research is particularly useful in exploring users' and professionals' experience, behaviour and practice, and for contributing to the definition of core nursing and health concepts. Both qualitative and quantitative research have their strengths and limitations. In the next chapter, we will explore how these two approaches and methods can be combined in the same study.

References

Ablett J R and Jones R S P (2007) Resilience and well-being in palliative care staff: a qualitative study of hospice nurses' experience of work. *Psycho-Oncology* **16**:733–40.

Alderson P (2001) *On Doing Qualitative research Linked to Ethical Healthcare*, Vol. 1 (London: Wellcome Trust).

Bailey C (2001) Revisiting qualitative inquiry: interviewing in nursing and midwifery research. *Nursing Times Research*, **6**, 1:551.

Baker C, Wuest J and Stern P N (1992) Method slurring: the grounded theory/phenomenology example. *Journal of Advanced Nursing*, **17**:1355–60.

Besser S J, Anderson J E and Weinman J (2012) How do osteoporosis patients perceive their illness and treatment? Implications for clinical practice. *Archives of Osteoporosis*, **7**, 1–2:115–24.

Blomberg A M, Hylander I and Tornkvist L (2008) District nurses' involvement in pain care: a theoretical model. *Journal of Clinical Nursing*, **17**, 15:2022–31.

Blumer H (1969) *Symbolic Interactionism: Perspective and Method* (Englewood Cliffs, NJ: University of California Press).

Bonia K, Twells L, Halfyard B, Ludlow V, Newhook L A and Murphy-Goodridge J (2013) A qualitative study exploring factors associated with mothers' decisions to formula-feed their infants in Newfoundland and Labrador, Canada. *BMC Public Health*, **13**:645.

Caelli K, Ray L and Mill J (2003) 'Clear as mud': toward greater clarity in generic qualitative research. *International Journal of Qualitative Methods*, **2**, 2:Art. 1.

Charmaz K (2006) *Constructing Grounded Theory: A Practical Guide Through Qualitative Analysis* (Thousand Oaks, CA: Sage).

Cicourel A V (1964) *Method and Measurement in Sociology* (New York: Free Press).

Cooper J, Hunter C, Owen-Smith A et al. (2011) 'Well it's like someone at the other end cares about you.' A qualitative study exploring the views of users and providers of care of contact-based interventions following self-harm. *General Hospital Psychiatry*, **33**, 2:166–76.

Cooper S and Endacott R (2007) Generic qualitative research: a design for qualitative research in emergency care? *Emergency Medicine Journal*, **24**, 12:816–19.

Corbetta P (2003) *Social Research: Theory, Methods and Techniques* (London: Sage).

Cowley S and Houston A M (2003) A structured health needs assessment: acceptability and effectiveness for health visiting. *Journal of Advanced Nursing*, **43**, 1:82–92.

Dunkley A J, Stone M A, Patel N, Davies M J and Khunti K (2009) Waist circumference measurement: knowledge, attitudes and barriers in patients and practitioners in a multi-ethnic population. *Family Practice*, **26**, 5:365–71.

Ekholm K, Gronberg C, Borjeson S and Bertero C (2013) The next of kin experiences of symptoms and distress among patients with colorectal cancer: diagnosis and treatment affecting the life situation. *European Journal of Oncology Nursing*, **17**, 2:125–30.

Escamilla Fresnadillo J A, Castaner Nino O, Benito Lopez S, Ruiz Gil E, Burrull Gimeno M and Saenz Moya N (2008) Reasons for therapy non-compliance in older patients taking multiple medication. [Spanish]. *Atencion Primaria*, **40**, 2:81–5.

Foucault M (1972) *The Archaeology of Knowledge* (London: Routledge).

Gadamer H G (1990) *Truth and Method*, 2nd rev. edn (New York: Crossroad).

Gilmet K and Burman M E (2003) Stroke perceptions of well laypersons and professional caregivers. *Rehabilitation Nursing*, **28**, 2:52–6.

Glaser B (1992) *Basics of Grounded Theory Analysis: Emergence versus Forcing* (Mill Valley, CA: Sociology Press).

Glaser B and Strauss A (1967) *The Discovery of Grounded Theory* (Chicago: Aldine).

Green J and Britten N (1998) Qualitative research and evidence based medicine. *British Medical Journal*, **316**:1230–32.

Hammersley M (ed.) (1993) *Social Research: Philosophy, Politics and Practice* (London: Sage).

Heidegger M (1962) *Being and Time*, trans. J Macquarrie and E Robinson (New York: Harper and Row).

Husserl E (1970) *Logical Investigations*, Vol. 2, trans. J N Findlay (London: Routledge and Kegan Paul).

Hutchinson S A (1993) People with bi-polar disorders quest for equanimity: doing grounded theory. In: P L Munhall and C Oiler Boyd (eds) *Nursing Research: A Qualitative Perspective* (New York: National League for Nursing).

Hutchinson S A (1998) An assessment guide for bi-polar disorders. [Unpublished]. Cited in: J M Morse, S A Hutchinson and J Penrod, From theory to practice: the development of assessment guides from quality derived theory. *Qualitative Health Research*, **8**, 3:329–40.

Im E-O (2010) Current trends in feminist nursing research. *Nursing Outlook*, **58**:87–96.

Johnson M, Long T and White A (2000) Arguments for 'British pluralism' in qualitative health research. *Journal of Advanced Nursing*, **33**, 2:243–9.

Keady J S (1999) The dynamics of dementia: a modified grounded theory. Bangor University of Wales, unpublished thesis.

Kearney M H (2001) Enduring love: a grounded formal theory of women's experience of domestic violence. *Research in Nursing and Health*, **24**, 4:270–82.

Kirkevold M (2000) Qualitative methods in the caring sciences: time for critical reflection and dialogue. *Scandinavian Journal of Caring Services*, **14**, 1:1–2.

Kleinman L, Buysse D J, Harding G, Lichstein K, Kalsekar A and Roth T (2013) Patient-reported outcomes in insomnia: development of a conceptual framework and endpoint model. *Behavioral Sleep Medicine*, **11**, 1:23–36.

Knight R, Shoveller J A, Oliffe J L et al. (2012) Masculinities, 'guy talk' and 'manning up': a discourse analysis of how young men talk about sexual health. *Sociology of Health and Illness*, **34**, 8:1246–61.

Laclau E and Mouffe C (1985) *Hegemony and Socialist Strategy: Towards a Radical Democratic Politics* (London: Verso).

Landman M (2006) Getting quality in qualitative research: a short introduction to feminist methodology and methods. *Proceedings of the Nutrition Society*, **65**, 4:429–33.

Leach L S and Mayo A M (2013) Rapid response teams: qualitative analysis of their effectiveness. *American Journal of Critical Care*, **22**, 3:198–210.

Learmonth E, Taket A and Hanna L (2012) Ways in which 'community' benefits frail older women's well-being: 'we are much happier when we feel we belong'. *Australasian Journal on Ageing*, **31**, 1:60–3.

Malinowski B (1922) *Argonauts of the Western Pacific* (London: Routledge & Kegan Paul).

Mazzei L A (2003) Inhabited silences: in pursuit of a muffled subtext. *Qualitative Inquiry*, **9**:355–68.

Merleau-Ponty M (1962) *Phenomenology of Perception*, trans. C. Smith (London: Routledge & Kegan Paul).

Merriam S B (1998) *Qualitative Research and Case Study Applications in Education* (San Francisco: Jossey-Bass).

Morse J M (1991) Qualitative nursing research: a free for all? In: J M Morse (ed.) *Qualitative Nursing Research: A Contemporary Dialogue* (Newbury Park, CA: Sage).

Morse J M (1999) Editorial: Myth 19: Qualitative inquiry is not systematic. *Qualitative Health Research*, **9**, 5:573–4.

Morse J M, Hutchinson S A and Penrod J (1998) From theory to practice: the development of assessment guides from quality derived theory. *Qualitative Health Research*, **8**, 3:329–40.

Munhall P L (1982) Nursing philosophy and nursing research: in apposition or opposition. *Nursing Research*, **31**, 3:176–7.

Nelson P, Cox H, Furze G et al. (2013) Participants' experiences of care during a randomized controlled trial comparing a lay-facilitated angina management programme with usual care: a qualitative study using focus groups. *Journal of Advanced Nursing*, **69**, 4:840–50.

Oakley A (1989) Who's afraid of the randomised controlled trial? Some dilemmas of the scientific method and 'good' research. *Women and Health*, **15**:25.

Patel B, Gorawara-Bhat R, Levine S and Shega J W (2012) Nurses' attitudes and experiences surrounding palliative sedation: components for developing policy for nursing professionals. *Journal of Palliative Medicine*, **15**, 4:432–7.

Penrod J and Morse J M (1997) Strategies for assessing and fostering hope: the hope assessment guide. *Oncology Nursing Forum*, **24**, 6:1055–63.

Phillips L and Jorgensen M W (2002) *Discourse Analysis as Theory and Method* (London: Sage).

Potter J and Wetherell M (1987) *Discourse and Social Psychology* (London: Sage).

Radcliffe-Brown A R (1964) *The Andaman Islanders* (New York: Free Press).

Robinson K M and VandeVusse L (2011) African American women's infant feeding choices: prenatal breast-feeding self-efficacy and narratives from a black feminist perspective. *Journal of Perinatal and Neonatal Nursing*, **25**, 4:320–8.

Root R (2009) Hazarding health: experiences of body, work, and risk among factory women in Malaysia. *Health Care for Women International*, **30**, 10:903–18.

Rubarth L B (2003) The lived experience of nurses caring for newborns with sepsis. *Journal of Obstetric, Gynaecologic and Neonatal Nursing*, **32**, 3:348–56.

Sandelowski M (1997) To be of use: enhancing the utility of qualitative research. *Nursing Outlook*, **45**:125–32.

Sandelowski M (2000) Focus on research methods: whatever happened to qualitative description? *Research in Nursing and Health*, **23**:334–40.

Sandelowski M (2010) What's in a name? *Research in Nursing and Health*, **33**:77–84.

Sartre J P (1993) Freedom and responsibility. In: W Baskin (ed.) *Essays in Existentialism* (New York: Kensington).

Saussure F de (1960) *Course in General Linguistics* (London: Fontana).

Seibold C, Richards L and Simon D (1994) Feminist method and qualitative research about midlife. *Journal of Advanced Nursing*, **19**:394–402.

Stern P N (1980) Grounded theory methodology: its uses and processes. *Image*, **12**, 1:20–3.

Strauss A and Corbin J (1990) *Basics of Qualitative Research: Grounded Theory, Procedures and Techniques* (Thousand Oaks, CA: Sage).

Thorne S, Kirkham S R and MacDonald-Emes J (1997) Interpretive description: a noncategorical qualitative alternative for developing nursing knowledge. *Research in Nursing and Health*, **20**:169–77.

Thorne S, Reimer Kirkham S and O'Flynn-Magee K (2004) The analytic challenge in interpretive description. *International Journal of Qualitative Methods*, **3**, 1:Art. 1.

Thunberg K A, Carlsson S G and Hallberg L R (2001) Health care professionals' understanding of chronic pain: a grounded theory study. *Scandinavian Journal of Caring Sciences*, **15**, 1:99–105.

Tod A M (2003) Barriers to smoking cessation in pregnancy: a qualitative study. *British Journal of Community Nursing*, **8**, 2:56–60, 62–4.

Traynor M (1996) Nursing documentation and nursing practice: a discourse analysis. *Journal of Advanced Nursing*, **24**:98–103.

van Nijnatten C and Heestermans M (2012) Communicative empowerment of people with intellectual disability. *Journal of Intellectual and Developmental Disability*, **37**, 2:100–11.

van Manen M (1996) Phenomenological pedagogy and the question of meaning. In: D. Vandenberg (ed.) *Phenomenology and Educational Discourse* (Durban: Heinemann).

Victorson D E, Anton S, Hamilton A, Yount S and Cella D (2009) A conceptual model of the experience of dyspnea and functional limitations in chronic obstructive pulmonary disease. *Value in Health*, **12**, 6:1018–25.

Wilson B, Harwood L and Oudshoorn A (2013) Moving beyond the 'perpetual novice': understanding the experiences of novice hemodialysis nurses and cannulation of the arteriovenous fistula. *Cannt Journal*, **23**, 1:11–8.

Yiu H Y, Chien W T, Lui M H and Qin B (2011) Information needs of Chinese surgical patients on discharge: a comparison of patients' and nurses' perceptions. *Journal of Advanced Nursing*, **67**, 5:1041–52.

5

Mixed Methods

Nursing is about the rational and the emotional.

Introduction

In the last two chapters, quantitative and qualitative research were presented as having different characteristics and purposes, although they also share some similarities. The debate about how different or similar they are and which one best serves the discipline of nursing has been going on for decades. More recently, the focus has shifted to the combination of quantitative and qualitative methods in the same study. In this chapter, we will explore the rationale for mixing methods and identify ways in which methods can be combined and the purposes for which this is done. We will also discuss the meaning of triangulation and the arguments for and against mixing methods from the two paradigms.

The quantitative–qualitative debate

For more than four decades, nursing has been discussing which of these two approaches has a more useful contribution to make towards developing and increasing its body of knowledge. The quantitative–qualitative debate is not confined to nursing and can be traced back to the two 'opposed Greek philosophical visions of human science that emphasise number (Pythagoras) and meaning (Socrates) as the essence of mind' (Wakefield, 1995). A revival of the debate about quantitative and qualitative research took place in the mid-nineteenth century when there was much argument about the scientific status of history and the social science (Hammersley, 1992).

The discussions have sometimes been at a lower level than one expects of intellectuals. Barber (1996) points out that qualitative research has been portrayed as 'noble, good and empowering', and quantitative methods as 'evil and oppressive'. On the other hand, qualitative research is often described as 'touchy-feely', story-telling and anecdotal. Referring to the field of education, Smith and Heshusius (1986) point out that, until the mid-1980s, the relationship between qualitative and quantitative researchers was one approaching 'mutual disdain'. Proponents of the two approaches have also been described 'as religious zealots who cannot perceive but one way to get to heaven' (Strickland, 1993).

The main (serious) arguments put forward for rejecting quantitative research are that it is limited in researching 'meaning', 'experience' and 'behaviour' (key concepts in understanding patients) and that it 'strips' data of their context. Qualitative research is criticised for being biased, subjective and lacking in reliability, validity and generalisability. In fact, each approach uses its own criteria to criticise the other. While there are some researchers who would totally reject one or the other approach, there are many who would acknowledge that both approaches have a contribution to make to nursing knowledge.

The following examples show how different questions can be addressed by different methods. Example A is about a study on social support and coping among people diagnosed with heart disease. The researcher may want to use quantitative methods to measure the presence and level of social support, the degree of coping and the relationship between these two variables. In example B, a researcher may want to conduct in-depth interviews to explore the meaning of social support, how it operates in practice and how it helps people cope. The choice of approach (qualitative or quantitative) depends on the type of data that the researcher requires in order to answer the research questions. Although qualitative research can still be used to answer the questions in example A, it is unlikely to satisfy those who require a degree of precision expressed in numerical and statistical terms. Similarly, the questions in example B, if studied by quantitative methods, would not satisfy those who want to understand what social support and coping mean for people with heart disease. Therefore it is the type of data the researcher seeks that determines the choice of methods.

A new perspective has been added to the quantitative–qualitative debate. Instead of discussing which approach is best and pointing out the differences, it argues that the two approaches should not be seen as dichotomous (divided into two opposing camps) but rather as sharing many similar characteristics (Hammersley, 1992). Those who argue for this position point out that both quantitative and qualitative researchers use numbers, that both approaches can be inductive and that some researchers on both sides even share the same vision of reality. Paley (2000) argues that the terms 'qualitative' and 'quantitative' refer 'not to different types of research, but to various tools . . . and nothing more'. (For a response to this position, see Sandelowski, 2000a.) Clark (1998) also points out that postpositivist research takes into account many of the concerns of qualitative researchers. In sum, some people argue that the differences between qualitative and quantitative approaches have been oversimplified (Hammersley, 1992); that there is a great deal of overlap between the two (Greenhalgh and Taylor, 1997); that the boundaries are fuzzy (Risjord et al., 2001); and that they should be seen as 'on a continuum with each approach at the opposite ends of the same pole' (Strickland, 1993).

The antagonism between the two approaches is, however, about more than methodology; it also has implications in terms of funding and status. It is a battle for the 'soul' of nursing research and about which one produces legitimate knowledge for nursing practice. This is one of the issues at the heart of evidence-based practice, which in its traditional form puts randomised controlled trials and measurable outcomes on a pedestal above qualitative research.

The quantitative–qualitative debate has to some extent been overtaken by a new development: the combination of quantitative and qualitative methods in nursing, health and social studies. According to Ozawa and Pongpirul (2013), mixed methods research has, in the last two decades, become increasingly popular as a third approach along with qualitative and quantitative methods. The increasing popularity of mixed method studies has given rise to a different but related debate, in particular on the reasons why they should or should not be mixed and the implications of mixing. We now turn to the main arguments for this new approach.

Rationale for combining quantitative and qualitative methods

Combining evidence from different sources and by different methods to make decisions is nothing new. In such fields as archaeology, navigation or forensic medicine, a number of methods and sources of data are used to answer single questions. For example, in archaeology when a skeleton is found, different data are collected in order to find out the time when the person died. Bones are examined (by visual and laboratory tests), samples of the soil are analysed, and clothing and other artefacts found near the body are examined to provide clues to construct (with the help of experts from different disciplines) a profile of the person to which this skeleton belongs. Roberts (2003), a palaeopathologist, explains that in order to interpret abnormalities in skeletons, a number of approaches including visual observation, radiography, histology and molecular methods of analysis are used. In the legal field, evidence from a number of sources such as witnesses' accounts, forensic tests and other circumstantial factors are considered in court. Together, they help the jury or the judge to decide whether or not the accused is guilty. Doctors and nurses, too, rely on information from a number of sources such as signs and symptoms, self-reports, X-rays and laboratory results when making a diagnosis or assessment.

Different methods bring different perspectives to what one studies. A single method is often incapable, on its own, of unravelling complex phenomena. Every method has its weaknesses. For example, interviewing people about what they eat does not necessarily describe what they actually eat. Observing them may be more accurate, but one observer (or even two) may miss important data. Observation itself may make people behave differently from usual. According to Östlund et al. (2011), mixed methods research uses the strengths and perspectives of each method, and recognises 'the existence and importance of the physical, natural world as well as the importance of reality and influence of human experience'. Nursing, in particular nursing research, uses approaches from the natural as well as the social sciences.

Those who oppose the use of qualitative and quantitative methods in the same study believe that the two paradigms cannot be reconciled. This is because the quantitative approach is based on a postpositivistic view that phenomena should be studied by methods that are objective, structured and standardised, while qualitative approaches tends to be semi- or unstructured, flexible and subjective. Their view of reality is also different. For a discussion of the methodological implications of mixing these two approaches, see Morgan (2007) and Fielding (2009). Some of these issues will be discussed later in this chapter.

Types and purpose of combining methods

Cresswell (2003) describes different designs that are used in mixed method studies: the concurrent triangulation design (in which qualitative and quantitative approaches are used to confirm, cross-validate or corroborate findings within a single study), the sequential exploratory design (with an initial phase of qualitative data collection and analysis, followed by a phase of quantitative data collection and analysis) and the parallel design (in which qualitative and quantitative approaches are used in parallel and have equal status).

From the literature, it seems that researchers have combined methods in a number of ways in order to achieve one or more of these objectives:

- To develop and enhance the validity of scales, questionnaires and other instruments.
- To develop, implement and evaluate interventions.
- To further explore or test the findings of one method.
- To study different aspects of the same topic.
- To explore complex phenomena from different perspectives.
- To confirm or cross-validate data.

Researchers can, of course, combine methods to achieve more than one of these purposes in the same study. For a fuller discussion on why and how researchers combine qualitative and quantitative sampling, data collection and analysis techniques, see Sandelowski (2000b).

Developing and enhancing the validity of scales and questionnaires

Qualitative methods, in particular semi-structured and in-depth interviews, focus groups and observations, are frequently used to develop and enhance the validity and reliability of quantitative scales and other measuring tools. Scales and questionnaires are often criticised for being 'researcher-oriented'. They tend to reflect researchers' values, their concerns and even their wordings. Qualitative methods are therefore ideal for generating items for these tools.

For example, to develop the Functional Assessment of Cancer Therapy (FACT) questionnaire for dermatological symptoms associated with epidermal growth factor receptor inhibitors (FACT-EGFRI-18), Wagner et al. (2013) reviewed the literature and conducted qualitative interviews with 12 experts and 20 patients and a quantitative survey, to identify the most important items to include in the scale. In another study, Jap et al. (2013) developed the Indonesian Online Game Addiction Questionnaire by drawing from earlier theories and previous research. To ensure 'appropriate expression of the items', they also conducted qualitative interviews and field observation.

Qualitative methods can be useful at every stage of scale development, validation and evaluation. Hanning et al. (2009) used 'Think aloud' techniques in cognitive interviews with 11 dietitian experts and 21 grade six students in a Canadian study to validate a web-based Food Behaviour Questionnaire.

There are numerous examples in the nursing literature of the use of qualitative methods in the construction, validation, implementation and evaluation of scales and questionnaires. This is an area where the integration of qualitative and quantitative methods seems to work well. Research Example 7 shows how a qualitative approach was used to develop a scale.

Research example 7

Using qualitative methods to inform scale development
Rowan and Wulff (2007)

Qualitative interviews were conducted to generate items for a scale to identify the reasons why people drop out of 'twelve steps' programmes (designed for those with alcohol and other drug addiction). The researchers believed that, apart from a literature review, qualitative interviews have the potential to produce more detailed and varied responses. The aim of the interviews was to generate a list of 'pros' and 'cons' to explain why people adhere (or not) to these programmes. From the list, seven themes emerged, and these were used to construct the seven domains of the scale.

The authors reported that the resulting scale had high reliability. They concluded that, after reading their paper, readers 'will have more of a transparent understanding of the process of using qualitative methods to create instruments for research'.

Developing, implementing and evaluating interventions

Quantitative methods within a randomised controlled trial design have traditionally been the premier method to evaluate the effectiveness of interventions. Practitioners and policy-makers put great emphasis on measurable outcomes on which to base their practice and develop policies. However, the need to develop outcomes that are patient-centred and the emphasis on involving patients in their own care have led to an increasing recognition of the value of qualitative research in intervention studies.

Quantitative methods on their own cannot answer questions such as why an intervention works for some people and not for others, and what types of intervention work best (from patients' perspectives). The Medical Research Council (2008), in its guidance for developing and evaluating complex interventions, acknowledges the contribution that qualitative methods such as focus groups, individual in-depth interviews and observations can make towards addressing some of these questions. In particular, qualitative research is suggested as potentially useful for developing and defining interventions that are patient-centred and for testing the underlying assumptions relating to an intervention. Ways in which interventions can be modified to suit different groups or types of people can also be studied by qualitative methods (Medical Research Council, 2008).

Crawford et al. (2002) also recognise the value and potential uses of qualitative research in 'exploring and describing the process and outcomes of psychological and other complex interventions used to treat mental disorders'. They suggest ways in which qualitative research can be of benefit in the pre-trial, during a trial and in the post-trial stages in the evaluation of complex interventions. They point out, however, that issues concerning the synthesis and interpretation of data are yet to be considered, in particular when one set of data (qualitative) challenges another (quantitative) or vice versa.

Using mixed methods to develop and evaluate interventions is not without its challenges. Farquhar et al. (2011) discusses the use of mixed methods in palliative care. They argue that mixed methods provide evidence from a variety of sources, enabling a better understanding of whether and how an intervention works (or does not work), and inform the design of subsequent studies. However, they warn that mixing methods may not always be appropriate, can be costly and can bring with it its own unique challenges in relation to data collection, integration in analysis and dissemination. For an example of the evaluation of the implementation of an intervention by combining a number of research methods, see Research Example 8.

A mixed method study to develop, implement and evaluate an intervention

Developing and evaluating the implementation of a complex intervention
Brady et al. (2011)

Brady et al. (2011) used a number of data sources to evaluate the implementation of 'a complex, multidimensional oral health care (OHC) intervention for people in stroke rehabilitation settings which would inform the development of a randomised controlled trial'. A questionnaire was used to collect data on the knowledge and attitudes of nursing staff immediately before and after receiving training to implement the intervention. Data on patients' profiles were collected at admission. Semi-structured interviews with staff and patients provided data on the feasibility of implementing the intervention.

Commenting on the use of multiple methods, the authors concluded that:

> By collecting both quantitative and qualitative data we were able to identify not only the comprehensive and complementary evidence relating to the implementation of a complex intervention that comprised of many components, but we captured information relating to the interactions (anticipated and unanticipated) between those components.

Research example 8

Exploring further the findings of one method by means of another

Qualitative methods can further explore quantitative findings to put them in context or to provide a more in-depth understanding. This is because, in researching large samples with structured methods such as questionnaires, it is not always possible to capture the particular contexts in which the responses are made. For example, in a study of 'the effects of mindful eating intervention for obese women', Kidd et al. (2013) measured their eating self-efficacy, mindful eating, depression, weight, body mass index, body fat percentage and blood pressure. The quantitative findings showed that the intervention was only effective in increasing their self-efficacy. When the authors explored these findings in a focus group with a smaller sample of women, they learnt more about the context in which data were collected. As they explain:

> [The women] also spoke about realizing during the 8-week intervention that they may have initially exaggerated their mindful eating, claiming that they were more mindful about eating than they actually were. That is, as the women read the workbook, learned about mindful eating, and practiced mindfulness exercises during the classes, they became aware of how mindlessly they had previously been eating and using food. If the women over-estimated mindful eating at baseline, this may explain the quantitative findings that the intervention had no effect on mindful eating.

In a survey on human immune deficiency virus (HIV), one of the items asked respondents if their relationship with their relatives had changed since being diagnosed with the disease. Most indicated that it had not. However, qualitative interviews revealed later that relationships did not change because they did not tell their relatives that they had HIV (Melby, 2010). Burch (1999) gives an example of the 'decontextualisation' of responses that may distort the score on a scale:

> Instruments in general use commonly asked questions about activities of daily living on the assumption that any limitation will be imposed by the physical inability to carry out the task in question. Thus whether one gets in or out of a car, an item in the Nottingham Extended Activities of Daily Living Scale, is assumed to be due to one's mobility. In reality, it may also be due to the fact that an older person or their carers cannot afford a car, cannot drive a car or that they are so isolated – by choice or compulsion – that they never have the opportunity to carry out this manoeuvre.

Individual interviews or focus groups with a smaller sample of respondents can help to clarify the results collected in the quantitative phase of a study. On the other hand, qualitative methods can reveal patterns, trends and relationships that can lead to the formulation of hypotheses. These can then be tested further by quantitative methods. For example, if qualitative interviews in phase 1 of a study identify gender differences in ways of coping among people with depression, this can be tested with a larger population by means of a survey. Research Example 9 shows how quantitative findings were further explored by means of qualitative methods.

A study using qualitative methods to further explore quantitative findings

The distress experienced by people with type 2 diabetes *West and McDowell (2002)*

West and McDowell (2002) explain:

> This study aimed to investigate the distress associated with type 2 diabetes, whether gender differences existed in the impact of type 2 diabetes and how men and women viewed dietary management. A multi-method, two-stage research approach was taken. Quantitative data were obtained using the Problem Areas in Diabetes (PAID) questionnaire, and no statistically significant gender difference was identified. Worrying about the future, the possibility of complications and feelings of guilt or anxiety when 'off-track' with diabetes management were sources of significant distress. Treatment mode, length of time diagnosed with diabetes and age were significant factors which impacted on the emotional distress experienced by the individual. A subsample of respondents took part in gender-specific focus group interviews which explored issues identified in the survey. Behavioural impact, emotional impact and fear of complications were major themes identified in the interviews. Views of the dietary management of diabetes were also explored within the focus groups and three broad categories identified: dietary restrictions, value judgments and the influence of others.

Studying different aspects of the same topic

Different aspects of the same topic can be explored by different methods in the same study. For example, in studying 'non-compliance with professional advice', the survey method can provide data from a large number of clients to explore the links between non-compliance and such variables as gender, occupation, education or age, and trends such as how often, when and in what circumstances people do not comply. At the same time, it is possible to use a qualitative method such as an in-depth interview to explore the meaning and experience of non-compliance of some of the respondents in order to gain an understanding of their way of thinking, their priorities, their motivations and their beliefs. In this way, a broader picture of non-compliance can emerge. It is not, and cannot ever be, the complete picture since there is more to compliance than these aspects described above. However, the findings will provide practitioners with valuable data to understand both the 'thinking' and 'experience' of participants, and the broader demographic profile of those who comply and those who do not.

With this type of combination of methods, it could appear that these are in fact two studies, each looking at different aspects of the same phenomenon (non-compliance). Researchers undertaking this type of study will have to explain why these two aspects were selected for study and how the two methods were integrated.

The use of different methods to study different aspects of the same phenomenon is illustrated in Research Example 10.

A study using different methods to explore different (but related) aspects of the same phenomenon

Public health education for midwives and midwifery students *McNeill et al. (2012)*

This mixed method study, which was in two phases, comprised a survey of 29 higher education institutions and nine focus groups.

The aim of phase 1 (the survey) was to explore the current provision of public health education within pre-registration midwifery curricula across the UK. The questions in the survey related to the nature of public health education in pre-registration midwifery curricula, with particular reference to topics such as the hours allocated, the importance of public health to midwifery and gaps or limitations.

The aim of phase 2 (focus groups with midwives and with midwifery students) was 'to ascertain their perspectives on how education around public health and inequalities relates to practice and service delivery'.

Comments

1   These two aims are different yet they relate to the same phenomenon (public health education for midwives and midwifery students). The participants in each phase were also different: lead midwives for education (phase 1) and midwives and student midwives (phase 2).

2. The results were analysed separately and then compared to get an overall picture of public health education for this group of health professionals. The use of these two methods helped the researchers to identify three clear issues that they believed would 'require significant consideration from the perspective of policy-makers, education providers, midwifery researchers and midwives in practice in order to maximise the public health role of the midwife moving forward'.

3   Comparing the data in this case was not for the purpose of finding out whether both methods produced the same results (or not), since the questions answered by each method were different. By comparing and combining the results, a larger, more complete view (from different stakeholders' perspectives) emerged of current provision and how things could be improved.

Exploring complex phenomena from different perspectives

To understand the complexity of concepts such as caring or the roles of health professionals requires data from a number of sources. To study the effects of care and services is equally daunting and often not possible using a single research method. For example, 'integrated care' is a complex concept that presents a challenge when one has to demonstrate its effectiveness. In designing an evaluation of such a programme, Greaves et al. (2013) recognise that the intervention has clinical, financial, strategic and political implications. To capture all these components, they used a mixed method approach including 'a quantitative approach measuring changes in service utilisation, costs, clinical outcomes and quality of care using routine primary and secondary data sources' and 'a qualitative component, involving observations, interviews and focus groups with patients and professionals'.

This type of approach is commonly used in evaluation studies. In order to carry out a 'holistic' evaluation, researchers seek data from the main groups involved in the service – patients, carers and health professionals – and by means of a variety of methods. There is no attempt to construct a consistent picture of patients', carers' and professionals' views. In fact, it is likely that each of these groups may perceive the service differently. See Research Example 11 for an example of a study combining multiple methods to study a complex phenomenon.

Using multi-methods to study complex phenomena

Person-centred interactions between nurses and patients during medication activities in an acute hospital setting *Bolster and Manias (2010)*

'Person-centred care' is a term commonly used in nursing, yet there are multiple interpretations of the term (Bolster and Manias, 2010). This can lead to different ways in which it is implemented in practice. Exploring person-centred care can be challenging, not least because, by observing practice, one cannot know the philosophy or theory that underpins it. On the other hand, self-reports of the use of person-centred care may not be reliable. Person-centred care should also be experienced by the person experiencing it. All these issues make the concept of patient-centred care a complex one to study with a single method.

Focusing on medication activities in an Australian metropolitan hospital, Bolster and Manias (2010) explored person-centred interactions between patients and nurses. They carried out 'naturalistic observations' in order to 'generate rich data'. Semi-structured interviews were conducted with participating nurses 'to increase the completeness of the data'. Patients were also interviewed to obtain information about their admission and length of stay, as well as about their medication.

The findings revealed that some nurse–patient interactions were consistent with person-centred care. However, there were 'discrepancies' between what nurses said they did and what they actually did. Some nurses perceived themselves as giving patient-centred care but this was not obvious in their practice.

Research example 11

Confirming or cross-validating findings

Two or more methods can be used simultaneously in order to answer the same question. It is thought that if the answers are similar, confidence in the validity of the findings is increased. These methods can all be quantitative, qualitative or a combination of both. For example, to find out what student nurses eat at lunchtimes, they can be asked to complete a questionnaire and they can be observed during lunch. If both methods reveal similar findings, the researcher will have greater confidence in the validity of the findings than if only one method were used. In a study of patient satisfaction with communication in surgical care, Meredith and Wood (1996) used a number of methods including qualitative interviews and observations, and a questionnaire. Their aim was to confirm qualitative findings through the quantitative method. Some of their findings were similar and some were different. For example, 'evidence that a long wait at the outpatient clinic led patients to take this dissatisfaction with them into the meeting was not forthcoming from the questionnaire survey' (Meredith and Wood, 1996).

To cross-validate findings, self-reports are often compared with biochemical measurements (for example, in studies on smoking) and instruments' scores are compared with data from semi-structured interviews (for example, in studies on quality of life). For an example of a study using qualitative and quantitative methods to answer the same question, see Research Example 12.

Research example 12

An example of triangulation

A mixed methods descriptive investigation of readiness to change in rural hospitals participating in a tele-critical care intervention *Zapka et al. (2013)*

In this study, a number of methods were used to explore 'readiness for change' in rural hospitals participating in a tele-critical care intervention'. As the authors explain:

> We evaluated 5 general domains and the related factors or topics of organisational context via key informant interviews (n=23) with hospital leadership and staff, compared these to data from hospital staff surveys (n=86) and triangulated data with investigators' observational reports.

There was general agreement in the findings between these three measures. Apart from providing opportunities to compare the findings, the use of multi-methods also provided 'a more comprehensive picture of health services than individual methods alone' (Zapka et al., 2013). They concluded that it was clear that the use of an exploratory mixed methods approach was valuable in the examination of domains and factors affecting the adoption and implementation of technology in small organisations.

In summary, researchers combine methods to achieve one of the following:

- complementarity
- completeness
- confirmation.

Complementarity is achieved when a different method from the one used in the main study is used to help in the construction and validation of tools, to develop, implement and evaluate interventions, and to put the findings in context. The methods in these types of studies are usually fully integrated and each one plays an important part in assisting (or complementing) the other methods by making their tools more valid or their findings more understandable. There is a division of labour, and each method has clear roles to perform. In this case, paradigms are not mixed, only the methods are.

When different methods are employed to look at different aspects of the same phenomenon, it is believed that a more complete picture is revealed than if only one method is used. This is similar to the construction of a whole picture by putting 'jigsaw pieces' together. Some research methods are more appropriate for the study of some aspects of phenomena than others. For example, a researcher aiming to offer a broad understanding of the problem of incontinence may carry out a survey on the incidence of incontinence, the types of incontinence and the demographic variables associated with it. She may also carry out in-depth interviews to explore patients' experience of incontinence. Each method provides an understanding of and insight into different aspects of the same phenomenon. These methods can be used side by side in the same study. Alternatively, they could be carried out as two separate studies. There is little danger of mixing paradigms.

Finally, researchers use different methods to answer the same question or study the same aspect of a phenomenon. If the findings are similar, confirmability is achieved and researchers may assume that their findings are valid. It is this type of combination of methods which is often described as triangulation. However, according to Fielding (2009), 'methodological combination cannot guarantee validity, but can provide a richer account'.

Triangulation

A number of terms are used interchangeably in the literature to describe the combination of methods in the same study. Some of the common ones are mixed methods, multiple methods, multi-method, methodological pluralism and triangulation. The latter is often an abused term to describe any study that uses more than one method or a study that combines qualitative and quantitative methods. From the examples given above, one can see that two or more methods can be used in the same study to do different, but related tasks. Therefore triangulation is one form of combining more than one method in the same study.

Triangulation has different meanings depending on the perspectives one adopts. In quantitative research, its purpose is to cross-validate the findings. Webb et al. (1966), representing this view, refer to triangulation as 'a series of complementary methods' to test a hypothesis. If the hypothesis is confirmed or rejected, then, according to Webb et al., it contains a degree of validity unattainable by a single method. This type of triangulation can involve methods within the same approach (quantitative) or from different approaches (quantitative and qualitative).

The view that triangulation is carried out for cross-validation or confirmation purposes is not universally shared (see, for example, Denzin, 1989; Sale et al., 2002). From a qualitative perspective, a variety of methods can be used in the same study, not to seek validity, but to gain in-depth understanding as each yields a different picture and slice of reality (Denzin, 1989).

In qualitative studies, researchers actively seek diversity and 'negative' cases in order to present phenomena in all their different facets and from different perspectives. Richness of data comes from diversity. When data from one method are different from those of another, it raises more questions, which can be further explored due to the flexible nature of qualitative enquiry.

Denzin (1989) defines triangulation as the combination of two or more theories, data sources, methods or investigators in the study of a single phenomenon. Kimchi et al. (1991), drawing on Denzin's work, list six types of triangulation:

- theory – an assessment of the utility and power of competing theories or hypotheses;
- data – the use of multiple data sources with similar foci to obtain diverse views about a topic for the purpose of validation;
- investigator – the use of two or more 'research-trained' investigators with divergent backgrounds to explore the same phenomenon;
- analysis – the use of two or more approaches to the analysis of the same set of data;
- methods – the use of two or more research methods in one study;
- multiple – the use of more than one type of triangulation to analyse same event.

For further discussion of the different types of triangulation, see Guion et al. (2011)

Implications of triangulation

Methods usually associated with different paradigms are increasingly being used in the same study. Not everyone agrees, however, that methods from different paradigms can be mixed in the same study as this can raise more questions than it can answer. Three outcomes are possible: the findings can be similar, inconsistent or divergent. What to do with findings that are inconsistent (some are similar, some are not) or divergent (not at all similar) is a serious problem. This is an issue that has received little attention in the research literature (Perlesz and Lindsay, 2003). As Maggs-Rapport (2000) explains, if multiple findings are produced by multiple methods, 'it may be impossible to make a case for the validity of one set of findings over another'.

Assessing the validity or worth of research findings in mixed methods studies depends on whether one uses quantitative or qualitative criteria (see Chapter 20). Those who believe that validity and reliability are achieved by being 'objective' and 'detached' will, by definition, believe that qualitative interviews are subjective, and therefore biased. It is not always possible for the same researcher to subscribe to quantitative and qualitative notions of what constitutes rigorous, unbiased and valid research. In practice, deciding which of the divergent findings are acceptable could depend on whether the researcher or the team are more quantitatively or qualitatively minded. It is likely that, within a postpositivist framework, the quantitative approach is the anchor or in a more dominant position than the qualitative one. On the other hand, qualitatively minded researchers can adopt the opposite view. In practice, it is probably rare that researchers reject the findings of one approach without seriously considering why the findings are divergent. It is possible that such differences can be explained by the characteristics of the researchers, the process of data collection, including the methods, and the context in which data are being collected and analysed. Such critical reflection is likely to raise further questions.

Researchers combining methods and approaches need to appreciate the context, nature and implications of the data obtained from different methods and not take them at face value. For example, data obtained in focus groups should be interpreted within the context of the group dynamics, the type of discussions that took place, the role of the researcher and how the participants perceived the whole exercise. This is different from that of 'one-to-one' interviews where privacy and intimacy provide the context in which the exchange takes place. The completion of self-administered questionnaires takes place in yet another context.

Combining methods and approaches should be a well thought-out process backed by a strong rationale discussing the purpose and benefits of such decisions and the choice of methods. Barbour (1999) points to 'the need to ensure that our combining of methods is driven by the research question rather than the perceived preference of funders for multi-method approaches or the diverse backgrounds of those who are collaborating'.

Summary

The quantitative–qualitative debate has been, to some extent, overtaken by discussions about the feasibility, benefits, limitations and implications of combining more than one method in the same study. The complex and multidimensional nature of nursing and health phenomena has led an increasing number of researchers to use a variety of methods and approaches, sometimes singly and sometimes in combination. This chapter has outlined the different types and purposes of combining methods to achieve complementarity, completeness and confirmation.

While some researchers find the combination of qualitative and quantitative approaches useful for complementary purposes, they reject the notion that these approaches can be used in the same study for validation or confirmatory purposes. In practice, when findings from qualitative and quantitative research are divergent, the methodological orientation of researchers often determines which sets of findings they can trust more.

Mixed methods studies are on the increase and are well accepted in nursing, health and social research. It is important that researchers are fully aware of why and how they combine methods and address the issues raised when the different methods do not produce similar findings. As Mechanic (1989) explains:

> In our efforts to understand our world around us we recognise many technical barriers, but we use the best methods we can … but it does us well to re-examine our assumptions periodically and to inquire more deeply about the meaning of the information which serves as a source of our interpretations of reality. By inquiring more carefully about what the data mean, we can also bridge gaps between the research culture of those committed to varying types of methods.

Useful sources on mixed methods include:

- Creswell (2003) *Research Design: Qualitative, Quantitative, and Mixed Methods Approaches*.
- Onwuegbuzie and Teddlie (2003) 'A framework for analysing data in mixed methods research'.

- Williamson (2005) 'Illustrating triangulation in mixed-methods nursing research'.
- Bryman (2006) 'Integrating quantitative and qualitative research: how is it done?'.
- O'Cathain et al. (2010) 'Three techniques for integrating data in mixed methods studies'.
- Gorard and Symonds (2010) 'Death of mixed methods?: or the rebirth of research as a craft'.
- Heyvaert et al. (2013) 'Critical appraisal of mixed methods studies'.

References

Barber J G (1996) Science and social work: are they compatible? *Research on Social Work*, **6**, 3:379–88.

Barbour R S (1999) The case for combining qualitative and quantitative approaches in health services research. *Journal of Health Services Research and Policy*, **4**, 1:39–43.

Bolster D and Manias E (2010) Person-centred interactions between nurses and patients during medication activities in an acute hospital setting: qualitative observation and interview study. *International Journal of Nursing Studies*, **47**, 2:154–65.

Brady M C, Stott D J, Norrie J et al. (2011) Developing and evaluating the implementation of a complex intervention: using mixed methods to inform the design of a randomised controlled trial of an oral healthcare intervention after stroke. *Trials*, **12**:168.

Bryman A (2006) Integrating quantitative and qualitative research: how is it done? *Qualitative Research*, **6**, 1:97–113.

Burch S (1999) Evaluating health interventions for older people. *Health*, **3**, 2:151–66.

Clark A M (1998) The qualitative–quantitative debate: moving from positivism and confrontation to post-positivism and reconciliation. *Journal of Advanced Nursing*, **27**:1242–9.

Crawford M J, Weaver T, Rutter D, Sensky T and Tyner P (2002) Evaluating new treatments in psychiatry: the potential value of combining qualitative and quantitative research methods. *International Review of Psychiatry*, **14**:6–14.

Creswell J W (2003) *Research Design: Qualitative, Quantitative, and Mixed Methods Approaches*, 2nd edn (Thousand Oaks, CA: Sage).

Denzin W K (1989) *The Research Act: A Theoretical Introduction to Sociological Methods*, 3rd edn (Englewood Cliffs, NJ: Prentice Hall).

Farquhar MC, Ewing G, Booth S (2011) Using mixed methods to develop and evaluate complex interventions in palliative care research. *Palliative Medicine*, **25**, 8:748–57.

Fielding N G (2009) Going out on a limb: postmodernism and multiple method research. *Current Sociology*, **57**:427–47.

Gorard S and Symonds J (2010) Death of mixed methods?: or the rebirth of research as a craft. *Evaluation and Research in Education*, **236**, 2:121–36.

Greaves F, Pappas Y, Bardsley M et al. (2013) Evaluation of complex integrated care programmes: the approach in North West London. *International Journal of Integrated Care*, **13**:e006.

Greenhalgh T and Taylor R (1997) Papers that go beyond numbers (qualitative research). *British Medical Journal*, **315**:740–3.

Guion L A, Diehl D C and McDonald D (2011) Triangulation: establishing the validity of qualitative studies. Department of Family, Youth and Community Sciences, Florida Cooperative Extension Service. Retrieved from http://edis.ifas.ufl.edu/pdffiles/FY/FY39400.pdf (accessed 2 November 2013).

Hammersley M (1992) Deconstructing the qualitative–quantitative divide. In: J Brannen (ed.) *Mixing Methods: Qualitative and Quantitative Research* (Aldershot: Avebury).

Hanning R M, Royall D, Toews J E, Blashill L, Wegener J and Driezen P (2009) Web-based Food

Behaviour Questionnaire: validation with grades six to eight students. *Canadian Journal of Dietetic Practice and Research*, **70**, 4:172–8.

Heyvaert M, Hannes K, Maes B and Onghena P (2013) Critical appraisal of mixed methods studies. *Journal of Mixed Methods Research*, **7**:302–27.

Kidd L I, Graor C H and Murrock C J (2013) A mindful eating group intervention for obese women: a mixed methods feasibility study. *Archives of Psychiatric Nursing*, **27**: 211–18.

Kimchi J, Polivka B and Stevenson J S (1991) Triangulation: operation definitions. *Nursing Research*, **40**, 6:364–6.

Jap T, Tiatri S J, Jaya E S and Suteja M S (2013) The development of Indonesian Online Game Addiction Questionnaire. *PLoS ONE*, **8**,4:e61098.

Maggs-Rapport F (2000) Combining methodological approaches in research: ethnography and interpretive phenomenology. *Journal of Advanced Nursing*, **31**,1:219–25.

McNeill J, Doran J, Lynn F, Anderson G and Alderdice F (2012) Public health education for midwives and midwifery students: a mixed methods study. *BMC Pregnancy and Childbirth*, **12**:142.

Mechanic D (1989) Medical sociology: some tensions among theory, method and substance. *Journal of Health and Social Behaviour*, **30**:147–60.

Medical Research Council (2008) Developing and evaluating complex interventions: new guidance. Retrieved from http://www.mrc.ac.uk/Utilities/Documentrecord/index.htm?d=MRC004871 (accessed 7 January 2014).

Melby V (2010) *Living with HIV in Ireland: Exploring the Challenges: Quality of Life, Social Support, Life Satisfaction and Psychosocial Adjustment – The Lived Experience* (Saarbrucken: VDM Verlag).

Meredith P and Wood C (1996) Aspects of patient satisfaction with communication in surgical care: confirming qualitative feedback through quantitative methods. *International Journal for Quality in Health Care*, **8**, 3:253–64.

Morgan D L (2007) Paradigms lost and pragmatism regained: methodological implications of combining qualitative and quantitative methods. *Journal of Mixed Methods Research*, **1**, 1: 48–76.

O'Cathain A, Murphy E and Nicholl J (2010) Three techniques for integrating data in mixed methods studies. *British Medical Journal*, **341**:c4587.

Onwuegbuzie A and Teddlie C (2003) A framework for analysing data in mixed methods research. In: A Tashakkori and C Teddlie (eds) *Handbook of Mixed Methods in Social and Behavioural Research*, pp. 351–83. (Thousands Oaks, CA: Sage).

Östlund U, Kidd L, Wengström Y and Rowa-Dewar N (2011) Combining qualitative and quantitative research within mixed method research designs: a methodological review. *International Journal of Nursing Studies*, **48**:369–83.

Ozawa S and Pongpirul K (2013) 10 best resources on … mixed methods research in health systems. *Health Policy and Planning*, doi: 10.1093/heapol/czt019.

Paley J (2000) Paradigms and presuppositions: the difference between qualitative and quantitative research. *Scholarly Inquiry for Nursing Practice: An International Journal*, **14**, 2:143–55.

Perlesz A and Lindsay J (2003) Methodological triangulation in researching families: making sense of dissonant data. *International Journal of Social Research Methodology*, **6**, 1:25–40.

Risjord M, Moloney M and Dunbar S (2001) Methodological triangulation in nursing research. *Philosophy of the Social Sciences*, **31**, 1:40–59.

Roberts C (2003) Palaeopathologist. In: J Turney (ed.) *Science, Not Art: Ten Scientists' Diaries* (London: Calouste Gulbenkian Foundation).

Rowan N and Wulff D (2007) Using qualitative methods to inform scale development. *Qualitative Report*, **12**:450–66.

Sale J E M, Lohfeld L H and Brazil K (2002) Revisiting the quantitative–qualitative debate: implications for mixed-methods research. *Quality and Quantity*, **36**:43–53.

Sandelowski M (2000a) Response to 'Paradigms and presuppositions'. The difference between qualitative and quantitative research. *Scholarly Inquiry for Nursing Practice*, **14**, 2:152–60.

Sandelowski M (2000b) Combining qualitative and quantitative sampling, data collection, and analysis techniques in mixed-method studies. *Research in Nursing and Health*, **23**:246–55.

Smith J K and Heshusius L (1986) Closing down the conversation: the end of the quantitative–qualitative debate among educational inquirers. *Educational Researcher*, **15**, 1:4–12.

Strickland O L (1993) Editorial: Qualitative or quantitative: so what is your religion? *Journal of Nursing Measurement*, **1**, 2:103–5.

Wagner L I, Berg S R, Gandhi M et al. (2013) The development of a Functional Assessment of Cancer Therapy (FACT) questionnaire to assess dermatologic symptoms associated with epidermal growth factor receptor inhibitors (FACT-EGFRI-18). *Supportive Care in Cancer*, **21**, 4:1033–41.

Wakefield J C (1995) When an irresistible epistemology meets an immovable ontology. *Social Work Research*, **19**, 1:9–17.

Webb E J, Campbell D T, Schwartz R D and Sechrest L (1966) *Unobtrusive Measures: Non-Reactive Research on the Social Sciences* (Chicago: Rand McNally).

West C and McDowell J (2002) The distress experienced by people with type 2 diabetes. *British Journal of Community Nursing*, **7**, 12:606–13.

Williamson G R (2005) Illustrating triangulation in mixed-methods nursing research. *Nurse Researcher*, **12**, 4:7–18.

Zapka J, Simpson K, Hiott L, Langston L, Fakhry S and Ford D (2013) A mixed methods descriptive investigation of readiness to change in rural hospitals participating in a tele-critical care intervention. *BMC Health Services Research*, **13**:33.

The Research Process and Ethical Issues

6

> **Opening thought** Ethics is in what we do, not in what we say we do.

Introduction

One of the first tasks in reading and evaluating a research study is to identify the actions and steps taken by the researcher in order to answer the research question. This chapter describes the research process in quantitative research and qualitative research and points out the differences between them. There are ethical implications at every stage of the research process. An outline of the guiding principles to safeguard patients' rights and safety is given.

The meaning of research process

The process of any activity is what happens from its inception to its end. The tasks and actions carried out by the researcher in order to find answers to the research question constitute the research process. Decisions are taken in choosing the tasks and the way in which they are carried out. A number of factors, including the researcher's beliefs and experience, and ethical considerations or resources, may influence these decisions. The thinking processes of the researcher, the assumptions made and the theoretical stance are also part of the research process. According to Denzin and Lincoln (1994), three interrelated activities define the research process: the articulation of the researcher's individual world view or basic belief system (in relation to the research domain), decisions on the theoretical perspective and strategies of enquiry, and decisions on methods of data collection and analysis.

Thus, although the research process is often described in terms of the tasks and actions undertaken, it also consists of the decisions and the thinking that underpins these decisions. Whatever the type of research carried out or the approaches used, the research process invariably consists of four main components:

- the identification of the research question;
- the collection of data;

- the analysis of the data;
- the dissemination of the findings.

To carry out these tasks, a number of other tasks may be performed. For example, in identifying the research question, a review of the literature and/or discussion with colleagues may be useful. Before data can be collected, a questionnaire or an interview schedule may have to be constructed. The research process, therefore, consists of all these tasks and the decisions made before and during the project.

The research process and the nursing process

The research process and the nursing process share some of the same characteristics. They are both problem-solving processes and both consist of a number of steps or stages. However, they differ in the goals they aim to achieve. The main purpose of the nursing process is to provide care to clients. In doing so, nurses gather information in order to assess the nursing problem and to evaluate the care given. The collection of such information is not always as formal as is the case in research. Data for research purposes must be collected more systematically. For example, when assessing clients, nurses can ask questions but do not have to use a tool such as a questionnaire with established validity and reliability in order to do so (although some do). The aim of research, on the other hand, is to find solutions to research questions, which may or may not contribute to better care for clients. Data for research purposes must be collected systematically and rigorously. Table 6.1 shows the main components of the nursing process and the research process.

The process in quantitative research

The research process is often described as having a number of stages and steps. Depending on the type of research, these stages are not necessarily linear (performed one after the other, in one direction only). There are important differences between quantitative and qualitative research in the way in which the research tasks are undertaken.

Table 6.1　The main components of the nursing and research process

Nursing process	Research process
Assessment	Identification of research problem
Planning	Collection of data
Implementation	Analysis of data
Evaluation	

The systematic and inflexible nature of quantitative research means that the research proceeds in a logical and sequential manner. The stages of the process in quantitative research can be broken down into a number of steps. The number of steps varies from author to author and with the design of the study. The difference in the number of steps is not important provided the main tasks are carried out and explained. The main stages of experimental and survey research are briefly described below. The process in quantitative research mirrors the scientific method used in the natural sciences (as described in Chapter 2). The chapters that follow will provide more detail and discussion on these topics.

Main stages of the research process

Identification and formulation of the research question

This is the first stage of a research project, when the researcher decides what is to be researched and formulates one or more questions. The next step is for the researcher to define the terms and concepts used in the research questions. A review of the relevant literature helps to clarify issues, informs the researcher of how others have formulated similar research questions and defines concepts. At the end of this stage, the research questions or hypotheses developed must be stated clearly and unambiguously.

Designing the study

Decisions will be taken in order to choose a design for the study and a conceptual framework (if appropriate), and to select or develop instruments to collect data (for example, questionnaires, interviews or observation schedules). This may be followed by the testing (or piloting) of these instruments in order to refine them (sometimes the whole study is piloted on a small scale to find out whether the project is feasible). At this stage of the process, the researcher will define the population from whom the data will be collected. Seeking access to them and obtaining ethical approval from the relevant ethical committees should begin well before the project is started. When all these preparations have been completed, data are ready to be collected.

Collection of data

This is the stage when the data are physically collected by sending out questionnaires, interviewing participants or extracting data from existing records. It is a time when outcomes are measured as part of experiments. It can be a long and arduous process culminating in large amounts of collected data, depending on the size of the project.

Analysis of data

In the final stage of the process, the researcher analyses, interprets and presents the findings. Prior to data collection, decisions about the type of analysis would have been taken. For example, when questionnaires are constructed, the researcher must decide whether (and what) statistical tests should be carried out and code the questionnaire accordingly.

Communicating the findings

When the data have been analysed, it is usual for the researcher to interpret the findings, discuss the limitations of the study, make recommendations for practice and further research, and present the study orally and/or in written form.

Conclusions

The stages described above are sometimes listed as a number of steps, as suggested below by Priest et al. (2006):

Step 1. Formulating the research question
Step 2. Reviewing the literature
Step 3. Designing the study
Step 4. Approval and access
Step 5. Data collection
Step 6. Data analysis and interpretation
Step 7. Presenting and disseminating the findings.

For an illustration of these different steps of the research process, see Priest et al.'s (2006) article on 'Understanding the research process in nursing'. These steps represent the tasks undertaken by the researcher or by others on her behalf.

In quantitative research, certain tasks must be carried out before undertaking others. For example, the research question or hypothesis must be clearly formulated before the data are collected. The research questions cannot be modified during the data collection phase, and analysis usually starts after the collection of data. According to Arber (1993), 'although the research process can be represented as a series of discrete stages, in practice a number of activities are generally in progress at the same time, for example, you can select a sample while designing the questionnaire and recruiting interviewers'. In randomised controlled trials (see Chapter 11), there is an implementation stage when the new intervention is administered. In action research, through consultation, participation and negotiation, the process is likely to undergo many changes and challenges before the project is completed. The design envisaged at the start is often modified several times throughout the process.

The process in qualitative research

The flexible nature of qualitative research is such that the research process takes on different forms. The stages of the research process may also differ from one qualitative study to another. As qualitative research comprises a variety of approaches and techniques, it is difficult to generalise about them. Chenail (2011) offers the following 10 steps for conceptualising and conducting qualitative research studies in a 'pragmatically curious manner':

Step One: reflect on what interests you.
Step Two: draft a statement identifying your preliminary area of interest and justifying its scholarly and/or practical importance.
Step Three: hone your topic focus.
Step Four: compose your initial research question or hypothesis.
Step Five: define your goals and objectives.
Step Six: conduct a review of the literature.
Step Seven: develop your research design.
Step Eight: conduct a self-assessment in order to determine what strengths you have that will be useful in your study and what skills you will need to develop in order to complete your study.
Step Nine: plan, conduct, and manage the study.
Step Ten: compose and submit your report.

Researchers using the qualitative approach may or may not define the research question prior to collecting the data. For example, in ethnographic studies (see Chapter 14), a broad topic is identified and the phenomenon on which the researcher finally focuses is decided during the data collection phase. Sometimes a thorough review of the relevant literature is carried out before the data are collected, and at other times no literature review is conducted as the researcher may not want to be influenced by what others have written. Regarding conceptual or theoretical frameworks, those using a grounded theory approach believe that hypotheses and theories are generated from the data collected. Therefore no attempt is made to use existing literature and conceptual frameworks, although there are cases where this happens.

Instruments may or may not be constructed in advance of data collection. In qualitative research, although questions can be written and asked of respondents, the researcher is part of the instrument of data collection. Some questions may be thought of and formulated on the spot and new perspectives explored. The researcher is at liberty to alter questions or omit questions asked of previous respondents. The designs of qualitative studies are flexible enough to accommodate these and other changes. The research enterprise is moulded to suit the phenomena being studied.

In qualitative research, the researcher can begin to analyse data as they are collected. Although formal analysis takes place when data collection has been completed, the researcher usually processes some of the data mentally or otherwise during fieldwork even before all the data have been collected. After data analysis, researchers can, and often do, go back to respondents to seek clarification and/or validation.

Do not be disheartened if at this stage you feel confused about some of the terms used. The rest of the book will clarify these terms and the topics mentioned here. In addition, a Glossary has been provided at the end of the book to help with a quick search of what they mean.

Understanding the research process

The research process is presented above as a framework for researchers to present their study and for readers to understand the reasons for the decisions taken and for the main tasks carried out. The research process is more than what is reported. For the purpose of articles or reports, the researcher breaks down the project into a number of parts or steps, which facilitates the reader's understanding of what has been done. The final publication is often a sanitised version, purified of the difficulties and frustrations encountered during the process, and almost never gives an insight into the trials and tribulations faced by the researchers. In reality, researchers go back and forth between these stages before the report is finally completed.

Publication conventions impose restrictions on how research studies are reported. Although, as pointed out earlier, some qualitative researchers do not consult or review the literature before collecting data, a literature review section invariably appears at the start of an article as if a review had been carried out at the start of the research. Journals adopt formats that they believe facilitate the reader's understanding. They invariably require research articles to have the following structure or sections: an introduction (which introduces the topic and gives a rationale for the study), a review of the selected literature, a description of the design, the main findings and a discussion of them. This extract from the *Journal of Advanced Nursing*'s (www.journalofadvancednursing.com) guide for contributors (2013) illustrates this point. For quantitative and qualitative research papers, the following headings are required:

Introduction
Background
Aim(s)
Design
Sample/participants
Data collection
Ethical considerations
Data analysis
Validity and reliability/rigour
Results
Discussion
Limitations
Conclusion.

As can be seen, this structure closely follows the stages of the research process mentioned above. There is a challenge on the part of the author to sift through all the details of the process and to present an account that is as succinct and brief and yet as comprehensible and complete as possible and in a language that clarifies rather than obfuscates.

Critiquing the research process

One of the first tasks in critiquing a research article is to attempt to describe the actions and tasks undertaken by the researcher. If the process is well described, you will have little difficulty in doing this. In some cases, however, the structure of the article may be such that you will need to 'tease out' what was actually done. It is for the benefit of readers that the research process is reported in a neat version. There is always a desire on the reader's part to know more than what is reported. While it is not possible for the researcher to describe in detail everything that happened, you must not be left with major questions unanswered. For example, if only the size of the sample is given and you are not provided with an explanation of how the sample was chosen, this will limit the extent to which the data can be generalised to other settings (see Chapter 15).

Some details are important in assessing the validity and reliability of data; some are not. For example, there are few implications for the data if the researcher had to make 10 telephone calls to a nurse manager in order to gain access to the respondents, but it is vital to know whether the nurse manager 'hand-picked' the respondents, thereby creating the possibility of bias in the sample. When reading a research article or report, it is essential for you to distinguish between information that is and is not relevant.

Ethical issues and the research process

There are ethical implications at every stage of the research process, including the choice of topic to research, the selection of the design and the publication of the findings. Even the decision of whether to research or not to research has ethical implications. By continuing to base practice solely on customs and traditions, consumers are denied the best possible care (Parahoo, 1991). Therefore, one can ask whether it is unethical not to examine one's practice.

Although this book is not about how to do research, nurses need to know the implications of research to be able to safeguard patients' rights and ensure their safety. Connolly (2003), pointing out that ethical issues should not be confused with methodological ones, explains that, 'research ethics involve a consideration of the conduct of researchers in relation to their own personal behaviour as well as how they relate to and treat others during their research'. They are also about abiding by the norms and standards of behaviour that researchers are expected to follow. Unfortunately, such basic principles as seeking informed consent from participants are often ignored. A systematic review of 489 studies (in a number of countries, including the USA and the UK), in school settings involving children and young people, reported that only 30 per cent reported seeking consent and 13 per cent sought consent from the children and young people themselves (Rees et al., 2007).

Connolly (2003) recognises that while most research is carried out according to high ethical standards, there are people who have experienced one or more of the following:

- being asked to participate in detailed interviews or focus group discussions while being told very little about the precise nature or focus of the research;
- not being shown any appreciation or recognition for the amount of time and effort they have given to the research;
- not being contacted again by the researcher(s) following their participation, and thus not knowing what has happened to the information they have shared;
- not being consulted or involved in any capacity in relation to the design and planning of the research that is being conducted about them;
- having no say about the way they are expected to participate in the research;
- being asked to participate in one study after another and yet seeing no change in their lives as a result of this;
- being asked to revisit and recount extremely stressful or traumatic experiences they have had and yet not being offered any help or support in terms of dealing with the distress that this may have caused them;
- perceiving that the research study they have participated in has led to a report being published that tends simply to reinforce existing stereotypes or other negative perceptions of them or their specific group or community;
- although they had been assured of anonymity by the researchers, finding that they or their particular group or community have consequently been identified.

Ethical principles in the conduct of research

There are six ethical principles (International Council of Nurses, 2003) that researchers and health professionals can use to protect patients or clients from harm. These principles apply to all types of research regardless of the format, setting, condition or types of participants. They are as follows:

- *Beneficence.* The research project should benefit the participating individual and society in general (by contributing to the pool of human knowledge). The benefit of participation is sometimes access to a new treatment not yet available to others. Participants are also likely to receive more attention and human contact than they might otherwise receive. On the other hand, when this attention is suddenly withdrawn at the end of the study, it can cause a feeling of isolation, which can be potentially harmful.
- *Non-maleficence.* Research should not cause any harm to participants. While the potential physical harm may be obvious, the psychological effects may not be as transparent.

- *Fidelity*. This principle is concerned mainly with the building of trust between researchers and participants. For example, if during a study researchers find that participants are in some way at risk, they should not put the need to complete the experiment above the participants' safety. Researchers are obligated to safeguard the rights of participants.
- *Justice*. This involves being fair to participants by not giving preferential treatment to some and depriving others of the care and attention they deserve. Participants' needs must come before the objectives of the study. Researchers must ensure that participants are treated fairly and that the power relation is not unfairly tilted in the researchers' favour.
- *Veracity*. To build trust between participants and researchers, the latter must tell the truth, even if this may cause participants not to take part in or to withdraw during the study. Being 'economical with the truth' can be a form of deception.
- *Confidentiality*. The confidentiality of the information gathered from and on participants must be respected. Giving consent to participate in a study does not mean giving researchers the right to consult the subject's medical notes as well. Researchers often ask nurses and doctors, but not the participants, for permission. The presentation of the findings can potentially identify participants or participating institutions. Researchers must take care not to inadvertently reveal information that participants may want to remain confidential.

The above six ethical principles have been synthesised into four rights of subjects considering participation in research: the right not to be harmed, the right of full disclosure, the right of self-determination (subjects' right to decide to take part or to withdraw at any time) and the right of privacy, anonymity and confidentiality (International Council of Nurses, 2003).

Nurses may not always have the necessary knowledge to decide whether a research study can be detrimental to the patients or clients invited to take part. Research ethics committees exist for the purpose of examining the ethical implications of such studies and for granting permission, when appropriate. The panel members should have a range of expertise necessary to carry out this task.

Ethical issues in quantitative and qualitative research

The six ethical principles apply to all types of research. However, each research approach and each study has its own ethical implications. There are some ethical issues that are more prominent in one type of design than in another. For example, in a quantitative study, participants can give informed consent prior to the study (although they have the right to withdraw). The data collection tools are unlikely to change. In qualitative studies, researchers often do not know how an interview is likely to unfold. Researchers cannot state in advance all the questions they may ask. Therefore asking for informed consent is a process rather than a one-off event.

The nature of qualitative research can seem harmless but as Alderson (2001) points out:

> qualitative research may seem like only talking to people, or observing them, or using written material they have provided. Surely this can do no harm, and have no side effects … Only talking, however, may have strong and possibly distressing effects. The ethics of consent do not simply relate to the legal dangers of being sued for physical harm; people have rights over their lives and beliefs and actions, and the use that is made of information about them.

Richards and Schwartz (2002) have listed four potential risks to research participants in qualitative studies: anxiety and distress, exploitation, misrepresentation and identification of the participant in published papers. Distress can be caused to participants in all types of research. Survey items can bring back traumatic memories or cause offence. However, in qualitative studies, the opportunities for sharing 'confidences' are greater than they are in quantitative research. Strategies such as 'probing' can sometimes put unnecessary pressure on participants to reveal intimate and personal details that they would have preferred to keep to themselves. Balancing 'harm' and 'benefits' in such interactions is not easy, especially when researchers are keen to obtain meaningful insights into people's lives. As Resnik (2011) explains:

> Although codes, policies, and principals are very important and useful, like any set of rules, they do not cover every situation, they often conflict, and they require considerable interpretation. It is therefore important for researchers to learn how to interpret, assess, and apply various research rules and how to make decisions and to act in various situations. The vast majority of decisions involve the straightforward application of ethical rules.

One must recognise that 'all research is potentially exploitative and researchers' motives can frequently be mixed' (Jones et al., 1995). In health and nursing studies, researchers are often health professionals. This can lead to a 'blurring' of roles, goals and motives. They should ensure that the need to obtain data (compounded by difficulties in recruiting participants) does not take precedence over patients' needs, wishes and rights. Another dilemma frequently faced by nurse researchers is when their participants perceive them as 'nurses' as well as, or instead of, researchers. In such cases, participants may disclose information that is not sought by the researcher, or the participant may seek advice or help with their problems or conditions. Researchers may also have to intervene when a participant's condition gets worse (see, for example, Fitzsimons and McAloon, 2004). In all these circumstances, the rights, well-being and safety of participants should take precedence over research objectives.

Participants' views can be misinterpreted in qualitative research. Some researchers may take transcripts or findings back to the participants for 'validation'. This can potentially cause distress to participants who may feel misrepresented. The small sample size in qualitative studies, and the use of 'quotes' to illustrate participants' views, can also potentially lead to the identification of participants in subsequent publications. Such problems of identification are not prominent in quantitative studies, where responses are presented in numerical forms. To reduce these risks, Richards and Schwartz (2002) recommend strategies such as 'ensuring scientific soundness, organising follow-up care where appropriate, considering obtaining consent as a process, ensuring confidentiality and taking a reflexive stance towards analysis'.

Robley (1995) explains how ethics affects all phases of the qualitative research process:

Decisions about what to study, which persons will be asked to participate, what methodology will be used, how to achieve truly informed consent, when to terminate or interrupt interviews, when to probe deeply, when therapy or nursing care supersedes research, and what and how case studies should be documented in the published results are all matters of ethical deliberation.

Both qualitative and quantitative research have ethical implications, but the differences in process and methods may lead to an emphasis on certain issues rather than others.

Research governance

Every society has a responsibility to protect the rights of its citizens and ensure their well-being and safety when they take part in research. This is enshrined in the Declaration of Helsinki on 'ethical principles to provide guidance to physicians and other participants in medical research involving human subjects', including human material or identifiable data (World Medical Association, 2008). The formal and informal regulations may vary from country to country, but the ethical principles governing the conduct of research should be the same.

The UK government has issued the governance arrangements for research ethics committees in England, Wales, Scotland and Northern Ireland (Department of Health, 2011). Similarly, other countries have their own laws and standards for the ethical conduct of research. Research ethics committees have a particular crucial role in implementing these standards.

The Department of Health (2011) defines a research ethics committee as 'a group of people appointed to review research proposals to assess formally if the research is ethical'. The role of the committee is to ensure that 'any anticipated risks, burdens or intrusions will be minimised for the people taking part in the research and are justified by the expected benefits for the participants or for science and society'. According to the Department of Health, 'this helps promote public confidence about the conduct of researchers and the dignity, rights, safety and well-being of research participants'; 'as a result, more people will be encouraged to take part in research'.

Achieving high-quality and ethically conducted research also depends on cooperation between a number of people and organisations. The following groups and organisations have key responsibilities: participants, researchers, research funders, research sponsors, universities, organisations providing care, healthcare professionals and professional organisations. Some have direct, and others indirect, responsibility.

Nurses' role as patients' advocates and as researchers

According to the Royal College of Nursing (RCN) Research Society Ethics Guidance Group (2004), 'nurses act in a range of roles in research – including carer, student, manager, investigator, research supervisor, sponsor, ethics or governance committee member'. Many of the people in the care of nurses are in vulnerable positions. According to the RCN Research Society Ethics Guidance Group (2009), the phrase 'people who are vulnerable' may encompass a multitude of different populations – for example, children, people with mental illness or learning disability, people with communication difficulties, prisoners or young offenders. The Ethics Guidance Group explains that:

> in varying degrees, other groups could also be considered to be vulnerable, such as people who are deaf or sight-impaired, or those individuals for whom English is not readily understood. In theory, any person who is receiving health care could be considered to be vulnerable.

For more discussion of the ethical principles for researching vulnerable groups, see Connolly (2003).

Nurses, as gatekeepers, have responsibilities towards those in their care and must balance the need to 'protect' their patients with the potential to influence the outcome of research. Redsell and Cheater (2001) explain that using 'intermediaries' to obtain consent from, and recruit, research participants can increase 'the risk of selection bias, may expose the practitioner to ethical difficulties and may compromise the external validity' of research findings.

'Informed consent', which is the cornerstone of ethically sound research (International Council of Nurses, 2003), is described as:

> a process by which researchers ensure that prospective participants understand the potential risks and benefits of participating in a study, they are informed about their rights not to participate, and they are presented this information in a manner that is free from coercion.

According to the RCN Research Society Ethics Guidance Group (2009), 'time should be provided for the participant to consider their involvement in the study and to ask questions' and that 'a consent form should be signed and witnessed'. Information should also be presented in a format, language and style that participants can understand. This means that researchers have to be particularly mindful of terminologies and jargons with which professionals are acquainted but that are not familiar to potential participants.

Giving informed consent is a process and not just a one-time event at the start of a project. As participants become more aware of the real implications of the study, they may decide that they need more information or they may decide to withdraw from the study. Their right to do so must take precedence over the need to complete the project. For an excellent example of the ongoing process of gaining consent, see Seymour and Ingleton (1999).

Researchers must be particularly aware of the vulnerability of some participants. Vulnerable populations include those who are physically and/or mentally incapable of giving informed consent. It also includes those 'confined' or 'captive' such as schoolchildren or prisoners who may not feel free to decline if access to them has been granted by someone in authority (International Council of Nurses, 2003). Others can be vulnerable by virtue of experiencing (or having experienced) physical and mental abuse or oppression.

Research ethics committees exist for the purpose of ensuring that the rights of all individuals are respected. However, health professionals, as advocates or researchers, must be sensitive to these issues, and must act according to the ethical principles outlined earlier in this chapter.

There is much discussion in the literature about specific issues related to obtaining informed consent from vulnerable people or their guardians (see, for example, Arraf et al., 2004, for ethics in palliative care research; Meaux and Bell, 2001, for children as research participants; Schmidt et al., 2004, for patients in emergency departments; and Ferguson, 2004, for learning disability research).

For further guidance on ethical issues in research, see:

- An Bord Altranais (2007) *Guidance to Nurses and Midwives Regarding Ethical Conduct of Nursing and Midwifery Research.*
- Royal College of Nursing Research Society Ethics Guidance Group (2009) *Research Ethics: RCN Guidance for Nurses.*
- The National Health and Medical Research Council, the Australian Research Council and the Australian Vice-Chancellors' Committee (2007) National Statement on Ethical Conduct in Human Research.
- Markham and Buchanan (2012) 'Ethical decision-making and internet research. Recommendations from the AoIR Ethics Working Committee (Version 2.0)'.

In this chapter, the ethical principles and related issues have been described. The ethical implications of research are discussed further in the relevant parts of the book, more specifically in relation to experiments, questionnaires, interviews and observations. The ethical implications of qualitative research are also further discussed in the chapters on phenomenology, grounded theory and ethnography.

Summary

The research process constitutes all the decisions and actions taken by the researcher. The process is normally reduced to a number of steps for the purpose of reporting. The stages and steps of the research process in quantitative research are more or less linear, while in qualitative research the steps are intertwined and it is possible to revisit previous stages during the project.

Research has many ethical implications, and both researchers and nurses can be guided by the six ethical principles outlined above. Patients' rights, well-being and safety should, at all times, take precedence over research objectives. Every country should have a research governance framework to provide guidance and to set up measures designed to ensure that research carried out is of good quality and ethically sound.

The format of the rest of this book will follow closely the stages of the research process.

References

Alderson P (2001) *On Doing Qualitative Research Linked to Ethical Healthcare* (London: Wellcome Trust).

An Bord Altranais (2007) *Guidance to Nurses and Midwives Regarding Ethical Conduct of Nursing and Midwifery Research* (Dublin: An Bord Altranais).

Arber S (1993) The research process. In: N Gilbert (ed.) *Researching Social Life* (London: Sage).

Arraf K, Cox G and Oberle K (2004) Using the Canadian Code of Ethics for Registered Nurses to explore ethics in palliative care research. *Nursing Ethics*, **11**, 6:600–9.

Chenail R J (2011) Steps for conceptualizing and conducting qualitative research studies in a pragmatically curious manner. *Qualitative Report*, **16**, 6:1713–30.

Connolly P (2003) Ethical principles for researching vulnerable groups. Office of the First Minister and Deputy First Minister in Northern Ireland. Retrieved from http://www.ed.ac.uk/polopoly_fs/1.71235!/fileManager/EthicsPr-Vulnerable.pdf (accessed 14 September 2013).

Denzin N K and Lincoln Y S (1994) Introduction: entering the field of qualitative research. In: N K Denzin and Y S Lincoln (eds) *Handbook of Qualitative Research* (Newbury Park, CA: Sage).

Department of Health (2011) *Governance Arrangements for Research Ethics Committees: A Harmonised Edition* (London: DoH).

Ferguson D (2004) Learning disability research: a discussion paper. *Learning Disability Practice*, **7**, 6:17–19.

Fitzsimons D and McAloon T (2004) The ethics of non-intervention in a study of patients awaiting coronary artery bypass. *Journal of Advanced Nursing*, **46**, 4:395–402.

International Council of Nurses (2003) *Ethical Guidelines for Nursing Research* (Geneva: ICN).

Jones R, Murphy E and Crossland A (1995) Primary care research ethics. *British Journal of General Practice*, **45**:623–6.

Journal of Advanced Nursing (2013) Empirical research – quantitative. Retrieved from http://onlinelibrary.wiley.com/journal/10.1111/(ISSN)1365-2648/homepage/empirical_research_-_quantitative.htm (accessed 13 September 2013).

Markham A and Buchanan E (2012) Ethical decision-making and internet research. Recommendations from the AoIR Ethics Working Committee (Version 2.0). Retrieved from http://aoir.org/reports/ethics2.pdf (accessed 15 September 2013).

Meaux J B and Bell P L (2001) Balancing recruitment and protection: children as research subjects. *Issues in Comprehensive Pediatric Nursing*, **24**, 4:214–51.

National Health and Medical Research Council, Australian Research Council and Australian Vice-Chancellors' Committee (2007) National Statement on Ethical Conduct in Human Research (Updated December 2013). Retrieved from http://www.nhmrc.gov.au/_files_nhmrc/publications/attachments/e72_national_statement_131211.pdf (accessed 7 January 2014).

Parahoo K (1991) Politics and ethics in nursing research. *Nursing Standard*, **6**, 6:36–9.

Priest H, Roberts P, Higginson G and Knipe W (2006) Understanding the research process in nursing. *Nursing Standard*, **21**, 1:39–42.

Redsell S A and Cheater F M (2001) The Data Protection Act (1998): implications for health researchers. *Journal of Advanced Nursing*, **35**, 4:508–13.

Rees R W, Garcia J and Oakley A (2007) Consent in school-based research involving children and young people: a survey of research from systematic reviews. *Research Ethics Review*, **3**, 2:35–9.

Resnik D B (2011) *What is Ethics in Research and Why is it Important?* National Institute of Environmental Health Sciences. Retrieved from http://www.niehs.nih.gov/research/resources/bioethics/whatis/ (accessed 14 September 2013).

Richards H M and Schwartz L J (2002) Ethics of qualitative research: are there special issues for health services research? *Family Practice*, **19**, 2:135–9.

Robley L R (1995) The ethics of qualitative nursing research. *Journal of Professional Nursing*, **11**, 1:45–8.

Royal College of Nursing Research Society Ethics Guidance Group (2004) *Research Ethics: RCN Guidance for Nurses*. London: Royal College of Nursing.

Royal College of Nursing Research Society Ethics Guidance Group (2009) *Research Ethics: RCN Guidance for Nurses* (London: RCN).

Schmidt T A, Salo D, Hughes J A et al. (2004) Confronting the ethical challenges to informed consent in emergency medicine research. *Academic Emergency Medicine*, **11**, 10:1082–9.

Seymour J E and Ingleton C (1999) Ethical issues in qualitative research at the end of life. *International Journal of Palliative Nursing*, **5**, 2:65–73.

World Medical Association (2008) Declaration of Helsinki: ethical principles for medical research involving human subjects. Retrieved from http//www.wma.net/e/policy/b3.htm (accessed 14 September 2013).

7

Literature Reviews

> We are bombarded with information, but are we better informed?
> Anon

Introduction

The purpose of research is to make a contribution, however small, towards understanding the phenomenon being studied and ultimately towards the total body of knowledge. Researchers can benefit from what has been done before and thereafter contribute something in return. The literature review serves to inform the various stages of a project and to put in context what is already known on the subject. There are different types of literature and different reasons why a literature review is carried out. In this chapter, the main purpose of reviewing the literature prior to and during a study will be explored. The increasing amount of information generated by research studies also needs to be systematically reviewed and summarised to facilitate practitioners in their use of research. The process of systematic reviews will also be outlined and discussed.

The meaning of literature

People are generally familiar with terms such as English or French 'literature'. In research terms, 'the literature' refers mostly to any published material, although reference is sometimes made to radio, television, the world wide web or other audiovisual media, such as slides, photographs and songs. What normally constitutes literature, however, is mainly books, journals, theses, reports, web material, newspapers, pamphlets and leaflets. These can be in hard copy or electronic format. Reference is sometimes also made to what has been said at a conference or to personal communications (face-to-face or telephone conversations, and letters).

Although the value of each of the different types of literature depends on what individuals derive from them, researchers place more value on some than on others. The value of each type of publication varies according to the type and quality of information it contains. The credibility of each type of information itself depends on how objective or subjective it is and whether or not it is verifiable. The nursing and health literature comes mainly in the forms of research papers, descriptions and discussions of practice, policies and issues, conceptual and theoretical papers, opinion articles and anecdotes.

Research information is generated by research studies and systematic reviews. It relates to the topic being researched, the methods of data collection and the findings. This type of information is highly valued by some as it is usually systematically and rigorously collected and analysed, and, in the case of quantitative research, may be verifiable.

Descriptive accounts of nursing practice can be found in nursing journals, especially professional ones. Although they contain valuable information, they tend to be subjective. Nonetheless, where little information is available, descriptive accounts, in particular when the author offers a critical and reflexive perspective, can be useful and informative. More importantly, they are vehicles for sharing experiences of practice between professionals and others.

Conceptual and theoretical discussions are the backbone of all disciplines. They take the form of an intellectual discussion of ideas. Although the views expressed are those of individuals, the arguments put forward must be structured logically and argued coherently for others to understand, contribute to and use.

Nursing and health journals often publish the personal opinions of practitioners, patients and academics. These opinions, based on experience and beliefs, are subjective, although the authors may back up their arguments by research and other evidence. The credibility of the information in a personal opinion article depends in part on how the arguments are developed and supported, and on the status of the author. The list of references or the absence of it, is an indication of how personal the opinion is or how much effort the author has made to relate her views to the available evidence.

There are many areas that remain unresearched or underresearched. Those reviewing the literature on such areas can only rely on anecdotes and personal accounts.

Primary, secondary and tertiary sources

The value of information also depends on whether it is reported first or second hand. Original publications are known as primary sources. Such publications as the Briggs Report (Briggs, 1972) and *Introduction to Nursing: An Adaptation Model* (Roy, 1976) are primary sources. Secondary sources are publications that report on the original work. *Callista Roy: An Adaptation Model* (Lutjens, 1991) is a secondary source because Lutjens reports on Roy's original work, published in 1976. Besides reporting on the original work, the authors may explain, comment on or discuss the original ideas. By doing this, secondary sources are sometimes useful in that they simplify, discuss and summarise the primary material. However, there is the possibility that the original work may be distorted, misinterpreted and selectively reported as the information is first filtered through the mind of someone else. Therefore, when reading secondary sources, the reader depends on a 'middle person' to accurately report what the original author(s) wrote. This is why primary sources are rated above secondary sources.

It is not always possible to review primary sources because some of these are out of print or not easily accessible, or the material is too 'hefty' and time-consuming to read. Although a secondary source may shed some light on the original material, it conveys the essence of the work and is not the work itself. When research projects are reported second hand, they can lack the details necessary to fully understand how the study was carried out. As far as possible, primary sources should be consulted. The reviewer has to make a judgement on how and when to use either of the sources. It is sometimes easier to quote Roy or the Briggs Report, for example, from a secondary source near at hand than to search for these quotes in the original works. However, if Roy's model is used as a conceptual framework in a study, it is inadmissible not to use the primary source. Reading the list of references at the end of a chapter or article will give you an idea of whether there is a reliance on secondary rather than primary sources.

Tertiary sources are databases and bibliographies. Databases in electronic versions are increasingly being used, especially as they provide instant access to large amounts of literature. This is further discussed later on in this chapter.

Assessing the value of publications

Let us now assess each type of publication according to the type of information it contains and its value as a source of material for a literature review.

Books

There are different types of nursing books (including e-books), such as, among others, general textbooks, books that contain a number of research projects and specialist books (for example, on stress or models of nursing). Books are good sources of material that can be used in a literature review. Textbooks provide some understanding of concepts and issues, but are limited in that they may cover a wide range of topics. Some textbooks make extensive reference to research, while others do so sparingly. There are also books that report exclusively on one research project or a number of projects. They provide useful information that can be used in literature reviews. It is worth noting, however, that by the time books are written, published and read, the research and statistical information they contain is already dated. A heavy reliance on books as sources of material for a review is a sign that the reviewer has missed what has recently been researched and written. Books are reviewed by 'experts' on the topic before publication. As such, they are credible sources of information. Their value also depends on how well researched they are and on their academic status.

Journals

The main sources of literature for researchers are journal articles, which are self-contained entities. This means that, unlike a chapter in a book, which should be read in relation to previous and later chapters, an article contains, in a few pages, all the messages the author wants to convey. Another advantage of articles over books is that they can be read quickly. Although on average it may take over a year from acceptance to publication, they are more 'fresh' than any other sources of information on research and other issues, excluding perhaps conference papers and personal communications. Many journals are publishing papers online before they appear in print form. There are also an increasing number of online journals such as the *Online Journal of Nursing Informatics*, the *Online Journal of Issues in Nursing* and the *BMC Nursing*.

A distinction is sometimes made between scholarly/academic and professional journals. Academic journals (for example, the *Journal of Advanced Nursing*) contain articles of high intellectual quality. These are written in a language and style that tend to appeal more to academics than practitioners. Professional or popular journals (for example, *Nursing Times*, *Nursing Standard* and *British Journal of Community Nursing*) are written mainly for practitioners, although they contain research papers as well. These tend to be more descriptive, seeking to identify practice implications, while academic journals are more abstract and put more emphasis on theory and research. The popular journals have a useful contribution to make, as Smith (1996) explains:

> The popular nursing journals aim to keep their readers regularly informed about up-to-date and topical professional developments, trends in nursing care and practice, news about individuals and the profession, and by providing conference reports. They also provide a marvellous forum for novice writers to air their views and to develop their writing and critical abilities in the correspondence columns and book reviews sections.

Journal articles submitted for publication are normally refereed; that is, they are sent to 'experts' who advise the journal on the feasibility of publication. The 'experts' are normally other authors, which is why this practice is referred to as 'peer review'. It helps to maintain standards in publishing and gives credibility and value to the published material as unsuitable articles are either rejected or sent back to the author for revision. On average, an article is sent by the journal editor to two reviewers, although some journals may require only one, and others three or more. Reviewers are not normally made aware of who the author is. Thus, a 'double-blind peer review' means that reviewers do not know who the author is, nor does the author know who the reviewers are.

Theses

Doctoral and other postgraduate theses are useful and credible sources of information. They should contain a thorough review of concepts, theories and research studies and also details of the research process and findings. Some doctoral theses are published as books (for example, McKenna, 1994: *Nursing Theories and Quality of Care*) or monographs (for example, Gott, 1984: *Learning Nursing*). Theses are examined, and the status of the information they contain is enhanced by this process. Theses can be accessed through inter-library loan, university repositories and other general online databases such as Intute (http://www.intute.ac.uk/), EthOS (http://ethos.bl.uk/), Index to Theses and the Networked Digital Library of Theses and Dissertations (http://www.ndltd.org/).

Research reports

Although doctoral theses follow a more or less prescribed format, research reports come in different sizes and forms of presentation. They tend to have a smaller literature review but focus instead on the data collection, findings, conclusions and recommendations. This is perhaps because sponsors, for whom research reports are primarily written, are more interested in the findings and their implications for policy and practice than they are in the literature review. Many of these research reports are also published in their original forms or as research articles. Research reports do not as a rule undergo a peer review process before publication, although they are subsequently scrutinised by researchers, clinicians and others. These projects are normally carried out by experienced researchers. An example of a research report is *Involving Older Age: The Route to Twenty-first Century Well-being* (Hoban et al., 2013).

Conference proceedings

The main reason to refer to, and review, conference proceedings is because the information is fresh and not yet published. Conference proceedings are in fact abstracts or summaries of papers submitted to conferences, and, as such, they contain only brief information. Their value is mainly in being 'hot off the press'. They are limited in that not enough details are available for the reader to evaluate the project. For example, the Royal College of Nursing Research Society organises annual research conferences and publishes summaries of all the papers presented at these conferences. Some presenters also make copies of their talk available to conference attendees.

Other forms of information

The value of newsletters, pamphlets and leaflets as sources of information is limited in that they are brief communiqués of news and comments. They only present information, with few opportunities for discussion and explanation. They also report much of their information second hand, although they have an advantage because they deal with topical issues. Leaflets and pamphlets from drug companies do contain useful information, but they can also be selective in their evidence, which they may produce in order to sell their products.

Blogs, Facebook and Twitter also contain potentially useful information for researchers and practitioners. While most of the postings are personal opinions, the debate and discussion that they generate can be insightful. Students writing assignments often use them to 'talk' about their experience or to ask for advice from others. The academic value of these online sources of information is, however, limited because the evidence tends to be of a personal nature.

Editorials and letters written to professional journals reflect the topical interests and concerns of practitioners and others, and express the views of the authors on topics they want to draw attention to. Their value lies in the fact that they are often the perceptions of practitioners who are working 'on the ground'. Newspapers and popular magazines also publish material related to health and nursing. They are interested in topical and sometimes 'sensational' issues and report the latest news on selected issues. The quality and credibility of the information depend on the author of the article and the type of newspaper or magazine.

Accessing information sources

All these sources of information can form part of a literature review. The researcher should cast her net wide in order to get an overview and ascertain the breadth of the phenomenon she is studying. The uses to which different types of information are put depends on what the reviewer wants to achieve. For example, if the reviewer wants to show that there is controversy over the benefits of Roy's model for the care of older people, she may refer to letters in the *Nursing Times* or the *Nursing Standard* to illustrate the point. However, she would have to look for discussions of models, in particular Roy's model, in academic books and journals. She would also need to search and review previous research on this issue, information that can be found mostly in academic journals and possibly in postgraduate theses.

Researchers must look for the most up-to-date, relevant and credible information they can find. In practice, this usually means relying more on academic/scholarly journals and books, research reports and theses than on professional journals, newspapers, leaflets and anecdotes.

Purpose of literature reviews

There are four common reasons why a literature review is carried out:

- to prepare for an essay or assignment;
- to increase understanding of a topic or issue;
- to inform a research project;
- for a systematic review.

To prepare for an essay or assignment

For students writing an essay or undertaking an assignment, the literature provides useful information that they can use for describing and discussing relevant issues. In this case, the essay or assignment is the outcome and the literature only serves to illustrate and discuss some of the ideas put forward. Sometimes the literature review is itself the assignment.

To increase understanding of a topic or issue

A literature review can also explore aspects of a phenomenon with the aim of increasing our understanding of it. For example, Davies (2004) carried out a literature review of 'parental grief'. As she explained:

> the aim of this review was to trace how theoretical perspectives on parental grief have changed over the last century and show how these influence therapeutic interventions with bereaved parents.

To inform a research project

Most researchers turn to the literature for ideas before or during a study. Many of those who start constructing a questionnaire find that they very quickly run out of questions to ask. Some learn later, to their cost, that they have omitted asking relevant and pertinent questions. The greatest feeling of frustration is to discover afterwards that the same research has already been carried out, and that, had this been known, 'reinventing the wheel' would have been unnecessary. More importantly, researchers find that they could have benefited from reading other similar studies, had they known about them prior to starting their own. There seems to be a natural tendency to get on with the project and start collecting data instead of (what could be seen as) 'wasting time reading the literature'.

A literature search and review serves to put the current study in the context of what is already known on the phenomenon. It should stimulate the researcher's thinking and can provide a wealth of ideas and perspectives. This is useful in helping to identify, refine and formulate questions. Research on the same or similar topics can, in many ways, be very informative and useful. Two questions researchers should ask are:

● What can the current literature contribute to my research?
● What can my research contribute, in particular, to the understanding of the phenomenon under investigation, and to knowledge in general?

In order to review the literature, a search must first be carried out. A literature search simply means locating and identifying the most up-to-date and relevant material. With the vast opportunities provided by online databases, it is crucial to possess the skills to search the literature efficiently and successfully. Most educational institutions organise sessions, often with the help of librarians, to introduce students to the art and science of searching the literature.

A literature review involves a critical reading of the selected literature to find out how it can be useful to the current research. From this review, a case can be made for the importance of the current research (in particular how it builds on current knowledge and what gaps it fills) and for justifying the design of the study. The scene is also set for comparing the current findings with those of similar studies. The review carried out by the researcher is much more than the written summary that appears in articles, or what is reported in theses and research reports. Much more literature is read and analysed than is discussed and presented.

The literature review, as part of a research project, should perform the following functions:

- provide a rationale for the current study;
- put the current study in the context of what is known about the topic;
- review relevant research studies carried out on the same or similar topics;
- discuss the conceptual/theoretical basis for the current study.

Providing a rationale for the current study

Researchers need to provide reasons for conducting their study. In doing so, they can try to convince readers that the study is of sufficient importance. Some give as many reasons as possible, perhaps in an attempt to convince the journal's editor and referees that the current research is important. Sometimes the real reason for doing research is because of the requirement of a course or because of the pressure on academics and others to publish. Ideas for research projects come mainly from one's observation of practice and/or from the literature.

The most frequently cited reason for doing a study is the lack of research on the particular aspect of the topic being researched. For example, Rutledge et al. (2013) explained that while fibromyalgia is a chronic widespread pain condition affecting 1–5 per cent of the population, many of whom are at risk of falling, there was no published research on this topic. They decided to carry out a study to explore the experiences of falling among people with fibromyalgia prior to developing a fall risk reduction intervention.

The reduction of morbidity and mortality, the prevention of illness and the economic and social costs of a particular illness or treatment are often cited as arguments for conducting a study. Abayomi and Hackett (2004), in their rationale for a study on the 'assessment of malnutrition in mental health clients: nurses' judgement vs. a nutrition risk tool', gave a number of reasons including the fact that 'malnutrition has a disabling effect on the NHS', and that 'up to 50% of hospital food in the United Kingdom (UK) is wasted, at a cost of £45 million a year'. They pointed out that previous studies evaluating the effectiveness of nutrition assessment tools have focused on physically ill people and not on those with mental illness. Using findings from previous studies, they explained that nutritional status affects recovery and that poor nutrition:

> can lead to increased risk of morbidity and death, impaired mental and physical function, apathy, depression, self-neglect, increased risk of complications, increased risk of pressure ulcers, reduced immune response, delayed wound healing, longer hospital stay and reduced quality of life.

Statistical data and research findings can provide valuable back-up for the arguments put forward by researchers for their studies. Another reason often given as rationale for a study is to inform the debate on controversial issues. For example, Jones et al. (2007) carried out a study to explore the experiences of nurse prescribing in a mental health setting in order to inform the debate on the 'controversial' issue of medication prescribing by mental health nurses in the UK.

The rationale for research projects often includes the need to evaluate the effectiveness of a particular practice or compare one nursing intervention with another. Questioning practice can provide ideas for research. For example, Fader et al. (2003) questioned the effects on skin care of prolonged wearing of incontinence pads by older people. As Fader et al. explained:

> based on current evidence, we cannot be confident that *less frequent* pad changing (resulting in *prolonged* skin contact with urine) does not compromise skin health, and there is a need to establish whether or not the night-time management of incontinence involving less *frequent* pad changing is justifiable.

Policy-related reasons are often cited as a rationale for research studies. Researchers may set out to investigate professionals' reactions to policies or recommendations. The need to evaluate the effects of particular aspects of policies, old and new, is frequently given as part of the reason for research being carried out.

In addition, researchers may simply want to replicate or follow up other studies. Whatever the reasons, the rationale for a study must be relevant, clear and convincing. It must be supported, where appropriate and possible, by research findings, statistical data and, in some cases, expert opinion.

Putting the current study in context

The literature review must place the present study in the context of what is already known about the topic. It should also, where appropriate, explain or discuss the concepts, variables and issues relevant to the research problem being investigated. In a study of factors influencing the job satisfaction of hospital nurses, the researcher should discuss the concept of job satisfaction. It is likely that she will compare and contrast various definitions and descriptions offered by others who have grappled with the concept, and choose the meaning she will give to job satisfaction in her study. She will also look for previous research findings and other conceptual/theoretical literature relating to factors affecting job satisfaction. If there is little or no literature relating to hospital nurses, the researcher will draw on literature on community nurses. Failing this, she could consult relevant research and non-research material relating to job satisfaction in other professions.

In reviewing the literature, the researcher will shed some light on what is already known about variables that may influence job satisfaction, such as gender, expectations, the nature of the job or pay. Although different researchers may approach this exercise in different ways, the key concepts, variables and issues must be explained, if not discussed.

Researchers have to be selective about what they present to readers. They cannot possibly write about everything known about the topic. They can only discuss material relevant to the case they want to make, but in doing so they must support their arguments with evidence and also present a balanced view in their discussion. Biases will be obvious when one-sided arguments are put forward, especially when readers are aware of counterarguments.

Carter and Tourangeau (2012) discussed a number of issues in their study of the retention of nurses in the National Health Service in the UK: government policies on recruitment and retention, the supply of registered nurses in the UK, the older age profile of those applying for training and those currently in employment, and the implications of the economic downturn on the nursing workforce.

Reviewing relevant research studies

In reviewing the literature, the researcher tries to identify research studies previously carried out on the topic. By comparing, analysing and summarising their focus, methodologies and findings, she can come to some conclusions on the state of research in this particular area. McCaughan et al. (2013) carried out a literature review for their study of the quality of life of men with prostate cancer. They reported that four different questionnaires measuring quality of life were used in the five studies they found, making it difficult to compare their findings. McCaughan et al. also noted that these five studies had small samples.

Researchers can build on the strengths of previous methodologies or adopt other strategies. The pitfalls of previous research can also be avoided. Perhaps one of the major benefits is to be able to make use of other researchers' tools, such as questionnaires or other measuring instruments.

Comparing the findings of similar studies is an important exercise in understanding the phenomenon being studied. Similar results may reinforce their validity, while contradictory ones may raise questions about, among others, the data collection and analysis methods. McCaughan et al. (2013) found that the few studies published on the quality of life of men with prostate cancer reported conflicting findings.

It is not important or necessary to discuss every previous research study in detail. How much the reviewer reports on or discusses depends on the particular points she wants to make. In literature reviews, the most common aspect of previous research reported is the findings. When the findings from similar studies are contradictory, a good reviewer should attempt to speculate on why this may be so. A close look at their methods, samples or data analysis would probably be required to explain the differences.

For example, one study looking at the health of carers of spouses with cancer found that only 10 per cent of carers consulted a general practitioner about their own health. Another similar study found that general practitioner consultation was 23 per cent. There may be good reasons why these findings are different. It could be that these studies were carried out in different populations with different types of cancer. Cultural differences as well as different healthcare systems may explain why consultation patterns vary. Alternatively, the explanation may also be found in the methods, response rates or data analysis. Whatever the reasons, the reviewer should not leave the reader to speculate on contradictory findings but must try to offer explanations, as it is the reviewer who has read these studies in detail. By reviewing previous studies, the researcher can explain what has been achieved so far and what contribution her study proposes to make, and also learn from the achievements and mistakes of other researchers.

Discussing the conceptual/theoretical basis for the current study

The purpose of research is to contribute to the pool of knowledge, and, as we found in Chapter 2, knowledge is organised, among other ways, in the form of theories. The use of conceptual frameworks or models is a step towards this contribution. Not all research uses a framework. However, a review of the literature will inform the researcher of what frameworks are available and how others have used them. In their study of factors that determine whether nurses intend to remain in employment, Carter and Tourangeau (2012) used a model consisting of eight thematic categories (including nurse characteristics, organisational support and practices, work rewards, and so on) to develop their questionnaire. The use of conceptual frameworks and models in nursing research is the subject of Chapter 8.

These functions of a literature review apply mainly to quantitative research. What is already known is then tested and built upon, which is why quantitative researchers, prior to starting their own research, need to know what has previously been done. In a qualitative study, the researcher does not want to be influenced by previous knowledge but she needs to know what contribution to knowledge she wants to make. She also needs to know enough about the subject she is researching. For example, if an ethnographic study of patient-centred care in a medical ward is carried out, the researcher must at least know what patient-centred care is. She may not be interested, at the initial stage, in the findings of other studies, but may later want to compare hers with others.

In practice, it is unlikely that qualitative researchers do not read the literature. They may have to be selective and read enough to enable them to carry out the study without being unduly influenced by previous research. Qualitative researchers may use existing conceptual frameworks or theories or may instead try to formulate their own from the data they collect. Finally, in quantitative research, the literature is reviewed and completed prior to data collection, whereas in qualitative research there is more flexibility. In practice, many quantitative and qualitative researchers continue to read and review the literature at any time in the research process, right up to the completion of the report or thesis. For a discussion of the role of literature review in a qualitative study, see Walls et al. (2010).

Critiquing the literature review

While a literature review primarily benefits those conducting the study, readers may want to know why the current study is important, what research, if any, has previously been carried out and what the researcher proposes to contribute. Books, theses and research reports give the authors ample scope to present extended literature reviews, while journal articles restrict them to a summary of the main arguments. The word-limit restriction should not, however, be used as an excuse for poor and inadequate reviews. The ability to present up-to-date, relevant information clearly, concisely and logically is crucial. The review should not be a collection of disparate, unconnected views or a series of quotes.

In critiquing a literature review, you may want to use the four functions described above as a framework to assess whether these four areas are covered. Is a rationale provided? If so, what is it? More than one reason for the study can sometimes be given. How convincing are these reasons? For example, in a study of 'attitudes of undergraduate nurses towards mental illness', the author stated that nurses' attitudes and values are of considerable importance. However, the only reason put forward for this was that 'they will be the leaders of tomorrow', undoubtedly a poor reason. Not only is the author making an assumption about 'undergraduates and leadership', but, more importantly, the relationship between 'attitudes and practice', which is more relevant, is not mentioned, let alone discussed.

Even when the rationale is convincing, the author needs to support it with such evidence as research findings, statistical data and, to a lesser extent, expert opinion. References to this evidence need to be relevant and up to date. Although statistical data take time to collect, analyse and publish, you must watch out for outdated figures. For example, in one study it was stated that 'there is a high incidence of incontinence in residential homes'. This was backed up by a reference dated 2004, while the article was written in 2014 – the incidence rate could have changed since the data were collected.

Does the author inform you of similar research studies carried out? You should not assume that no previous research exists when the author does not mention it. It is incumbent on the researcher to provide a brief critical overview of previous research. Making selective references to one or more studies whose findings may be favourable to her cause can only bring charges of bias against the author. Readers may be aware of the existence of contradictory findings or counterarguments.

A detailed critical review of all previous research may be boring and inappropriate. The author should guide you to make sense of the focus, methodologies and findings of other studies, rather than just describe them. Where necessary, inconsistent or contradictory findings must be explained. Prior to writing the review, it is the task of the reviewer to read, digest, compare and analyse most of the relevant material, and draw general conclusions.

If the current research study proposes to adopt approaches and methods different from those of previous research, you will be left wondering, if you are not told, which approaches and methods were previously used and why they have been discarded. When critiquing a literature review, you must identify information that is often omitted yet is crucial to your understanding of the review.

You must also find out whether important issues and concepts are dealt with adequately. It is unfair to expect the author to present a discussion of everything related to the topic. However, if, for example, in a study investigating the 'health promotion strategies of health visitors', the concept of 'health promotion' is not explored, you may find it difficult to understand what constitutes health promotion for the author. You would also like to know what health promotion strategies are and, briefly, what the state of knowledge on them is.

As explained earlier, it is important to pay attention to the publication dates of the literature referred to in the review. It is difficult to generalise about what constitutes a 'dated' reference. If you read the nursing literature frequently, you will be aware of areas that are well researched. If you find that references are more than 5 years old, you can ask yourself whether there is more recent literature on the topic. It is up to the author to mention why the literature she refers to is 'dated'. You must also take into account that it can take time for an article, once accepted for publication, to be published. You should also question the author's reliance on secondary sources if this is the case.

Not every literature review fulfils the four functions mentioned above. In practice, the author focuses on one or more of these and pays less attention to the others. This choice depends on the case she wants to put across. Provided crucial information – such as a discussion of concepts relevant to the study and information about previous studies – is not omitted, the review may be adequate. You must also look out for assumptions and generalisations. In a study of 'psychiatric nurses' attitudes and behaviours towards patients in acute wards', the authors make the assumptions in the literature review that 'the management approach in acute psychiatric care needed to be changed' and that 'nurses working in these settings needed to have greater skills in rehabilitation and health promotion'. No evidence was offered to support either of these two statements. The study itself did not set out to investigate management approaches or the skills of psychiatric nurses.

It is unfair to be overcritical of literature reviews, especially in journal articles where the authors are limited for space. Not every issue, concept or research study can be discussed in depth. If the information is not there, you can ask yourself whether the lack of it affects your understanding of the study. If it does, it is a good indication that this information should have been included in the review. A good literature review provides you with essential, relevant information to put the current study in context of existing knowledge and research available on the topic.

Systematic reviews

The emphasis on evidence-based practice (see Chapter 21) has focused attention on 'systematic reviews', which involves searching, appraising and summarising the available evidence for practice. The glut of information, coupled with competing demands on practitioners' time, means that it is difficult for them to keep abreast of the mass of information that they are faced with on a daily basis. We continue to produce knowledge, much of which gets lost in the sea of information. Like the sea, information is a valuable resource, and unless we learn how to harness it and make use of it, we can drown in it.

Evans and Pearson (2001) explain that the findings of the systematic review 'frees the decision maker from reliance on the mass of published primary research'. In any case, most practitioners do not have the resources and expertise to search and appraise the large number of studies that are relevant to their practice. In their busy world, summaries of findings or evidence are more helpful.

A systematic review can be defined as the rigorous and systematic search, selection, appraisal, synthesis and summary of the findings of primary research studies in order to answer a specific question. The process of systematic reviews from question formulation to the summary of evidence should be transparent and, therefore, potentially replicable. The rationale and actions of the systematic reviewer should be clear for readers to assess the reliability, validity and relevance of the review for their practice. The term 'systematic' refers to the system adopted by the reviewer, which details the parameters set (for example, the time-frame in which studies are selected), the method of appraisal (for example, the tools used to evaluate the quality of the studies) and the method of synthesis (for example, qualitative summaries or statistical calculations).

Systematic reviews can be broadly termed as 'research on research'. This is sometimes called secondary research because it does not collect new information (primary research) but makes use of the findings of previous research. Table 7.1 makes a comparison between primary research and systematic reviews.

Table 7.1   Comparison of primary research and systematic reviews

Primary research	Systematic reviews
Choose a topic and formulate a question, objectives or hypothesis for which data are to be collected	Choose a topic and formulate a question, objectives or hypothesis in order to begin a systematic search
Select a sample or population and study site(s)	Select databases and set inclusion/exclusion criteria for the selection of studies/other evidence
Choose data collection methods (e.g. questionnaires, interviews or observations)	Search the literature and extract relevant, valid and reliable information and collect data from articles (through critical appraisal) using of a checklist of questions
Analyse the data collected	Analyse and synthesise the findings of the selected (methodologically sound) studies
Draw conclusions from the analysis of data	Draw conclusions from the findings of the review

In contrast, a non-systematic literature review is normally broad. The questions for which evidence are sought may not be stated or may be unclear. The method of selecting items for review is not always transparent, nor is the method of appraisal. Readers are unsure how the review was carried out. A non-systematic review, often called a 'narrative' or 'descriptive' review, can be 'haphazard and biased, subject to the idiosyncratic impressions of the individual reviewer' (Mulrow, 1994).

The terms 'systematic review' and 'meta-analysis' are sometimes used interchangeably. However, meta-analysis is one form of systematic review. Meta-analysis has been defined as 'a mathematical synthesis of the results of two or more primary studies that addressed the same hypothesis in the same way' (Greenhalgh, 1997b). Meta-analysis is a term normally used to describe a process of combining and summarising the statistical findings of a number of clinical trials.

The association of systematic reviews with randomised controlled trials (RCTs) comes mainly from those who believe that there is a hierarchy of study designs for studies of effectiveness in which systematic reviews of RCTs provide the best evidence. In this hierarchy, evidence from other research approaches and designs, including qualitative ones, is not as highly regarded as is evidence from RCTs. This view, however, is not shared by all and is indeed contested (Nutley et al., 2012). The York Centre for Reviews and Dissemination (CRD; 2009) explains that there is growing recognition of the valuable contribution that qualitative research can make to effectiveness reviews. For a useful discussion of the practical issues in conducting systematic reviews of qualitative studies, see Lloyd Jones (2004). Nutley et al. (2012) also provide an insight into what constitutes 'good evidence'.

'Meta-synthesis' (Jensen and Allen, 1994; Sandelowski et al., 1997) and 'meta-ethnography' (Noblit and Hare, 1988) are terms that have been used interchangeably to describe the techniques or methods used to search, appraise and synthesise (combine) the findings of qualitative studies. This type of review is carried out to compare and combine the findings of qualitative studies in order to describe phenomena or to develop theories. The task of appraising and synthesising qualitative studies is made more difficult because of the 'widely varying theoretical perspectives and diverse analytical approaches' used in these studies (Dixon-Woods and Fitzpatrick, 2001). Examples of qualitative meta-syntheses include 'Experiences of kidney failure' (Schick Makaroff, 2012) and 'experiences of poststroke fatigue' (Eilertsen et al., 2013).

Sandelowski et al. (1997), Thorne et al. (2004) and Campbell et al. (2011) provide useful discussions and insights on the value, methodology and limitations of qualitative systematic reviews.

The systematic review process

As with primary research, there are a number of key steps that have to be followed when undertaking a systematic review:

- Formulate/select the questions, aims, objectives or hypotheses.
- Define the outcome and intervention.
- Set inclusion/exclusion criteria.
- Search the evidence.

- Select items to review.
- Appraise the evidence.
- Synthesise the evidence.
- Conclude and make recommendations.

Formulating questions for a systematic review

No systematic review can take place without a question, an aim or a hypothesis. According to Pearson (2004) 'a sound, systematic review rests on a well defined review question'. These have to be clear and unambiguous. Questions for reviews can come from one's practice or professional interest. Systematic reviews are associated with clinical practice, mainly because they are an integral component of evidence-based practice. However, a systematic review is a technique or design to answer a range of questions, including non-clinical ones. Below are examples of questions for which systematic reviews have been carried out.

- From Laird and Coates (2013) 'Systematic review of randomized controlled trials to regulate glycaemia after stroke':

    The primary aim of this systematic review was to evaluate the available evidence on the effectiveness of tight glucose regulation intervention for clinical outcome of adults admitted to hospital with acute stroke. The secondary aim was to present a narrative synthesis of the key issues that pertain to glucose monitoring, protocol adherence, and adverse incidents, to inform nurses in clinical decision-making.

- From Ling et al. (2012) 'Do educational interventions improve cancer patients' quality of life and reduce pain intensity? Quantitative systematic review':

    The aim of the review was to evaluate the effect of patient education on pain intensity and pain interference, as well as on the quality of life of cancer patients.

These examples show that more than one question can be formulated, and that they have to be focused and realistic as well. The broader the review question, the more difficult it can be to conduct the review and reach conclusions.

Defining outcome and interventions

Outcome measures in reviews of effectiveness of interventions have to be operationally defined. In particular, the outcome measures of 'effectiveness' have to be clearly stated. For example, in a review on 'nursing interventions for smoking cessation' (Rice and Stead, 2008), the principal outcome was smoking cessation rather than a reduction in withdrawal symptoms or a reduction in number of cigarettes smoked. Nursing intervention was defined as the provision of advice, counselling and/or strategies to help patients quit smoking.

Setting inclusion/exclusion criteria

The questions and the available resources determine to a great extent the scope of the review. Therefore inclusion and exclusion criteria are set to define the boundaries of the review. These criteria must be justified, and their implications for the validity of the review must be recognised. For example, if the evidence is searched manually from selected journals, or if only English-language publications are considered, the findings will have limitations as it is possible that significant evidence may be missed. The generalisability of the findings depends on how inclusive or exclusive the review is in its identification and selection of evidence. For example, in a review of 'psychosocial interventions for men with prostate cancer', Parahoo et al. (2013) set the following inclusion and exclusion criteria for selecting interventions:

individual or group interventions, whether delivered via telephone, at home or during clinic visits (or a combination of these) by lay or trained personnel (or a combination of both) were included. Interventions based solely on distribution of leaflets or other informational material (without an input from trained or lay personnel) were excluded.

Searching the evidence

The aim of a systematic review is to answer the review question. For this answer to be credible, every effort to locate all relevant studies must be made. The resources and skills to do so often determine how successful reviewers will be in identifying all the relevant literature.

The most common format in which research findings are presented is the journal article. Abstracts (a brief summary outlining relevant information) of these articles are compiled in registers, known as databases, which are available online or as CD-Roms. Three of the most relevant and useful databases for nurses are the Cumulative Index to Nursing and Allied Health (CINAHL), MEDLINE and Allied and Complementary Medicine (AMED). CINAHL is a comprehensive research database that provides the full text of over 760 journals of nursing and allied health and full text for more than 275 books/monographs dating back to 1937. It also provides access to healthcare books, nursing dissertations, selected conference proceedings, standards of professional practice, educational software and audiovisual materials in nursing. MEDLINE covers the international literature from 5,400 journals published worldwide from 1946 on biomedicine, including the allied health fields and the biological and physical sciences, humanities, and information science as they relate to medicine and healthcare. Subirana et al. (2002), who compared the efficiency of MEDLINE and CINAHL in identifying references, concluded that searches on nursing-related subjects should combine CINAHL and MEDLINE in order to obtain the best results. There are other databases relevant to nurses, including CANCERLIT, which is produced by the US National Cancer Institute and which covers all aspects of cancer therapy. PsycINFO is another database that contains citations and summaries in the field of psychology with particular reference to medicine, psychiatry, nursing and other related disciplines.

Reviewers rely mainly on databases. However, depending on a number of factors, including which journals are included in the database and how articles are indexed, it may not be possible to identify all the relevant literature. Some literature is published in house, and some researchers do not publish their projects. These studies are known as the 'grey literature'. They are important to include in the review. Hopewell et al. (2007) reviewed research studies that have investigated the impact of the grey literature in the meta-analysis of randomised trials of healthcare interventions. They concluded that 'published trials are generally larger, and may show an overall greater treatment effect than grey trials'. According to Hopewell et al., 'reviewers need to ensure they identify grey trials in order to minimise the risk of introducing bias into their review'.

Reference lists of published papers and manual searches of relevant journals can also be useful. Databases, the grey literature, reference lists and manual searches are all important sources of literature that should be accessed, where possible, in the process of a systematic review. Searching computerised databases successfully is a skill that requires training and experience. The use of appropriate search terms is the key to the successful identification of relevant material. Each database has information on how to search the literature. Librarians can also be helpful in advising how to access them or what courses are available for training. There are a number of useful resources to help you in this process (see, for example, Greenhalgh, 1997a). In the extract below, Petticrew et al. (2002a) describe how they searched and identified the literature for their review of the 'influence of psychological coping on survival and recurrence in people with cancer'.

> *Search strategy* – Following systematic review guidelines we searched several databases for published and unpublished studies (in any language) on the association between progression of cancer, recurrence or survival, and psychological coping: Medline 1966–June 2002, PsycINFO 1887–June 2002, ASSIA 1987–June 2002, Embase 1980–June 2002, Cancerlit 1966–June 2002, Dissertation Abstracts 1975–June 2002, the NLM gateway (accessed 21 June 2002), and CINAHL 1982–June 2002. We searched bibliographies and reviews and contacted key individuals and authors for additional unpublished information when necessary.

Knowing what sources of information to access and how to access them are key requisites for locating the evidence.

Selecting items to review

The search for literature will identify relevant and non-relevant items. The reviewer's next task is to select only those that meet the inclusion criteria. Reading the abstracts or summaries of the selected items will quickly determine which items should be included. Sometimes, however, abstracts may not be clear or may not provide adequate or relevant information for reviewers to make a decision. This can be done when the full article is accessed.

Appraising the evidence

Before synthesising the findings of the selected items, the quality of these studies must be appraised since not all studies are valid and reliable. There are a number of tools or checklists available to help in this process. The CASP (Critical Appraisal Skills Programme) has developed a number of tools that are available and free for personal use at http://www.casp-uk.net/find-appraise-act/appraising-the-evidence/. Other references for checklists include Treloar et al. (2000) and Greenhalgh (1997a). The Cochrane Reviewers' handbook (http://www.cochrane.org/resources/handbook/index.htm) can also be useful. The appraisal of research studies is explained further in Chapter 20.

To avoid subjectivity in the use of these tools, it is usual for two or more reviewers to carry out the appraisal independently and to compare the results. Differences can be resolved and a consensus can be reached. Only items that meet the quality criteria set by reviewers are included in the next stage of the review.

Synthesising the findings from selected studies

The aim of data synthesis is to collate, combine and summarise the findings of studies selected for inclusion in the review (CRD, 2009). There are different ways in which these findings can be synthesised depending on whether the reviewed studies are RCTs, non-RCTs, quantitative studies, qualitative studies or those combining qualitative and quantitative studies.

For a meta-analysis of RCTs, the aim of the synthesis is to find out if there is a difference between the intervention groups and the control groups in terms of the pre-selected outcome measures. These could be 'the difference in number of days in which a condition is treated with a new drug when compared with a placebo', 'the risk of developing infection (in the two groups) following two types of wound care' or 'the incidence of relapse between two different treatments'. These are normally expressed in terms of the odds ratio (the ratio of the odds of an event in the intervention group to the odds of an event in the control group), the relative risk (the ratio of risk in the intervention group to the risk in the control group) or the mean difference (the difference between the mean scores, for example of quality of life) of the two groups. These are only some of the measures in which the synthesised data can be presented.

The findings of the selected studies are not just added up and averaged. Weightings can be given according to the size and the quality of individual studies. Larger studies and those judged to be of higher quality can be given more 'weight'.

The heterogeneity (variability in the characteristics of the sample of individual studies) and 'publication bias' (the likelihood that RCTs which show that the interventions had little or no effects were not published) are two of the other factors that can be taken into account when the results of the studies are combined. Statistical techniques to carry out these calculations and test the accuracy of the results are well developed (for more details, see CRD, 2009). Many people may find it difficult to interpret data on 'odds ratio', 'relative risk' or 'number needed to treat'. The latter term means the number of people who should be treated before one person can benefit from the treatment. Therefore the findings should also be summarised and presented in a prose form that is easier to understand.

The synthesis of qualitative studies requires a more descriptive and narrative approach since the findings are normally presented in the form of themes. The process is similar to the analysis of data from a number of interview scripts. However, when the populations in these studies are not similar and the approaches are diverse, the reviewer may be faced with difficult decisions, especially if the findings are divergent too. The variety of qualitative approaches (ethnography, phenomenology, grounded theory, and so on) and their different theoretical underpinnings make it difficult for qualitative findings to be compared, combined and summarised. Many of the methods are still at a developmental stage (CRD, 2009). However, there is some guidance for those who undertake such reviews (see, for example, Noblit and Hare, 1988; Sheldon, 2005; Sandelowski and Barroso, 2006; Pope et al., 2007; Garside 2008).

Concluding and making recommendations

Systematic reviews are carried out in order to appraise and synthesise the available evidence in answer to a specific question. Readers are eager to know what the conclusions are and how they can use the findings in their practice. Reviewers, by virtue of appraising a number of studies, can also comment on the quality of the evidence and make recommendations for future research. For example, after reviewing seven randomised trials on acupuncture for depression, Mukaino et al. (2005) concluded that 'the evidence from controlled trials is insufficient to conclude whether acupuncture is an effective treatment for depression, but justifies further trials of electroacupuncture'. Conclusions and recommendations in systematic reviews should be based on the findings and should be made with care as they may subsequently influence practice.

Systematic and exploratory reviews

The increasing emphasis on the need for literature reviews to be systematic and rigorous has raised concerns about other types of review that do not rigorously follow the process of systematic reviews. Does every literature review have to be systematic? If you want to know whether there is evidence that 'discharge preparation' reduces anxiety among older patients in hospitals, the review has to be valid and reliable, otherwise the results will be contested. Every step of the review, from the formulation of the question to the conclusions, has to be explained and justified. Readers can thus judge the rigour with which the review was carried out and decide whether the conclusions are credible or not.

On the other hand, if you want to use the literature to explore and discuss a particular concept such as 'discharge anxiety', you have the freedom to use the literature to explain your perspective on the topic. It is no more than a 'well-researched' essay, but it serves the purpose of giving readers an insight into 'discharge anxiety', and, as such, has a valuable contribution to make to practitioners' knowledge. The quality of the review depends on how you draw from the existing literature, and on the strength and nature of your arguments. It is not possible or even desirable that every bit of literature on 'discharge anxiety' is searched and reviewed. You must, however, demonstrate an adequate awareness of the relevant literature on the subject, and not be biased in selecting only literature that supports your views.

Validity and reliability of reviews

Practitioners rely on the summaries of systematic reviews to provide valid and reliable evidence. There are some built-in safeguards that could, to some extent, reassure practitioners. For example, the Cochrane Collaboration, the CDR based at the University of York (UK) and the Joanna Briggs Institute (based in Australia) are dedicated to achieving the highest standards in systematic reviews and allocate 'Kite Marks' to the reviews that they endorse. Yet a systematic review (Olsen et al., 2001) of the quality of 53 Cochrane reviews first published in issue 4 of the Cochrane Library in 1998, reported:

> No problems or only minor ones were found in most reviews. Major problems were identified in 15 reviews (29%). The evidence did not fully support the conclusion in nine reviews (17%), the conduct or reporting was unsatisfactory in 12 reviews (23%), and stylistic problems were identified in 12 reviews (23%).

They concluded that while the Cochrane Library remains a key source of evidence about the effects of healthcare practice, there is always room for improvement. Olsen et al. suggest that 'users should interpret reviews cautiously, particularly those with conclusions favouring experimental interventions'.

Petticrew et al. (2002b) carried out a similar exercise with 480 systematic reviews on the Database of Abstracts of Reviews of Effectiveness (DARE) at the University of York (UK) and reported, among other things, that only half (52%) of the reviews had systematically assessed the validity of the included studies and that most systematic reviews were unlikely to be comprehensive.

These 'reviews of reviews' were conducted more than a decade ago, and systematic reviewing has experienced a great deal of development since then. Methods to access, search, appraise and synthesise evidence have been developed at a level of sophistication that could have hardly been expected within such a short time. Yet despite being referred to as a 'science', the systematic review is still subject to a number of validity and reliability threats. Bias related to publication, searching, appraising, synthesising and concluding can all affect the final product. Practitioners do not normally have the skills and experience of these reviewers to begin to cast doubt on the results (often couched in statistical terms) and the conclusions of systematic reviews. They are dependent on reviewers (another set of experts!) to provide them with valid and reliable evidence.

Appraisal of systematic reviews

Although most nurses and other health professionals cannot be expected to carry out systematic reviews, they should be able to appraise or evaluate these reviews. Not all reviews are prepared by, or in collaboration with, the Cochrane Review Groups, the Joanna Briggs Institute or the CRD. Reviews have to be appraised before their recommendations can be applied to practice. The following checklist is offered as a framework for appraising systematic reviews. It is based on the steps of systematic reviews outlined earlier in this chapter.

1 Are the questions for the review clearly stated?
2 Are the terms or concepts operationally defined? This will help you decide whether you understand the terms used in the review question in the same way as the reviewers do.
3 What are the inclusion and exclusion criteria? This has implications for the generalisability of the findings.
4 What databases and other sources were accessed? This will inform you of the extensiveness of the search.
5 What terms and combination of terms were used in the search? Are they adequate?
6 How were the items (studies) in the review appraised? If a checklist was used, is it rigorous?
7 How was the evidence combined or summarised?
8 What were the conclusions?
9 What were the limitations of the review?
10 Overall, do the findings of the review help or confuse you?

A clear and unambiguous question and transparency in how the search was carried out, how the selected studies were appraised and how the conclusions were reached are all crucial for readers to assess the validity and reliability of the findings, and their relevance to, and usefulness in, their particular practice. For more details on how to appraise systematic reviews, see JBIEBNM (2000) or Abalos et al. (2001).

The main purpose of a literature review is to show why the current study is needed and where it fits into the overall body of knowledge on the phenomenon being researched. Additionally, the review sets the scene by discussing the relevant issues and concepts in, and related to, the research question, objectives or hypotheses. In designing their studies, researchers can draw upon the theoretical and research literature available.

There are different types of literature, and the information they contain varies according to the type of publication. Researchers must as far as possible consult, and refer to, reliable and credible sources. This invariably means research-based literature, although there is other valuable information in the non-research literature as well. Primary sources should be consulted and reported where possible. A literature review, as part of

Summary

a research study, can have four functions and they can be used as a framework for critiquing reviews.

In this chapter, the purpose and process of systematic reviews were discussed. The process consists of formulating clear questions, searching relevant databases, appraising the quality of relevant studies and summarising their findings. Finally, a checklist to appraise systematic reviews was provided.

References

Abalos E, Carroli G, Mackey M E and Bergel E (2001) *Critical Appraisal of Systematic Reviews: The WHO Reproductive Health Library*, No 4 (WHO/RHR/01.6) (Geneva: World Health Organization).

Abayomi J and Hackett A (2004) Assessment of malnutrition in mental health clients: nurses' judgement vs nutrition risk tool. *Journal of Advanced Nursing*, **45**, 4:430–7.

Briggs A (1972) *Report of the Committee on Nursing* (London: DHSS).

Campbell R, Pound P, Morgan M et al. (2011) Evaluating meta-ethnography: systematic analysis and synthesis of qualitative research. *Health Technology Assessment*, **15**: 43.

Carter M R and Tourangeau A E (2012) Staying in nursing: what factors determine whether nurses intend to remain employed? *Journal of Advanced Nursing*, **68**, 7: 1589–600.

Centre for Reviews and Dissemination (2009) *Systematic Reviews: CRD's Guidance for Undertaking Reviews in Health Care* (York: University of York, CRD).

Davies R (2004) New understandings of parental grief: literature review. *Journal of Advanced Nursing*, **46**, 5:506–13.

Dixon-Woods M and and Fitzpatrick R (2001) Qualitative research in systematic reviews. *British Medical Journal*, **323**, 7316:765–6.

Eilertsen G, Ormstad H and Kirkevold M (2013) Experiences of poststroke fatigue: qualitative meta-synthesis. *Journal of Advanced Nursing*, **69**, 3:514–25.

Evans D and Pearson A (2001) Systematic reviews of qualitative research. *Clinical Effectiveness in Nursing*, **5**:111–19.

Fader M, Clarke-O'Neill S, Cook D et al. (2003) Management of night-time urinary incontinence in residential settings for older people: an investigation into the effects of different pad changing regimes on skin health. *Journal of Clinical Nursing*, **12**, 3:374–86.

Garside R (2008) A comparison of methods for the systematic review of qualitative research: two examples using meta-ethnography and meta-study. Exeter: Peninsula Postgraduate Health Institute, Universities of Exeter and Plymouth, PhD thesis.

Gott M (1984) *Learning Nursing* (London: Royal College of Nursing).

Greenhalgh T (1997a) *How to Read a Paper* (London: BMJ Publishing Group).

Greenhalgh T (1997b) Papers that summarise other papers (systematic reviews and meta-analysis). *British Medical Journal*, **315**:672–5.

Hoban M, James V, Beresford P and Fleming J (2013) *Involving Older Age: The Route to Twenty-first Century Well-being* (Cardiff: Royal Voluntary Service).

Hopewell S, McDonald S, Clarke MJ, Egger M (2007) Grey literature in meta-analyses of randomized trials of health care interventions. *Cochrane Database of Systematic Reviews*, Issue 2:MR000010.

JBIEBNM (2000) Appraising systematic reviews, changing practice Sup. 1. Retrieved from http://connect.jbiconnectplus.org/ViewSourceFile.aspx?0=4311 (accessed 7 January 2014).

Jensen L A and Allen M N (1994) A synthesis of qualitative research on wellness–illness. *Qualitative Health Research*, **4**, 4:349–69.

Jones M, Bennett B, Lucas B, Miller D and Gray R (2007) Mental health nurse supplementary prescribing: experiences of mental health nurses, psychiatrists and patients. *Journal of Advanced Nursing*, **59**, 5: 488–96.

Laird E A and Coates V (2013) Systematic review of randomized controlled trials to regulate glycaemia after stroke. *Journal of Advanced Nursing*, **69**, 2:263–77.

Ling C C, Lui Y and So W K W (2012) Do educational interventions improve cancer patients' quality of life and reduce pain intensity? Quantitative systematic review. *Journal of Advanced Nursing*, **68**, 3:511–20.

Lloyd Jones M (2004) Application of systematic review methods to qualitative research: practical issues. *Journal of Advanced Nursing*, **48**, 3:271–8.

Lutjens L R J (1991) *Callista Roy: An Adaptation Model* (Newbury Park, CA: Sage).

McCaughan E, McSorley O, Prue G, Parahoo K, Bunting B, Sullivan J O and McKenna H (2013) Quality of life in men receiving radiotherapy and neo-adjuvant androgen deprivation for prostate cancer: results from a prospective study. *Journal of Advanced Nursing*, **69**, 1:53–65.

McKenna H P (1994) *Nursing Theories and Quality of Care* (Aldershot: Avebury).

Mukaino Y, Park J, White A and Ernst E (2005) The effectiveness of acupuncture for depression – a systematic review of randomised controlled trials. *Acupuncture in Medicine*, **23**, 2:70–6.

Mulrow C (1994) Rational for systematic reviews. *British Medical Journal*, **309**:597–9.

Noblit G W and Hare R D (1988) *Meta-Ethnography: Synthesizing Qualitative Studies* (London: Sage).

Nutley S, Powell A and Davies H (2012) *What Counts as Good Evidence?* (St Andrews: University of St Andrews, School of Management, Research Unit for Research Utilisation).

Olsen O, Middleton P, Ezzo J et al. (2001) Quality of Cochrane reviews: assessment of sample from 1998. *British Medical Journal*, **323**:829–32.

Parahoo K, McDonough S, McCaughan E et al. (2013) Psychosocial interventions for men with prostate cancer. *Cochrane Database of Systematic Reviews*, Issue 12:CD008529.

Pearson A (2004) A response to 'The effectiveness of public health nursing: the problems and solutions in carrying out a review of systematic reviews'. *Journal of Advanced Nursing*, **47**, 1:109–10.

Petticrew M, Bell R and Hunter D (2002a) Influence of psychological coping on survival and recurrence in people with cancer: a systematic review. *British Medical Journal*, **325**:1066.

Petticrew M, Wilson P, Wright K and Song F (2002b) Quality of Cochrane reviews is better than that of non-Cochrane reviews. *British Medical Journal*, **324**, 7336:545.

Pope C, Mays N and Popay J (2007) *Synthesizing Qualitative and Quantitative Health Evidence: A Guide to Methods* (Maidenhead: Open University Press).

Rice V H and Stead L F (2008) Nursing interventions for smoking cessation. *Cochrane Database of Systematic Reviews*, Issue 1:CD001188.

Roy C (1976) *Introduction to Nursing: An Adaptation Model* (Engelwood Cliffs, NJ: Prentice Hall).

Rutledge D N, Martinez A, Traska T K and Rose D J (2013) Fall experiences of persons with fibromyalgia over 6 months. *Journal of Advanced Nursing*, **69**, 2:435–48.

Sandelowski M, Docherty S and Emden C (1997) Qualitative metasynthesis: issues and techniques. *Research in Nursing and Health*, **20**:365–71.

Sandelowski M and Barroso J (2006) *Handbook for Synthesizing Qualitative Research* (New York: Springer).

Schick Makaroff K L (2012) Experiences of kidney failure: a qualitative meta-synthesis. *Nephrology Nursing Journal*, **39**, 1:21–9, 80.

Sheldon T A (2005) Making evidence synthesis more useful for management and policymaking. *Journal of Health Services Research and Policy*, **10**, Suppl. 1:1–5.

Smith J P (1996) Editorial: The value of nursing journals. *Journal of Advanced Nursing*, **24**:1–2.

Subirana M, Sola I, Garcia J M et al. (2002) Importance of the database in the literature research: the first step in a systematic review. [Spanish]. *Enfermeria Clinica*, **12**, 6:296–300.

Thorne S, Jensen L, Kearney M H, Noblit G and Sandelowski M (2004) Qualitative meta-synthesis: reflections on methodological orientation and ideological agenda. *Qualitative Health Research*, **14**, 10:1342–65.

Treloar C, Champness S, Simpson P L and Higginbotham N (2000) Critical appraisal checklist for qualitative research studies. *Indian Journal of Pediatrics*, **67**, 5:347–51.

Walls P, Parahoo K and Fleming P (2010) The role and place of knowledge and literature in grounded theory. *Nurse Researcher*, **17**, 4:8–17.

8 Research and Theory

> He who loves practice without a theory is like the sailor who boards a ship without a rudder and compass and never knows where he may cast.
>
> Leonardo da Vinci

Introduction

In science, research is one of the main processes by which data are collected to support, reject or modify theories, or to develop new ones. Researchers often use theories implicitly or explicitly to underpin their studies. Others formulate their own hypotheses and theories from observations.

The development of any profession or discipline depends on the accumulation of a body of knowledge. Theories play an important part in this process by making the link between knowledge and practice. In this chapter, we will explore the meaning of theory and examine its relationship to knowledge, research and practice.

What is a theory?

The term 'theory' is often defined in relation to 'practice', as when, for example, a teacher describes in the classroom the process of giving an injection, as opposed to students actually giving injections to patients. Theory, in this sense, means dealing with a topic (in this case the administration of an injection) in an abstract way. Everyday conversations are full of theories. For example, people have their own theories of why working-class children are poor achievers at school or why there is an increase in crime. These lay theories (from non-experts) differ from scientific theories because the latter must go through a process of falsification or verification before they are accepted, at least for a while, before new data come to light to modify or replace them with new theories. The theory that the earth was flat was replaced when new observations made scientists think again. Many scientific theories began life as speculations (see Chapter 2). In the absence of empirical evidence (as observed by the human senses), the best that people could offer was speculation. Even today, many of the theories about 'space' and 'black holes' are speculations, even though great strides have been made in the science of astronomy.

Theories are merely interpretations of phenomena. They are not the definitive explanation as they may in time be rejected or modified. There may also be competing theories to explain the same phenomenon. For example, the theory about the origin of man in the Bible's book of Genesis is different from Darwin's theory of human evolution.

Morse (1992) sums up the nature of theories thus:

> Theories are not fact. They are not the truth. They are tools. They are merely abstractions, conjectures, and organisations of reality, and as such, are malleable, changeable, and modifiable. There are historical examples of theory adopted as doctrine that with the benefit of hindsight look ridiculous and even silly to our sophisticated eyes. As a theory is changeable, anyone has the privilege of making modifications, for on the day that theory is believed and accepted as fact, science will cease to advance.

Defining a theory

There are a number of definitions of 'theory'. At its most basic, theory explains the occurrence of phenomena. To do this, it has to explain the relationship between variables or concepts. To borrow an example from the field of physics, 'an expansion in a bar of metal occurs when it is heated'. The phenomenon of expansion is therefore explained by the relationship between 'metal' (one variable) and 'heat' (another variable). After a number of observations, it can be deduced (concluded) that when heat is applied to a bar of metal, it will cause the latter to expand.

In offering an explanation of why a phenomenon occurs, a theory must also predict that each time the variables happen to be in the same relationship, the same results will be obtained. In other words, the theory of metal expansion predicts that each time heat is applied to metal, the latter will expand. These explanatory and predictive functions of a theory are expressed in Kerlinger and Lee's (2000) definition:

> A theory is a set of interrelated constructs (concepts), definitions and propositions that present a systematic view of phenomena by specifying relations among variables, with the purpose of explaining and predicting the phenomena.

From these two definitions, it is clear that a theory is made up of a number of concepts that form not one but a set of interrelated propositions or hypotheses. Thus, from the above example, the theory of metal expansion comprises a number of propositions, mainly that:

- metals are made up of atoms;
- the structure of atoms is changed by heat;
- heat causes atoms to expand.

In each of these propositions or hypotheses, there are a number of concepts (metals, atoms, heat and expansion). A concept is a label, expressed as a word or phrase, that summarises the essence of a phenomenon (Fawcett, 2012). The relationship between concepts, propositions and theory can be explained in a simplified way by stating that a theory is made up a set of propositions, and each proposition is made up of concepts. Without concepts, there are no theories; this is why concepts are referred to as the 'building blocks' of theories (Waltz et al., 2010). Therefore, the importance of operationalising concepts (see Chapter 9) for the development or testing of theories cannot be overemphasised.

Fawcett (1999) finds that definitions which emphasise that a theory must state relationships between variables are too restrictive, as they exclude descriptive theories. She defines theory as 'a set of relatively concrete and specific concepts and the propositions that describe or link those concepts'.

Types of theory

Moody (1990) identifies three types of theory: descriptive, explanatory and predictive. She refers to 'descriptive theories' as the most basic type of theory. According to her:

> They describe or classify specific dimensions or characteristics of individuals, groups, situations, or events by summarizing the commonalities found in discrete observations. They state 'what is'. Descriptive theories are needed when nothing or very little is known about the phenomenon in question.

While description and classification are important parts of the scientific process (as described in Chapter 2), they would not, according to positivists, constitute theories in themselves, because they do not seek to explain the causes of phenomena. On the other hand, qualitative researchers do not see theories in the social sciences as necessarily having explanatory and predictive functions. They believe in the uniqueness of individuals and situations, and while they seek to find commonalities between different and similar situations, some are concerned not with explaining why things happen but with what actually happens, from the respondents' perspectives.

Explanatory theory is described by Moody (1990) as one which specifies:

> relations between dimensions or characteristics of individuals, groups, situations, or events. These theories explain how a phenomenon is related to another. They can be developed only after the phenomenon has been explored and described, that is, only after descriptive theories have been developed or validated.

It is clear that explanatory theories are seen as a 'step up' from descriptive theories in the scientific process of theory development. Few researchers would be content to know only what happens; most would probably want to know why these things happen, without necessarily seeking to find general laws to explain human behaviour.

Predictive theories, according to Moody (1990):

move beyond explanation to the prediction of precise relationships between dimensions or characteristics of a phenomenon or differences between groups. This type of theory addresses cause and effect, and 'why' changes occur in a phenomenon. Predictive theories may be developed after explanatory theories have been formulated.

This type of theory is normally developed in the natural sciences (where 'cause and effect', as for example between chemicals, is more easily established) and aspired to by positivists, in the social sciences. It is likely, however, that most research in the social sciences falls within the first two categories: descriptive and explanatory. Both nursing practice and nursing research use theories from the natural sciences (for example, biology, chemistry and physiology) and the social sciences (for example, sociology, psychology and philosophy).

Levels of theory

Another way of describing and classifying theories is in terms of levels. Three levels – grand theory, middle-range theory and laws – will be described here.

Grand theory

These are broad and abstract ideas put together to give a vision of a phenomenon. Examples of 'grand theories' include Darwin's theory of evolution, Marx's theory of social structure and Freud's theory of human motivation. These theories are based on the synthesis of the theorist's own ideas and those obtained from other sources. They are examples of 'armchair' theorising, although, as in the case of Darwin and Freud, some experiments were carried out. Philosophers have for centuries formulated grand theories describing and explaining such phenomena as morality or human nature.

Grand theories tend to be all-encompassing of the phenomenon they describe. The Marxist theory of social structure comprises ideas, among others, about the relationship between those who produce (workers) and those who own the means of production (capitalists), the evolution and existence of social classes historically and cross-culturally, and ideology and its role in maintaining the status quo. Marx's theory is contained in many books and cannot be adequately described here. As can be seen, this type of theory comprises a multitude of other theories. Because they are broad conceptualisations, they have also been termed 'conceptual frameworks'.

Nursing theories tend to fall in the category of grand theories. Most of them offer broad conceptualisations of nursing. Fawcett (1999) describes nursing as having at least seven major conceptual models, including Johnson's behavioural system model, King's interacting systems framework, Levine's conservation model, Neuman's systems model, Orem's self-care framework, Rogers' science of unitary beings and Roy's adaptation model. Walker and Avant (1988) believe that the grand theories of nursing 'have made an important contribution in conceptually sorting out nursing from the practice of medicine by demonstrating the presence of distinct nursing perspectives'.

Middle-range theories

Grand theories themselves cannot be empirically tested as they contain too many theories and propositions. Other researchers can take some of these propositions and develop smaller, more manageable theories with fewer concepts, and can be more specific about the relationship between them. These middle-range theories (Merton, 1967) fit the definition of scientific theories, as discussed in Kerlinger's definition given earlier. Layder (1993) explains that 'middle range theories describe the relations between empirically measurable variables ... which can therefore be "tested" against empirically observed evidence'.

Examples of middle-range theories that are frequently used in nursing research include 'experiencing transitions' (Meleis et al., 2000), the 'theory of planned behaviour' (Ajzen, 2001) and 'becoming a mother' (Mercer, 2004).

Laws

Laws in science (or scientific laws) are statements of cause and effect, established by research evidence, that can predict with consistent accuracy the relation between phenomena. One of the most popularly known scientific law is Einstein's theory of relativity ($E = mc^2$), which stipulates the relationship between energy, mass and the speed of light. This theory played a part in producing nuclear energy, including the atom bomb. There are, however, other less famous examples of scientific laws such as Boyle's law (about the relationship between the pressure and volume of a gas) or electromagnetic laws.

As explained earlier, the purpose of theory in the view of positivists is not only to explain, but also to predict and control phenomena. Since nursing deals with human beings in a social and cultural context, it is unlikely that laws, in the way described above, can be developed. Instead, middle-range theories, clearly defined and tested, comprehensive and of value to practitioners, remain the goal to be aspired to.

Practice, research and theory

You may think at this point that all this is too 'theoretical' (i.e. abstract) or that theories are of interest and use only to academics. You may also wonder how theories in fact contribute to the accumulation of knowledge. Consider the following example. Suppose nurses in one hospital observe that patients rarely follow their advice on healthy eating. They may speculate or find out by reading the research literature that the following factors are associated with this type of behaviour: lack of motivation, lack of incentive and poor nutritional knowledge. Nurses in other hospitals, clinics or nursing homes may also have similar problems. They may find that this type of non-compliant behaviour is associated not only with lack of motivation, but also with the patients' age, social class or personality. In addition, non-compliance with dietary advice is not restricted to one country or culture:

nurses in African or Asian hospitals may face similar problems. For them, a lack of nutritional knowledge, the influence of the family and local food customs may stand in the way of implementing a healthy diet.

Thus, casual observations, speculations and research findings together point to a multitude of factors that may be associated with non-compliance with dietary advice. These factors together constitute what can be called an accumulation of facts. A researcher may try to make sense of all these data by describing the non-compliant behaviour and by classifying these factors into, for example, individual factors (age, gender), psychological factors (motivation, incentive, personality), social factors (family influence, social class background, local customs) and economic factors (earnings, cost of food). Additionally, the researcher may compare this type of non-compliant behaviour with others, such as failure to act on advice on smoking, breast self-examination or the wearing of seat belts. The outcome of this process may be a descriptive theory describing and classifying non-compliant behaviours and the factors associated with them.

Researchers can also contribute by investigating more closely the relationship between some of these factors and non-compliant behaviour. Thus, not only has a large amount of knowledge been accumulated on non-compliant behaviours, but attempts have also been made to make sense of it. The researcher processes the mass of information available from various groups of people in different situations who experience the same phenomena. However, she may not be content with explaining specific situations but is rather more ambitious and may seek to explain non-compliant behaviours in general. By moving from the specific to the general, the researcher becomes the theorist.

Having identified the problem in the first place, nurses all over the world can thereafter benefit from such a theory to guide their practice. Many nursing practices, such as choosing an injection site, rehydrating a patient, giving information to patients prior to surgery and helping people to quit smoking, are based on physiological, sociological or psychological theories.

Theories are not always invented in ivory towers. It is true that they can be formulated through the process of speculation, but most theories are based on observations by people in various situations and settings. The relationship between practice and theory is symbiotic, in that each one feeds on the other to their mutual advantage. The practice setting presents questions and problems, while observations and theories help to make sense of these. Practitioners can thereafter apply them to their practice and, in so doing, help to provide information that can be used to support, reject or modify them; and so the process continues. Moody (1990) explains the relationship between theory and practice:

> Theorizing is not reserved for academicians – good practitioners are often some of the best theorists in that their hunches provide the basis for developing propositions that can be empirically tested.

Some theorists may try to draw general principles from observations of non-compliant behaviours in order to predict and prevent such behaviours in the future.

Others may see theories only as showing a range of possible factors associated with this type of behaviour, thereby increasing their understanding of this particular problem. Theories, in this case, are expected to guide nurses' actions rather than to prescribe them. For more discussion of the importance of theory to practice, see Colley (2003).

Theory and research

Research is the process by which evidence is provided in order to support, reject or modify theories and develop new ones. Thus, research has theory-testing and theory-generating potential. Science needs research (the process) to achieve its outcome (theories). As explained in Chapter 2, there are two main routes by which research can make this contribution: deduction and induction. Theory-testing research adopts the deductive approach, while theory-generating research uses the inductive one.

Theory-testing research

Theory-testing research is mainly in the positivist tradition and is characteristic of middle-range theories. Layder (1993) explains how theory is tested in research through the deductive process:

> a testable hypothesis or proposition is logically deduced from an existing set of assumptions. The empirical data that is then collected either confirms or disconfirms the original hypothesis or propositions.

Only hypotheses or propositions drawn from a theory, and not the theory itself, can be empirically tested through research. For example, Skinner's theory (Skinner, 1938) of positive reinforcement (which occurs when a pleasant consequence follows a particular response, strengthening that response and therefore making it more likely to happen) is stated in an abstract form and has to be translated into real-life situations for it to be tested. An example of a proposition or hypothesis that can be derived from nursing practice based on Skinner's theory (Skinner, 1938) is: 'there are fewer drop-outs among patients who are praised about their weight loss in the early sessions of a weight loss programme than among those who are not'. By collecting and analysing data to support or reject this hypothesis, a researcher is at the same time putting Skinner's theory to the test. In this case, 'praising weight loss' is the positive reinforcement and 'fewer drop-outs' is the response.

One proposition or hypothesis is hardly enough to test a theory. Many more from different situations would have to be drawn and tested. The theory of planned behaviour, as mentioned above, is an example of a theory from which many hypotheses have been developed and tested, relating to such phenomena as 'nurses' intention to use a computerized platform in the resuscitation unit' (Malo et al., 2012), 'nurses' intention to integrate research evidence into clinical decision-making' (Côté et al., 2012) and 'monitoring blood pressure' (Nelson et al., 2013).

Theory-generating research

Much credit for pioneering the theory-generating role of research in the social sciences is given to Glaser and Strauss (1967). They pointed out that theory generation had been hampered by an overemphasis on testing existing theories, which were often limited in explaining reality as they were based not on observation but on speculation.

Glaser and Strauss (1967) saw the generation of theories from observation as a preliminary stage before they could be tested by quantitative methods later, thus acknowledging the dual functions of research as theory generating and theory testing. They, however, put more emphasis on the role of research in generating theories since, according to them, the inductive process is capable of producing more relevant theories. Glaser and Strauss also agreed with positivists that the role of research 'is to enable explanation of behaviour, prediction and control'. This view is not shared by all qualitative researchers, many of whom see the aim of research as describing how phenomena are perceived, rather than explaining, predicting and controlling phenomena. Layder (1993) believes that there is a place, in qualitative research, for theory generation and for approaches that 'seek to develop theory' and 'employ systematic methods of study'. According to him, 'there is no reason for the two to be seen as competing approaches'.

Since it is believed that theories can be generated by the collection of data, many researchers feel the pressure to invent or discover a theory each time they carry out a qualitative study. Theories do not grow on trees. They are the result of much intellectual and physical labour and patience. What most small research projects can hope to achieve is to describe and clarify concepts. This in itself contributes to knowledge and practice and is a worthwhile enterprise that can thereafter be built upon.

Finally, as explained in Chapter 2, few theories are formulated without some prior observations, conscious or unconscious, systematic or informal, made by the theorists or derived from the observations of others. Similarly, theories derived from qualitative data can be influenced by the researcher's knowledge (of existing theories among others) and experience, despite the conscious effort not to allow these to influence the research process. As Morse (1992) aptly puts it:

> Although most researchers agree that a conceptual framework should not be used in qualitative research and that prior knowledge of the topic should be 'bracketed', we would be fooling ourselves if we thought that qualitative enquiry was divorced from established knowledge.

Sandelowski (2010) also pointed out we may not be aware that we are using theories when we describe a phenomenon (for example, talking about miscarriage as 'loss').

Conceptual frameworks in quantitative research

Not all quantitative research is theory testing. The purpose is often to find answers to particular localised problems. For example, a survey of newly qualified midwives' knowledge of breastfeeding can be carried out to identify gaps in their knowledge, with a view to improving midwifery education in their school. Or patients can be interviewed to discover their views about the care they receive in a particular hospital. In both cases, researchers may only be interested in finding answers to their specific research questions. However, the link with previous knowledge (which includes theories, research findings, expert opinions and descriptive accounts of practice) is important because researchers can learn from it and, in return, contribute to it. Without reference to existing knowledge, the study and its findings will exist in isolation from other similar work or studies. To increase and enhance our understanding of phenomena, we must build upon our present knowledge. One cannot, however, 'build upon' if one does not know what already exists. Volumes have been written on phenomena of interest to nurses, such as compliance, patient satisfaction, quality of life, social support, patient teaching, stress, bereavement, physical development and so on. Some of these have more than one theory dedicated to them. By making use of the relevant ones in their studies, researchers can help to test them in practice.

While reading research articles, you may have come across a sentence stating that 'a conceptual framework is used to underpin this study'. The *Oxford Dictionary* defines 'framework' as 'frame, structure, upon or into which casing or contents be put in', and 'underpin' as 'support from below with masonry … strengthen'. This reference to building and construction can equally apply to research. One can say that the function of a conceptual framework is to provide a structure that can strengthen the study. The nursing process is an example of a conceptual framework; it has four components (concepts): assessment, planning, implementation and evaluation. These components represent the structure to which nurses attach the contents (such as the information gathered in the process of assessing a patient). Thus, the nursing process can be used as a conceptual framework in a study of nursing care.

A conceptual framework for a research study can be derived from conceptual definitions, models or theories. For example, in a study of 'student nurses' views of health', the researcher can use the World Health Organization (1946) definition of health as physical, mental and social well-being to underpin her study. These three components provide a guide to the researcher for the areas of health on which to base her questions. She could have chosen Smith's (1981) 'progressive model of health which has four levels: clinical, role performance, adaptive and eudomonistic', on which Kenney based her study of 'the consumer's view of health' (Kenney, 1992). Our researcher could then base her questionnaire or interviews on each of these components. Alternatively, she could combine both definitions and provide her own conceptual framework.

The nursing research literature reveals a number of ways in which researchers make the link between previous knowledge and their own studies. For example, Demarré et al. (2012) studied the 'knowledge and attitude of nurses and nursing assistants in Belgian nursing homes regarding pressure ulcers'. They used a psychological theory to justify their focus on beliefs and attitudes. As they explain:

Cognitive theories support the importance of knowledge and attitudes in relation to behaviour. Azjen (2005) stated that behaviour is affected by intentions, derived from attitudes, subjective norms and perceived behavioural control and beliefs. These beliefs are, in turn, affected by background factors such as education, knowledge and experience (Azjen, 2005). Education, knowledge and individual skills are suggested to lead to favourable intentions by affecting both behavioural beliefs and control beliefs (Azjen and Gilbert Cote, 2008).

Demarré et al. (2012) also used a questionnaire consisting of 26 items relating to the aetiology, classification, nutrition, risk assessment and preventive measures to reduce the amount/duration of pressure and shear. Each of these components of the questionnaire is based on theories or explanatory models. For example, pressure ulcers develop (aetiology) when capillaries supplying the skin and subcutaneous tissues are compressed enough to impede perfusion, leading ultimately to tissue necrosis (Lyder and Avello, 2008). Therefore researchers use theories (implicitly or explicitly) in a number of ways in their studies.

A study that has no identified conceptual framework but which draws on the existing literature, especially research findings, is that of Woodward (1995) on 'psychosocial factors influencing teenage sexual activity, use of contraception and unplanned pregnancy'. According to the author, findings from the literature search into factors that influence teenage sexual behaviour and the use of contraceptives formed the basis of her study. The link with previous knowledge is made clear. For example, in her literature review, Woodward discusses previous work by Bury (1986), who stated:

contraception may be more effectively and consistently used in established teenage relationships. This may be due to the increased communication about sex and contraception that exists in stable relationships as well as the anticipation of when sexual intercourse will occur.

Implicit in this statement is the hypothesis that 'increased communication can lead to more effective and consistent use of contraception'.

Although she does not mention a conceptual framework, Woodward (1995) bases her questions on existing research findings. She is in fact testing some of the ideas or proposals put forward by others. The findings of her study on 61 teenagers were used to support, reject or make suggestions on what was previously known about the subject. She has thus placed her study in the context of a wider discussion on psychosocial factors influencing teenage sexual activity. Woodward's conclusion makes this implicit:

The findings of this study demonstrate that there is no simple model of teenage sexual or contraceptive behaviour which would assist in developing strategies to stem the continuing rise of unplanned pregnancy in the teenage years. Further studies to investigate the effects of family discord, unemployment and perception of future life prospects on use of contraception and unplanned pregnancy in their teenage years emerged as important areas for future research.

As the questionnaire is based on the existing literature, Woodward's findings contribute to the general debate on the phenomenon she investigates.

An example of a study based on a conceptual framework is that of Mock et al. (2007) on 'mitigating fatigue in cancer patients'. The Levine conservation model (Levine, 1973) was adopted 'because it includes principles that help explain cancer-related fatigue and support exercise as a potential intervention for the fatigue'. This model informed the whole design and research process, as explained by Mock et al. (2007):

> Once the Levine Conservation Model was chosen to guide this study, the study varia-
> bles were carefully selected to be congruent with the model, as were the tools used for
> data collection and the intervention being tested. This approach ensured that appro-
> priate outcome variables were used in the evaluation, which includes measurement of
> the four components of this particular model. Also, it became clear that all four compo-
> nents should be addressed in implementing the intervention, as well as in interpreting
> the study data.

Conceptual frameworks in qualitative research

There are at least three ways in which conceptual frameworks have a role in quali-
tative research. These are to develop conceptual frameworks or theories, to use conceptual frameworks to justify the design or approach of the study, or to use frameworks or theories to analyse and interpret data.

As qualitative researchers adopt an inductive approach, their main aim is to develop descriptions, conceptual frameworks and theories out of data. Many of the descriptions are in the form of themes that researchers use to give us insight into phenomena. For example, in a study of 'Sharing control of appointment length with patients in general practice' (Sampson et al., 2013), the authors reported that key themes that emerged for patients included 'the impact of the shift in power and the impact of introducing the issue of time', and for doctors, 'important themes that emerged were impacts on the provider, on the doctor–patient relationship, and on the consultation'. These findings and their implications for practice were discussed in the context of existing literature.

Others would go further and use their findings to develop a conceptual frame-
work. For example, Carter et al. (2004), in a study of the priorities of people living with a terminal illness, carried out qualitative interviews with 10 participants. From the data, they identified 30 categories that were put into five interrelated themes, as shown in Figure 8.1. Other researchers are able thereafter to use these as a conceptual framework for their studies. Practitioners, too, may find this framework useful for their practice. For another study in which themes were integrated into a concep-
tual framework, see Cross et al. (2013).

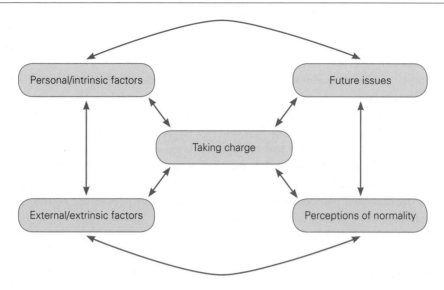

Figure 8.1   Living with dying

Source: Carter et al. (2004). Reproduced with kind permission from John Wiley and Sons Ltd.

The ultimate aim of qualitative research is to develop theories. As Reeves et al. (2008) explain:

> Theories provide complex and comprehensive conceptual understandings of things that cannot be pinned down: how societies work, how organisations operate, why people interact in certain ways. Theories give researchers different 'lenses' through which to look at complicated problems and social issues, focusing their attention on different aspects of the data and providing a framework within which to conduct their analysis.

Grounded theory is one qualitative approach whose expressed aim is to develop substantive theories (see Chapter 13). An example of such a theory comes from a study of 'how hospitalized patients with gastro-intestinal problems going through diagnostic workups experience and handle the situation' (Giske and Gjengedal, 2007). The authors developed a substantive theory of 'preparative waiting' to explain this process.

The function of the inductive process in qualitative research is summed up by Morse (1992), who states:

> the inductive process of qualitative methods provides a powerful means for us to develop and to modify theory, to examine the conceptual basis of our discipline as well as our own beliefs, and to (cautiously) move the discipline forward. Because in qualitative research theory is developed from data (rather than from the library) and is verified, it is usually quite solid. Sometimes, it is even surprising as new directions are identified and old concepts challenged.

Qualitative researchers often use conceptual frameworks and theories to underpin the particular approaches they take in their studies. The choice of a Husserlian or a Foucauldian approach means that the theories of Edmund Husserl or Michel Foucault are used to guide the design of the study, including the analysis and interpretation of data.

Finally, it is not uncommon for qualitative researchers to use one or more frameworks to interpret their data. For example in a study of 'patients' interpretations of a counselling intervention for low back pain', Angel et al. (2012) used Ricoeur's (a phenomenologist) method as well as Bury's concept of chronic illness (Bury, 1982) as a theoretical framework to analyse their qualitative interview data. In another study, the theory of planned behaviour was used to explore 'beverage consumption behaviours among adults' (Zoellner et al., 2012).

Evaluating the use of conceptual frameworks in research

You can start this exercise by identifying the links that the researcher makes with previous knowledge. This may not be made explicit, as explained earlier. If previous knowledge is used, you can find out whether or not reference is made to conceptual definitions, theories, models, research findings or other material. In some cases, the researcher may refer to some or all of these in the same study. More important, however, is how researchers use previous knowledge to guide their study. It often happens that one or more theories or research findings are mentioned without any indication of how (if at all) they are integrated into the study. For example, there may be no indication of how the research questions were derived. In some cases, a theory is mentioned to embellish the study and raise its 'academic status' without any intention of integrating it into the study.

When research findings, conceptual definitions or theories are used to underpin a study, the researcher must justify her choice. There is sometimes more than one theory to explain the same phenomenon. For example, researchers have a choice between the health belief model and the theory of reasoned action to explain patient compliance with health advice. Similarly, if there is more than one conceptual definition of 'stress', why does the researcher choose one as opposed to another? The choice must be objective and appropriate.

To justify the claim that a conceptual framework underpins a particular study, the framework should, as explained earlier, guide every stage of the research process from the literature review to the analysis of data. You must therefore find out how the framework is reflected in the research questions or hypotheses and in the data collection and analysis methods.

The study must also 'feed back' to the conceptual framework on which it is based if it is to contribute to knowledge in general. You should look for discussions on how the current findings relate to the conceptual framework or other theories (even when these were not discussed earlier in the literature review). Unfortunately, this is not a frequent practice among researchers.

To contribute fully to existing knowledge, nurse researchers must, on the basis of their findings, make clinical, methodological and theoretical recommendations.

Summary

In this chapter, we have explored the meaning, types, levels and functions of theories. The relationship between knowledge, theory, practice and research has been further examined. We have also looked at some examples of how researchers make use of previous knowledge, especially research findings and theories, to underpin their quantitative studies. Those adopting a qualitative approach often choose not to be influenced by existing knowledge but instead aim to generate their own concepts and theories. Nevertheless, they can still discuss their findings in the context of existing theories and research findings.

Not all research studies have an identified conceptual framework, and not all researchers believe they need one. To contribute to the pool of knowledge, researchers must not only make use of what is already known, but also test it in practice. This deductive process must not, however, occur at the expense of the efforts of others who seek to increase our understanding of phenomena by searching for new and fresh perspectives.

References

Angel S, Jensen L D, Gonge B K, Maribo T, Schiøttz-Christensen B and Buus N (2012) Patients' interpretations of a counselling intervention for low back pain: a narrative analysis. *International Journal of Nursing Studies*, **49**, 7:784–92.

Ajzen I (2001) Perceived behavioural control, self-efficacy, locus of control and the theory of planned behavior. *Journal of Applied Social Psychology*, **321**:665–83.

Azjen I (2005) *Attitudes, Personality and Behaviour*, 2nd edn (Milton-Keynes: Open University Press/McGraw-Hill).

Azjen I and Gilbert Cote N (2008) Attitudes and the prediction of behaviour. In: W Crano and R Prislin (eds) *Attitudes and Attitude Change* (New York: Psychology Press).

Bury M (1982) Chronic illness as biographical disruption. *Sociology of Health and Illness*, **4**, 2:167–82.

Bury J (1986) Teenage and contraception. *British Journal of Family Planning*, **12**:11–14.

Carter H, MacLeod R, Brander P and McPherson K (2004) Living with a terminal illness: patients' priorities. *Journal of Advanced Nursing*, **45**, 6:611–20.

Colley S (2003) Nursing theory: its importance to practice. *Nursing Standard*, **17**, 46:33–7.

Côté F, Gagnon J, Houme P K, Abdeljelil A B and Gagnon M-P (2012) Using the theory of planned behaviour to predict nurses' intention to integrate research evidence into clinical decision-making. *Journal of Advanced Nursing*, **68**, 10:2289–98.

Cross V, Leach C M J and Fawkes C A (2013) Patients' expectations of osteopathic care: a qualitative study. *BMC Complementary and Alternative Medicine*, **13**:122.

Demarré L, Vanderwee K, Defloor T, Verhaeghe S, Schoonhoven L and Beeckman D (2012) Pressure ulcers: knowledge and attitude of nurses and nursing assistants in Belgian nursing homes. *Journal of Clinical Nursing*, **21**:1425–34.

Fawcett J (1999) *The Relationship of Theory and Research*, 3rd edn (Philadelphia: F A Davis).

Fawcett J (2012) Thoughts on concept analysis: multiple approaches, one result. *Nursing Science Quarterly*, **25**: 285.

Giske T and Gjengedal L E (2007) 'Preparative waiting' and coping theory with patients going through gastric diagnosis. *Journal of Advanced Nursing*, **57**, 1:87–94.

Glaser B and Strauss A (1967) *The Discovery of Grounded Theory* (Chicago: Aldine).

Kenney JW (1992) The consumer's view of health. *Journal of Advanced Nursing*, **17**:829–34.

Kerlinger F and Lee H B (2000) *Foundations of Behavioral Research* (New York: Harcourt).

Layder D (1993) *New Strategies in Social Research* (Cambridge: Polity Press).

Levine M E (1973) *Introduction to Clinical Nursing*, 2nd edn (Philadelphia: F A Davis).

Lyder C H and Ayello E A (2008) Pressure ulcers: a patient safety issue. In: Malo C, Neveu X, Archambault P M, Émond M and Gagnon M-P (2012) Exploring nurses' intention to use a computerized platform in the resuscitation unit: development and validation of a questionnaire based on the theory of planned behavior. *Interactive Journal of Medical Research*, **1**, 2:e5.

Malo C, Neveu X, Archambault P M, Émond M and Gagnon M-P (2012) Exploring nurses' intention to use a computerized platform in the resuscitation unit: development and validation of a questionnaire based on the theory of planned behavior. *Interactive Journal of Medical Research*, **1**, 2:e5.

Meleis A I, Sawyer L M, Im E, Hilfinger Messias D K and Schumacher K (2000) Experiencing transitions: an emerging middle range theory. *Advances in Nursing Science*, **23**, 1:12–28.

Mercer R T (2004) Becoming a mother versus maternal role attainment. *Journal of Nursing Scholarship*, **36**, 3: 226–32.

Merton R (1967) *On Theoretical Sociology* (New York: Free Press).

Mock V, St Ours C, Hall S et al. (2007) Using a conceptual model in nursing research – mitigating fatigue in cancer patients. *Journal of Advanced Nursing*, **58**, 5:503–12.

Moody L E (1990) *Advancing Nursing Science through Research* (Newbury Park, CA: Sage).

Morse J (1992) Editorial: The power of induction. *Qualitative Health Research*, **2**, 1:3–6.

Nelson J M, Cook P F and Ingram J C (2013) Utility of the theory of planned behavior to predict nursing staff blood pressure monitoring behaviours. *Journal of Clinical Nursing*, doi: 10.1111/jocn.12183.

Reeves S, Albert M, Kuper A and Hodges B D (2008) Why use theories in qualitative research? *British Medical Journal*, **337**: 631–4.

Sampson R, O'Rourke J, Hendry R et al. (2013) Sharing control of appointment length with patients in general practice: a qualitative study. *British Journal of General Practice*, 63:e185–91.

Sandelowski M (2010) What's in a name? *Research in Nursing and Health*, **33**:77–84.

Skinner B F (1938) *The Behavior of Organisms* (New York: Appleton-Century-Crofts).

Smith JA (1981) The idea of health: a philosophical enquiry. *Advances in Nursing Science*, **3**, 3:43–50.

Walker L O and Avant K C (1988) *Strategies for Theory Construction in Nursing* (East Norwalk, CT: Appleton & Lange).

Waltz C, Strickland O L and Lenz E (2010) *Measurement in Nursing and Health Research*, 4th edn (New York: Springer).

Woodward V M (1995) Psychosocial factors influencing teenage sexual activity, use of contraception and unplanned pregnancy. *Midwifery*, **11**:210–16.

World Health Organization (1946) *Constitution* (Geneva: WHO).

Zoellner J, Krzeski E, Harden S, Cook E, Allen K and Estabrooks P A (2012) Qualitative application of the theory of planned behavior to understand beverage consumption behaviors among adults. *Journal of the Academy of Nutrition and Dietetics*, **11**, 11:1774–84.

Research Questions and Operational Definitions

Judge a man by his questions rather than by his answers.

Voltaire

Introduction

The formulation of research questions is fundamental to the research process. It helps the researcher to clarify in her mind those questions which need to be answered. These can be formulated in a variety of formats, which often reflect the type of research carried out and the personal preference of individual researchers. Additionally, the terms and concepts used by the researcher must be defined in ways that can be understood by others who read the article or report. This chapter will help you to understand this important stage of the research process.

Formulating research questions

Research starts with a problem, which is often broad and multifaceted. For example, if there is an increase in the incidence of pressure ulcers on a particular ward, the nurse researcher faced with this problem may ask several questions, such as:

- Is there a relationship between nursing care and the incidence of pressure ulcers?
- Is there a policy on the prevention and treatment of pressure ulcers?
- Is this policy effective?
- How does the current prevention practice compare with a new form of practice on another ward with a similar group of patients?
- Do nurses have the necessary knowledge and skills to prevent and treat pressure ulcers?

It is not possible, especially in a small project, to address all these issues. The researcher may have to settle for one or two of these questions and focus on them. The literature review can play an important part in narrowing the problem down to manageable proportions. By reviewing what has been written on the topic and how others have approached similar studies, the researcher is better informed about what needs to be done. The final choice of which aspect of the problem to focus upon depends on a number of factors, including the researcher's skills and interest, the lack of research on the topic and the available resources.

The next step in quantitative research is for the researcher to state clearly what the purpose of the study is.

Aim or purpose of the study

The aim or purpose of the study is formulated so that researchers and readers are clear about what is being researched. Although the aim of most research is ultimately to improve practice, the aim of a study, in research terms, relates to the particular question(s) for which data can be collected. For example, the aim of the above study could be 'to find out if there is a relationship between nursing care and the incidence of pressure ulcers' on a particular ward. The long-term goal of a study may be to improve a particular practice, but the latter depends on more than research findings. Only in action research (see Chapter 10) do researchers aim to answer research questions and make changes (such as improving practice) at the same time. More often than not, the purpose of a study is stated earlier on in the article, but when this does not happen readers sometimes have to look for it. The 'aim' is itself broad and needs a further explanation of how it is to be achieved. It should be further subdivided into specific questions, objectives or hypotheses.

Research questions

Research is about finding answers, and in order to do this questions must be posed. The purpose or aim of a study is usually formulated as a statement that begs many questions. For example, in the study 'Urinary incontinence and sexual function in pre-menopausal women' (Serenko et al., 2010), the purpose of the study was to 'explore the relationship between urinary incontinence and female sexual function in pre-menopausal women' and the research questions were:

1 What is the severity of urinary incontinence in premenopausal women with urinary incontinence?
2 What is the level of sexual function in premenopausal women with urinary incontinence?
3 What is the relationship between urinary incontinence and sexual function in premenopausal women with urinary incontinence?

As you can see, the aim only broadly hints at the topic to be studied. The research questions elaborate on the exact questions that the researchers want to study. By asking specific questions, the researcher has given more details about what the purpose of the study is. However, the above questions are not exactly or necessarily the questions that the participants in the study will be asked. These questions only provide a basis or framework from which further and final questions can be formulated in order to construct the tool of data collection, for example a questionnaire. The broad research questions that emerge out of the purpose of the study must not be confused with detailed questions that the respondents are asked to answer.

Formulating the purpose or aim of a study in the form of questions is useful in helping to clarify exactly what the study is about, and sets the parameters of the research project. It focuses the researcher's and the reader's mind on the task in hand.

Research objectives

Another way of detailing the purpose or aim of a study is in the form of objectives. Like research questions, objectives are set by the researcher in order to explain in some detail what the study is expected to achieve. For example, a study of 'Equality of employment opportunities for nurses at the point of qualification' (Harris et al., 2013) aimed to explore the relationship between ethnicity and employment at the point of qualification within one large city. The objectives were:

1 To describe the characteristics (for example, age, gender and ethnicity) of the newly qualified nursing workforce completing diploma and degree qualifications at the September 2009 (autumn intake September 2006) and February 2010 (spring intake February 2007) time points from eight universities within the city.
2 To describe the first post gained after qualification and all posts undertaken within 3 months of qualification in terms of grade, setting, nature and duration of contracts and geographical distribution.
3 To explore the employment patterns of the newly qualified nurses from the eight universities, including differences between ethnic group, age, gender, branch of nursing (that is, adult, child, mental health and learning disabilities), level of achievement in both academic and nursing practice skills and time of intake (that is, autumn and spring intake).

Hypotheses

Instead of asking questions or setting objectives, some researchers may go further in proposing what the answer to their main research question might be, and then set out to look for evidence to support or reject their 'hunch'. In everyday life, people make educated guesses for why certain things or events happen. For example, the increase in the number of crimes committed by children is often blamed on violent behaviour in television programmes. Nurses hypothesise about the phenomena they deal with. For example, they may attribute the high incidence of pressure ulcers in obese patients to their weight, or blame constipation in older people on their lack of exercise. Some of these guesses may be influenced by their beliefs and experiences, and what they have read or heard.

Researchers, too, make educated guesses about the phenomena they investigate. However, unlike other people, they have to collect data in order to support or reject their guesses. By proposing that there may be a relationship between pressure ulcers and obesity, the researcher is putting forward a hypothesis. By its very nature, a hypothesis is a tentative statement since the researcher is merely making an assumption before data are collected. A hypothesis can be defined as a tentative statement, in one sentence, about the relationship, if any, between two or more variables. A variable is anything that varies or can be varied. An example of a hypothesis is 'lack of exercise causes constipation in older people'. To be complete and comprehensive, a hypothesis must include three components: the variables, the population and the relationship between variables.

Variables

In the above example, 'exercise' and 'constipation' are the two variables for which a relationship is stated. In this case, it is a causal relationship because one (exercise) is assumed to cause the other (constipation). The variable 'exercise' can be varied (changed): older people can take more or less exercise. The other variable, 'constipation', may vary according to the presence or absence of exercise. The variable causing the change is referred to as the independent variable, and the one which is changed is known as the dependent variable. One way to remember which is which is to view the dependent variable as the one that depends on the other to be changed. These and other types of variables are further discussed in Chapter 11.

The population

For a hypothesis to be complete, the population to which the phenomenon is related must be stated. For example, in the above hypothesis, the population is older people. Later on, more information or a definition of older people (that is, the age group, the clinical area in which they are cared for or their gender) will be required to enable readers to identify more specifically the population to whom the hypothesis applies.

Relationship between variables

A hypothesis is a statement that normally specifies the relationship between variables. This relationship can be positive, inverse or of difference. Here are some examples:

- positive – the more food people consume, the more obese they become;
- inverse or negative – the more information given to patients preoperatively, the less anxiety they experience postoperatively;
- difference – patients who exercise during the day sleep longer at night than those who do not.

Hypotheses are not only about cause and effect. Sometimes they point out that there is a relationship between two or more variables without any explanation of the exact nature of this relationship. This type of hypothesis is known as 'associative'. An example of an associative hypothesis is: 'there is a relationship between the amount of daily protein consumed and success in examinations'.

Evidence to support or reject hypotheses can be obtained through the collection of data and by statistical analysis. Hypotheses for research purposes are stipulated in two main formats: the null hypothesis (H0) and the alternative hypothesis (H1). An example of a null hypothesis is that there is no relationship between portion size of meals and obesity. When a null hypothesis is not supported by research evidence, it gives rise to an alternative hypothesis. In this case, if the null hypothesis is rejected, the alternative hypothesis is that 'there is a relationship between food portion and obesity'. The null hypothesis is usually the one used because it is a simpler one than a hypothesis that specifies that there is a relationship.

When a null hypothesis is tested, the results are expressed in terms of whether it is supported or rejected. However, it does not follow that because the null hypothesis is rejected, the alternative hypothesis is accepted. It merely shows that there is not enough evidence to support the null hypothesis. The new, alternative hypothesis has itself to be put to the test in further studies.

Hypotheses can also stipulate the relationships between more than two variables. These complex hypotheses are stated because, in real life, a number of factors or variables work together in order to produce an effect. Although it is common knowledge that high-fibre diets can prevent constipation, other factors such as mobility and fluid intake can also be implicated. By controlling mobility and fluid intake in an experiment focusing solely on fibre, the researcher creates an artificial situation. To make the experiment more like real life, the researcher may decide to study a number of variables at the same time. A hypothesis for this study may read as follows: 'Lack of dietary fibre and low fluid intake cause constipation among older people'. The independent variables are dietary fibre and fluid intake, and the dependent variable is constipation. See Research Example 13 for a study testing a hypothesis.

An example of a hypothesis

Psychological morbidity in catheterized prostate-enlarged men in a Nigerian hospital *Ilesanmi and Adejumo (2009)*

In this study, the hypothesis was: 'There will be no significant relationship between length of time with a catheter in situ and a client's psychological well-being'.

The independent variable is 'length of time with a catheter in situ'. The dependent variable is 'psychological well-being'.

The population is 'clients' (defined in this study as 'patients with obstructing prostatic enlargement who had indwelling urethral catheters and were attending the urology outpatient clinic'. The relation between these two variables is 'no significant relationship' (null hypothesis).

Research example 13

Finally, a hypothesis is either supported or rejected but not 'proven', because there may be many reasons or factors other than the independent variable that account for the results (see Chapter 11). Research findings must always be treated with caution.

The PICO formula is commonly used to formulate questions related to intervention studies and systematic reviews. The letters in the formula stand for:

- P: population/disease (characteristics, condition, etc.);
- I: intervention (for example, exposure or a new treatment);
- C: comparison: (for example, the usual treatment, placebo or other intervention);
- O: outcome: (symptom relief, recovery duration, better diagnosis, etc.).

For example, in the question 'Is psychotherapy more effective in reducing depression in young women in the postpartum period than antidepressant medication?', the population is 'young women in the postpartum period' (the exact age group as well as the postpartum period will need to be stipulated further), the intervention is 'psychotherapy' (psychotherapy will need to be defined), the comparison is 'antidepressant medication', and the outcome (effectiveness) is an acceptable reduction in depression (with what constitutes 'acceptable' needing to be stipulated).

In formulating questions, objectives or hypotheses, a number of terms or concepts are used. The next step in the research process is for these concepts (effectiveness, psychotherapy, reduction in depression, and so on) to be defined so that readers (fellow researchers, practitioners and others) may be aware of the precise meaning of these terms and so that they can assess whether these definitions are adequate for use in the study.

Ambiguities arise in the use of concepts in everyday language. Such familiar terms as 'happiness', 'love', 'coping' or 'human rights' give rise to a multitude of definitions. A common and agreed understanding of these and other terms that we use can greatly enhance communication.

Operational definitions

If someone is asked whether she is happy, the answer is quite often: 'It depends on what you mean by happiness.' We are supposed to have a common understanding of what the term 'happiness' means. Yet when it comes to conveying such meanings to others, this can be quite difficult.

In nursing practice, too, we use a vast number of terms and concepts (for example, 'pressure ulcer', 'fatigue', 'coping' or 'pain'). Professionals have to develop a common understanding of these terms to facilitate communication between themselves and with their clients. The definition of terms and concepts that nurses and other health professionals use is central to their practice. Without a consensus of what these mean, and in particular how they can be observed, nursing practice would be 'chaotic'. For example, a term like 'depression' may mean different things to different people. However, if nurses, as a professional group, are involved in assessing and treating this condition, they need to have a consensus of what it means and how it can be assessed. Thus, whole books are dedicated to exploring, assessing, measuring and treating depression. Nonetheless, our knowledge of some of the concepts used in everyday nursing practice still lacks clarification, let alone definition.

Legg et al. (2011), in their comments on a literature review of interventions for carers in stroke, were concerned about the fundamental lack of an operational definition of what is meant by informal care. As they explain:

> Without a clear specified set of characteristics, it is impossible to know who has been recruited into studies, who to apply the results of studies to or whether the study has been adequately designed to answer the research question it sets out to address. Frequently, the role of carer is self defined or is based on a relatively loose definition (for example, 'A person who lives with the patient and has the closest contact') but this is not the equivalent to the identification of those who actually provide care.

If you think of research as an 'operation' or 'procedure', an operational definition in a research study is the way in which the terms and concepts are defined for the purpose of the study. Although there is a universal understanding of what the term 'nurse' is, the way in which 'nurse' is defined in a particular study depends on the context of the study. Researchers may define 'nurse' (for the purpose of the study) as only those qualified in the last 5 years or those working in hospitals or in particular clinical areas. Without this definition, it is not possible for readers to know whom the researcher is referring to. This information is crucial for deciding whether the study is rigorous enough and to whom the findings are generalisable. The more precise and adequate the description and definition of the nurses in the sample, the easier it is for readers to know the exact population from whom data are collected. Researchers, therefore, set inclusion and exclusion criteria in order to define their samples. For example, in a study by Lin et al. (2013) on 'fatigue and Internet addiction', the participants (nurses) were defined as:

> female registered nurses from a regional teaching hospital with 958 hospital beds located in southern Taiwan. Exclusion criteria for the participants included: (1) non-clinical nurses; (2) duration of the current job of less than 3 months; (3) on maternity leave; (4) on unpaid leave; and (5) on vacation leave at the time of survey.

Samples are relatively easy to define compared with other phenomena such as 'pressure ulcers' or 'drowsiness'. Researchers carrying out a study of the prevalence of pressure ulcers in a number of hospitals must ensure that the definition of the term 'pressure ulcer' is clear to everyone taking part in the study (that is, those carrying out the observations) and those appraising the study. They can use the European Pressure Ulcer Advisory Panel and National Pressure Ulcer Advisory Panel's (2009) four stages/categories of pressure ulcers:

- category/stage I: non-blanchable erythema;
- category/stage II: partial thickness;

- category/stage III: full-thickness skin loss;
- category/stage IV: full-thickness tissue loss.

Each of these categories is further described for health professionals and others to be able to identify, assess and differentiate between them. The descriptions of these categories/stages are useful for researchers and practitioners undertaking observations to establish the prevalence of pressure ulcers in their clinical areas.

Even then, what constitutes 'blanchable and 'non-blanchable' erythema is not as straightforward when one has to identify them. Sterner et al. (2011) carried out a study to establish inter-rater reliability between blanching and non-blanching erythema as assessed by two independent assessors. They reported that 'both visual inspection and the finger-press test were unreliable methods of differentiating between reactive hyperemia and Category I pressure ulcers in the sacral area'. One of their conclusions was that 'further research regarding precision in differentiating between Category I pressure ulcers and blanchable erythema should be carried out'.

Other phenomena that nurses deal with, such as 'coping', 'comfort' or 'fatigue', are even more difficult to define operationally in research studies, mainly because they are not directly observable. Dictionary definitions are often of little use. One needs, as much as possible, to fully understand a phenomenon before it can be measured. For example, if a researcher wants to measure chronic fatigue, she needs to understand the concept in all its different manifestations, what gives rise to it, its main attributes or characteristics, how it differs from similar concepts (such as depression) or whether it is a process, an outcome or both. This type of exploration is known as conceptual analysis, the outcome of which is a conceptual definition. Conceptual analyses are carried out mainly for the purpose of clarifying concepts that practitioners use in their practice. They are useful for researchers who can use them for defining concepts and as conceptual frameworks in their studies.

To fully explore, analyse and describe a concept, a number of sources and methods are used. Those doing concept analysis draw mainly upon the literature, the experience of practitioners, case studies and research. The conceptual definitions that emerge as a result of this type of analysis contribute towards a fuller understanding of concepts. Such definitions can never fully capture the meaning of concepts. Trendall (2000), who carried out a concept analysis of 'chronic fatigue', concluded that while the exercise assisted with the understanding of the concept and future research, the complexity of chronic fatigue was still evident.

Although conceptual definitions shed more light on the use and meaning of concepts, they are not operational definitions as they do not specify what must be done in order to measure or assess them. Wang (2004), after completing a conceptual analysis of functional status, defined it as:

activities performed by an individual to realize needs of daily living in many aspects of life including physical, psychological, social, spiritual, intellectual, and roles. Level of performance is expected to correspond to normal expectation in the individual's nature, structure and conditions.

If a researcher wants to measure functional status using this conceptual definition, she has to operationalise it for use with specific populations and in specific conditions. Fortunately for researchers, tools have been developed to measure these concepts. For example, the functional ability of children and young people with myalgic encephalopathy can be measured by the Moss Scale (Moss, 2005).

To summarise, operational definitions are important in order to convey to readers the precise and specific meaning researchers give to the terms or concepts used in a study.

Evaluating operational definitions

There are a number of criteria that can be used to evaluate the efficacy of operational definitions. The main ones (adapted from a list from Waltz et al., 2010) include clarity, precision, validity, reliability and agreement/consensus.

Clarity

If the operational definition is not clear, it cannot be put into practice. The process of operational definition is precisely to reduce a complex or abstract concept into simple instructions that can be understood in the same way by everyone.

Gobbens et al. (2012) reviewed the literature and consulted experts to develop an operational definition of 'frailty'. They defined it as 'a dynamic state affecting an individual who experiences losses in one or more domains of human functioning (physical, psychological, social), which is caused by the influence of a range of variables and which increases the risk of adverse outcomes'. However, the physical, psychological and social components of human functioning needed to be operationally defined as well. In this study, the components of frailty selected for this study were strength, nutrition, endurance, mobility, physical activity, balance, cognition, sensory functions (hearing, visual acuity), mood (depressive functions, anxiety), coping, social relations and social support. One can see the steps taken to translate a 'conceptual definition' into an 'operational definition', thereby making it more clear to readers how the concept of frailty was measured.

Precision

Operational definitions must be as precise as possible, so that a degree of consistency is achieved when they are put into operation in the study. Below are three operational definitions, with varying degrees of precision, of the family carers of people with stroke:

- A caregiver was defined as the main person (other than a health, social or voluntary care provider) helping with activities of daily living and advocating on behalf of the patient (Kalra et al., 2004).

- To be included in the study, carer participants had to be unpaid (informal) carers looking after stroke survivors in either their own or the carers' homes. Carers were identified by survivors, staff or carers themselves (Greenwood and Mackenzie, 2010).
- The carer was defined as: 'a primary and current caregiver of a person with stroke for at least a 6-month duration since the person's initial discharge from the rehabilitation program; (b) responsible for coordinating and providing the caring actions and/or resources required by the person with stroke; (c) a resident in the same home environment as the care recipient; and (d) most knowledgeable about the domain of inquiry and expressed the norms and values of the culture under study. They had a family income that was at or below the current poverty level, received federal, state, and/or county financial health care assistance, and had no private health care insurance for the care recipient; they had an urban residence that could be verified by zip code' (Pierce, 2001).

All three definitions served the purpose of the particular study. However, by being precise and as detailed as possible, operational definitions offer readers the opportunity to compare whether the population in the study is similar to their own client group(s) and whether the findings can be generalised to (used in) their own settings.

Validity

To be valid, the operational definition must represent what it is supposed to represent. There is a danger in translating a broad conceptual definition into a number of constituent parts that it may not represent the concept being defined. One can ask whether, in fact, when a researcher sets out to measure a particular concept, she actually measures that concept or something else. As Wilson (1989) explains:

> there is a logical gap between the concept with which the researcher begins and the subsequent research. To take an absurd (but, believe it or not, real life) example, researchers interested in what makes happy marriages decided to assess a marriage as happy if the partners called each other 'darling' more than a certain number of times a day. As many married couples know, one can say 'darling!' *con amore*, or through clenched teeth: as a candidate for a reasonable way of verifying, or explicating the concept 'happily married', this is a non-starter.

One of the common ways of operationalising such conditions as schizophrenia or depression is to rely on medical diagnosis. Although it saves the researcher the effort of providing her own definitions, using medical diagnoses as operational definitions is not without problems. If, in a study measuring the 'level of social support available to chronic fatigue syndrome (CFS) sufferers, the latter are defined as persons diagnosed by their general practitioners as having CFS', it is possible that some general practitioners may overdiagnose, underdiagnose or misdiagnose CFS. Some people with CFS may not even have consulted a general practitioner anyway.

Therefore, in some instances, the validity of using medical diagnoses as operational definitions is questionable.

Another aspect of the validity of an operational definition is its appropriateness for the specific population for whom it is formulated. Concepts may have different meanings for different groups due to social, cultural, geographical, gender and age differences. For example, such a concept as 'touch' or 'bereavement' can be manifested and interpreted differently in different cultures or even according to gender.

Reliability

The question to ask about the reliability of an operational definition is whether it will be consistently interpreted (in the same way) by all those who have to use it. Sometimes two or more researchers carry out observations in the same study; they must be able to interpret operational definitions in the same way. In the above example of research into pressure ulcers, Sterner et al.'s (2011) study demonstrated that inter-rater reliability was low when two researchers tried to differentiate between 'blanchable' and 'non-blanchable' erythema. Misinterpretation of definitions could lead to the under- or overreporting of phenomena, thereby giving inaccurate results on which subsequent decisions on nursing practice might depend.

Agreement/consensus

For some terms such as 'students' or 'patients', researchers can offer their own definitions to suit their studies. No consensus or agreement is necessary for the term, provided that the researcher makes it very clear how the population is defined and that the definition is not absurd. On the other hand, there are concepts such as 'anxiety' or 'stress' for which there must be a consensus for their definitions, otherwise the validity of the findings will be seriously in question. To achieve consensus, operational definitions must reflect the concept in all its complexities and must be informed by the current state of knowledge on the concept. To gain consensus, researchers may provide a rationale for their definitions.

In some cases, researchers use operational definitions from previous studies. This allows for comparisons of the findings to be made and may lead to further refinement of the definition. The drawback of this is that sometimes no fresh contribution towards defining concepts is offered.

Operationalising concepts that figure in research questions, objectives or hypotheses is an important but often difficult part of the research process in quantitative research. It is not possible to offer absolutely perfect operational definitions, nor is it possible to offer further definitions of each of the terms that operational definitions generate. The problem with definitions is explained below by Bertrand Russell (1918):

It is rather a curious fact in philosophy that the data which are undeniable to start with are always rather vague and ambiguous. You can, for instance, say: 'There are a number of people in this room at this moment'. This is obviously in some sense undeniable. But when you come to try and define what this room is, and what it is for a person to be in a room, and how you are going to distinguish one person from another, and so forth, you find that what you have said is most fearfully vague and that you really do not know what you meant.

Research questions in qualitative research

Different approaches within qualitative research mean that one cannot generalise about them. Purists, however, would see qualitative research as inductive rather than deductive. With the inductive approach, hypotheses and theories are expected to emerge out of the data. In phenomenological research, the researcher collects data from the respondent's perspective, and formulating questions or hypotheses at the start of the study is therefore not appropriate. However, in order to focus the study, some broad aims or questions are formulated. For example, in a qualitative study exploring 'reflection as a process embedded in experienced nurses' practice' (Asselin et al., 2013), the aim and research question were formulated as follows:

> The aim of this study was to provide an in-depth description of how experienced acute care staff nurses perceive and use reflection in clinical practice. The research question was: How does the experienced nurse reflect on clinical practice situations?

Although aims, research questions or objectives can be set, qualitative researchers tend to use these as broad areas on which to focus.

In some qualitative studies, however, broad questions are not set in advance, although researchers choose a starting point to focus on certain aspects of a phenomenon. During fieldwork (when researchers are out there collecting data), they may be more attracted to some aspects of the phenomenon than others. The ethnographic approach, which uses participant observation as its main data collection method (see Chapter 14), provides the opportunity for starting with a broad topic and thereafter focuses on a particular aspect. In phenomenological studies (Chapter 12), it is also possible for researchers to select broad topic areas that they want to cover, but they may find their attention drawn to certain specific issues. Although the purpose of the study or broad questions are reported at the start of qualitative research articles, one cannot be certain that they were in fact the original aspects on which the researchers set out to focus.

In quantitative research, the measurement of concepts, whether in surveys or experiments, is central to the research process, and therefore these concepts require precise operational definitions. In qualitative research, the respondents' conceptualisation of the phenomenon is often the outcome of the study. In a study of 'Making decisions about delirium' (Agar et al., 2012), the findings showed how delirium was operationally defined by participants. According to purists, the researcher's conceptualisation of the problem is 'bracketed' to prevent it from influencing respondents.

It is possible to find qualitative studies in which concepts are operationally defined. In a study on 'The process and consequences of institutionalizing an elder',

Dellasega and Mastrian (1995) offer these operational definitions of the following concepts: 'specific stressors', 'family members' and 'decision-making/placement'. As they explain:

> In this study, specific stressors were defined as emotionally difficult events and feelings that were described by subjects in connection with the decision-making process, the placement process, or both. Family members were a spouse, a sibling, or a child of an elderly nursing home resident who was intimately involved in the decision-making or placement process and who consented to be interviewed. Decision making/placement was defined as considering alternatives and making choices that led to admission of an elder to a skilled nursing facility.

These definitions are broad and serve to explain the areas on which the researchers focused. They are not operational definitions in the 'quantitative' sense as they do not specify how these concepts are to be precisely measured; they merely delineate the areas of study. They are sometimes called 'inclusion' or 'exclusion' criteria. They specify who/what to include or exclude from the study.

In quantitative research, all questions must be decided in advance. This assumes that researchers know what questions to ask or the attributes of the phenomenon to be observed. However, it is possible that by just talking to or observing respondents, we come across new ways of thinking on certain topics. The view often taken by qualitative researchers is that not only do we not know the answers, but also we do not always know what questions to ask.

Qualitative researchers work with the assumption that operational definitions fail to capture the essence of what is being studied. For example, such a concept as 'intelligence' is reduced to being measured by a set of responses to a questionnaire called an intelligent quotient test. By defining the attributes or symptoms, we can miss the essence of the phenomena we seek to study. The dilemma of operational definitions is aptly expressed by Bertrand Russell (1918):

> Everything is vague to a degree you do not realise till you have tried to make it precise, and everything precise is so remote from everything that we normally think, that you cannot for a moment suppose that is what we really mean when we say what we think.

Critiquing research questions and operational definitions

It is important to identify the purpose of the study, the research questions, objectives or hypotheses. Sometimes these are not reported under their respective headings; more often, readers have to tease out what they are. In one experimental study published in a reputable journal, the hypotheses were stated in the 'findings' sections. Readers cannot fully evaluate the methodology (and the literature review) that comes earlier in the article if they do not know what hypotheses or objectives are set.

Additionally, do not be surprised if the objectives are presented as aims (the distinction between these terms was made earlier in this chapter) or the conceptual definitions as operational definitions, as frequently happens. Terminologies do not always convey exactly what researchers did; they have to provide the relevant information clearly and precisely. It is essential for you to be clear about what questions are posed, how the variables are defined for the purpose of the study, what the researchers did to find answers to the questions and what the findings to these questions are. One useful exercise is to divide a page into three columns, and list the research questions in column 1, the method of data collection in column 2 and the findings in column 3. In this way, you can find out whether the purpose of the study, as expressed through research questions, objectives or hypotheses, has been achieved. It is not unusual to find that not all the research questions set at the beginning of an article are dealt with in the results and discussion sections. New findings unrelated to the original research questions sometimes creep into the results and can surprise you.

To assess the value of operational definitions in quantitative research, you can use the five criteria discussed in this chapter: clarity, precision, validity, reliability and agreement/consensus. Although specific questions and operational definitions are not normally stated in qualitative research, the article or report must give a clear account of the broad area of study, the concepts investigated, the methods used and the findings.

Summary

In quantitative research, the formulation of the purpose of the study, research questions and operational definitions is a crucial part of the research process. These facilitate the readers' understanding of the nature and magnitude of the task undertaken by the research. They inform readers of what the study is about, what is being measured, assessed or explored and how. Research is a private enterprise that is made public for it to contribute to existing knowledge.

Reporting research questions and operational definitions facilitates the communication between researchers and those who subsequently read and use the report.

Most qualitative researchers only formulate broad questions or identify a broad area of study. During the study, questions emerge as the researcher learns more about the area and decides what to focus on. Concepts constructed from the data can thereafter be operationalised.

References

Agar M, Draper B, Phillips P A et al. (2012) Making decisions about delirium: a qualitative comparison of decision making between nurses working in palliative care, aged care, aged care psychiatry, and oncology. *Palliative Medicine*, **26**, 7:887–96.

Asselin M E, Schwartz-Barcott D and Osterman P A (2013) Exploring reflection as a process embedded in experienced nurses' practice: a qualitative study. *Journal of Advanced Nursing*, **69**, 4:905–14.

Dellasega C and Mastrian K (1995) The process and consequences of institutionalizing an elder. *Western Journal of Nursing Research*, **17**, 2:123–40.

European Pressure Ulcer Advisory Panel and National Pressure Ulcer Advisory Panel (2009) *Prevention and Treatment of Pressure Ulcers: Quick Reference Guide* (Washington DC: National Pressure Ulcer Advisory Panel).

Gobbens R J, van Assen M A, Luijkx K G and Schols J M (2012) Testing an integral conceptual model of frailty. *Journal of Advanced Nursing*, **6**, 9: 2047–60.

Greenwood N and Mackenzie A (2010) An exploratory study of anxiety in carers of stroke survivors. *Journal of Clinical Nursing*, **19**, 13–14:2032–8.

Harris R, Ooms A, Grant R et al. (2013) Equality of employment opportunities for nurses at the point of qualification: an exploratory study. *International Journal of Nursing Studies*, **50**, 3:303–13.

Ilesanmi R and Adejumo P (2009) Psychological morbidity in catheterized prostate-enlarged men in a Nigerian hospital. *International Journal of Urological Nursing*, **3**, 3: 104–14.

Kalra L, Evans A, Perez I et al. (2004) Training carers of stroke patients: randomised controlled trial. *British Medical Journal*, **328**:1-5.

Legg L, Quinn T and Langhorne P (2011) Assessing and helping carers of older people. Retrieved from http://www.bmj.com/rapid-response/2011/11/03/assessing-carers-assessing-carers-research (accessed 2 September 2013).

Lin S C, Tsai K W, Chen M W and Koo M (2013) Association between fatigue and Internet addiction in female hospital nurses. *Journal of Advanced Nursing*, **69**, 2:374–383.

Moss J (2005) Development of a functional ability scale for children and young people with myalgic encephalopathy (ME)/chronic fatigue syndrome (CFS). *Journal of Child Care*, **9**, 1:20–30.

Pierce L L (2001) Coherence in the urban family caregiver role with African American stroke survivors. *Topics in Stroke Rehabilitation*, **8**, 3:64–72.

Russell B (1918) The philosophy of logical atomism. In: R C Marsh (ed.) (1971) *Bertrand Russell: Logic and Knowledge* (London: George Allen & Unwin).

Serenko A, Morrison B and Suresky J (2010) Urinary incontinence and sexual function in pre-menopausal women. *International Journal of Urological Nursing*, **4**, 2:80–6.

Sterner E, Lindholm C, Berg E, Stark A and Fossum B (2011) Category I pressure ulcers: how reliable is clinical assessment? *Orthopaedic Nursing*, **30**, 3:194–207.

Trendall J (2000) Concept analysis: chronic fatigue. *Journal of Advanced Nursing*, **32**, 5:1126–31.

Waltz C, Strickland O L and Lenz E (2010) *Measurement in Nursing and Health Research*, 4th edn (New York: Springer).

Wang T J (2004) Concept analysis of functional status. *International Journal of Nursing Studies*, **41**, 4:457–62.

Wilson J (1989) Conceptual and empirical truth: some notes for researchers. *Educational Research*, **31**, 3:176–80.

10 Research Designs

> If we are to achieve things never before accomplished we must employ methods never before attempted.
>
> Francis Bacon

Introduction

The next step in the research process after the literature review and the formulation of the research questions is planning or designing strategies for the collection and analysis of data. In practice, while the aims and objectives or hypotheses are being formulated, the researcher must also give prior thought to the possible design to be used to avoid setting unachievable objectives. The literature review should help the researcher to identify research designs and related issues in similar studies. Researchers have coined a number of terms to describe research designs in quantitative research and qualitative research, with which you should become familiar if you are to fully understand the research process. Such terms as 'prospective', 'longitudinal', 'cross-sectional' or 'ex post facto' may mean little at present; this chapter will explain these and other terminologies commonly used in order to enhance your understanding of research articles and reports.

Research design

The term 'research design' means a plan that describes how, when and where data are to be collected and analysed. The design of a study comprises the following aspects:

- the approach (qualitative, quantitative or both, with or without a conceptual framework);
- the method(s) of data collection and the ethical considerations;
- the time, place and source of the data;
- the method of data analysis.

However, a design does not only specify the steps and actions to be taken; it also represents the thinking, beliefs and strategies of the researcher(s) and the logic of the enquiry.

The terms 'design', 'methods' and 'methodology' are sometimes used interchangeably. Methods of data collection are the tools (for example, questionnaires or scales) and techniques (for example, interviews or observations). Methodology is the study of methods.

Selecting a design

In order to meet a study's aims and objectives, researchers must select the most appropriate design. In practice, selection of the design depends largely on the beliefs and values of the researcher (she may, for example, place particular value on the quantitative approach), the resources available (cost, time, expertise of the researcher), how accessible the respondents are and whether the research is ethically sound. Resources often influence the choice of questionnaires over interviews. While such practices may be acceptable, readers must bear in mind that there is no short cut to knowledge. Making compromises and selecting strategies other than the most appropriate has implications for the validity and reliability of the data.

The purpose and types of quantitative research

One can group quantitative studies into three overlapping categories: descriptive studies, correlational studies and causal studies. In quantitative descriptive studies, researchers aim to describe phenomena about which little is known. Descriptive studies tend to answer questions such as: What is the attrition rate of students on a particular course? What is the pattern of alcohol consumption among third-year student nurses? What is the bed occupancy rate in an intensive care unit? What is the attitude of health visitors towards teenage mothers? In quantitative descriptive studies, researchers use measurements to answer these questions (see Chapter 3). From the data, patterns or trends may emerge and possible links between variables can be observed, but the emphasis is on the description of phenomena. For an example of a quantitative descriptive study, see Research Example 14.

Correlational studies (Research Example 15) seek deliberately to examine or explore links between variables. The purpose is often to develop hypotheses that can be tested later in experiments, if feasible. The term 'exploratory' is sometimes used to denote descriptive or correlational studies. To some extent, all research explores phenomena.

Research designs depend on the research questions. For example, a descriptive study of postoperative stress may reveal how people experience stress, what factors they perceive as causing or relieving their stress and how they cope with it. Such a study may also give an indication that patients who are given information prior to surgery are less stressed afterwards. A correlational study can be carried out to collect data specifically to examine the connection between the two or more variables (for example, information and stress). A questionnaire may be administered to a large number of patients to find out whether there is a difference in the self-reported levels of postoperative stress between those who received information and those who did not.

A quantitative descriptive study

Pilot survey of domestic abuse amongst pregnant women attending an antenatal clinic in a public hospital in Gauteng Province in South Africa *Modiba et al. (2011)*

The rationale of this study was the lack of data on domestic abuse against pregnant women who were attending an antenatal clinic in South Africa.

Mobida et al. (2011) collected data on:

- the incidence of domestic abuse in a cohort of women attending an antenatal clinic;
- the common factors associated with the domestic abuse of these women; and
- the factors that contributed to domestic abuse.

Descriptive statistics were used to present sociodemographic data and the prevalence of domestic abuse.

Comments

In descriptive studies, researchers usually attempt to find whether there is a relationship between demographic factors (for example, age, gender and education) and the problem/issue (for example, domestic abuse). In this study, no statistically significant association was found between the prevalence of abuse and the sociodemographic profile of these pregnant women.

A correlational study

Association between fatigue and Internet addiction in female hospital nurses
Lin et al. (2013)

The aim of this study was to explore the association (correlation) between fatigue and internet addiction among female nurses. Lin et al. (2013) justified the focus on fatigue on the basis that it negatively affects the health of nurses and compromises the safety of patients.

The key finding was that internet addiction was significantly associated with fatigue levels among these nurses. Data were also collected on a number of other variables such as 'shift rotation' and 'regular self-medication'. Lin et al. (2013) reported that both these variables were found to be associated with higher levels of fatigue.

Although correlational studies may seek to establish links between variables, no firm conclusions can normally be drawn. For example, in the previous correlational study of information and postoperative stress, the researcher had no control over the information given and had to rely retrospectively on the respondents' reports. To be able to make more definite statements about the relationship between preoperative information and postoperative stress, an experimental design may be used, in which the researcher controls or manipulates the information given and measures the level of stress while trying to control for other factors that may influence postoperative stress. The next chapter gives examples of various types of experiments.

Descriptive and correlational studies, perhaps the most common forms of research in nursing, are no less important or difficult than experimental ones. All research studies require rigour, and all have a contribution to make that can be assessed by the 'added understanding' they bring to the phenomenon being investigated. Although research is described here as having three neat, distinct categories, studies may in practice combine elements from each of them. It is not unusual, therefore, to find descriptive studies that are also correlational.

Types of research designs

There is no consensus among researchers on the classification of designs (Castles, 1987); what seems to emerge is that, broadly speaking, there are three types of design:

- experimental (including quasi-experimental)
- survey
- case study.

Experiments examine and establish causal links between variables. In its basic form, an experiment consists of a researcher introducing and manipulating a variable (for example, information-giving prior to surgery) and measuring its effects, if any, on another variable (for example, postoperative stress), while making sure that there is no interference from other variables (for example, drug intake or information from other sources). In quasi-experiments, the researcher has less control over certain variables than in a true experiment.

A survey is a research design to collect information from whole populations or from groups or clusters of people about their views, beliefs, attitudes, expectations and behaviour. In a postal survey of 'factors associated with dementia care practices among community health nurses', the information that Huang et al. (2013) wanted to collect is reflected in the following aims:

> (i) to investigate the dementia care practices among district nurses, home health care nurses and care managers; (ii) to compare the knowledge level, attitude, level of confidence, and the type of dementia care practices among these different types of community health care nurses; and (iii) explore the factors that influence these dementia care practices.

Sometimes the entire population is surveyed (as in the case of a census), or a representative sample may be drawn. The main methods of data collection in surveys are questionnaires, structured interviews and semi-structured interviews, although observations can also be used, as in a survey on dressing practices or pressure sores. Survey methods are discussed in Chapter 16.

The survey is also a choice design for descriptive and correlational studies. As explained earlier, links between variables suggested by data from descriptive studies can be followed up in correlational studies. Correlational studies using the survey design aim to establish links without introducing an intervention. A survey can be carried out to find whether or not there is a link between lung cancer and people who smoke. The survey may comprise a large number of smokers and non-smokers. Data may show that indeed those who smoke have a higher prevalence of lung cancer. In this case, the researcher did not introduce 'smoking' to a group of people, but simply investigated the link after the smoking had taken place. Such a design is also known as ex post facto or 'after the fact'. In correlational studies, researchers commonly collect demographic details such as age, occupation, gender and educational background and seek to establish links between these and other characteristics of respondents, such as their beliefs and behaviours.

Case studies focus on specific situations. Using this design, the researcher studies individuals, groups or specific phenomena. Creswell (1994) explains that, in case studies, the researcher 'explores a single entity or phenomenon ("the case") bounded by time and activity (a program, event, process, institution, or social group) and collects detailed information by using a variety of data collection procedures during a sustained period of time'. However, in a large study, a multi-case study approach can also be used. For example, in a study of 'Patient safety in healthcare preregistration education curricula', Cresswell et al. (2013) collected data from eight medicine, nursing, pharmacy and physiotherapy university courses.

The case study design lends itself well to both quantitative and qualitative approaches. For example, a researcher may evaluate a particular health promotion programme or find reasons why some women do not comply with advice from midwives at an antenatal class using by means of qualitative interviews and questionnaires.

The cases on which researchers focus need not necessarily be unusual; they can, and often are, typical of others. Using the case study approach, data can be collected in the past, present or future. For example, a researcher may investigate the events that led to the closure of hospital X in 1980 by interviewing some of those who were involved in the closure and by studying newspaper and television reports of what happened at the time. A researcher can also 'follow' a group of mothers from the time they give birth to 18 months afterwards, to find out about infant feeding practices.

While surveys involve large populations and use samples for the purpose of generalising their findings, case studies tend to be more specific, in-depth and holistic. In Cresswell et al.'s (2013) qualitative case studies of eight university courses, they 'collected policy and course documentation; interviews and focus groups with educators, students, health service staff, patients and policy makers; and course and work placement observations'. The emphasis is on understanding a particular case or group of people, although the data gathered may be useful for other similar cases. See Taylor (2013) and Sangster-Gormley (2013) for more discussion on case studies research.

Experiments, surveys and case studies broadly describe the main research designs in social, health and nursing research. There are also different types of experiment, survey and case study, as will be shown later in this chapter and in the next. Not all research fits neatly into this classification, as, for example, the Delphi technique. The purpose of classification, however crude, is to simplify things and thus facilitate understanding. It has few implications for the reliability and validity of the data if a survey is wrongly described as a case study. What is crucial is for researchers to explain the research process in detail for readers to understand what was done. However, confusion can be created if the right terminologies are not used.

Variations on research designs

Not all experiments, surveys and case studies are the same. Some surveys collect data on one occasion only; others do so at intervals. Case studies can investigate current as well as past phenomena; some experiments may have only two groups, while others may have three or more. Research designs can be further classified according to their data sources (longitudinal and cross-sectional, retrospective and prospective) and their functions (evaluative or comparative). Other variations include the Delphi technique and action research.

Longitudinal and cross-sectional studies

Some nursing phenomena evolve over time, and it seems appropriate that data should be collected at intervals in order to capture any change that may take place. For example, people coming to terms with the loss of a spouse may go through different phases of bereavement. Collection of data at 3- or 6-monthly intervals from the time of bereavement until up to 2 years afterwards would probably provide a better picture of the bereavement process than would the collection of data on only one occasion. People's attitudes, beliefs and behaviours may change over a period of time. A researcher may be interested in studying the impact of patient education on the subsequent behaviour of post-myocardial infarction patients. It is possible that, a month after the infarction, patients may be following nurses' advice, but there is no guarantee that this behaviour will be sustained.

Researchers who want to know whether the effects of patient education are sustained will have to collect data at intervals over a period of time. Such a design is called longitudinal (Research Example 16). It is appropriate for phenomena that change over time. The intervals at which data are collected must be justified, and this should be on the basis that they are the most appropriate times to capture the phenomena under investigation. The term 'cohort' is used to describe the same group of respondents who are 'followed' over a period of time. Thus, if a class of students takes part in a longitudinal study to find out how their careers progress over the next 10 years, this class constitutes a cohort. This type of design is also called 'cohort study'. Two or more groups can also be 'followed' for comparative purposes. One of the problems with cohort studies is the likelihood of a 'cohort effect'. This is described as the effects on a particular cohort as a result of sharing common life experiences. The particular time and context in which a cohort live and interact may influence the attitudes, beliefs and behaviour of those in the cohort.

One of the main problems with longitudinal studies is that some of those supplying the data (the participants) may drop out of the project. This is referred to as 'mortality' or 'attrition'. Respondents may actually die, but more often they withdraw or cannot be traced. This affects the original composition of the sample and may have implications for the generalisability of the findings. If the project lasts for several years, it is not unusual for the original researchers to cease to be involved in the project, often as a result of a career move.

Research example 16

A prospective, longitudinal study

Quality of life in men receiving radiotherapy and neo-adjuvant androgen deprivation for prostate cancer *McCaughan et al. (2013)*

The quality of life of men with prostate cancer was measured at 4–6 weeks post-radiotherapy and at 6 and 12 months thereafter. A longitudinal design was used because radiotherapy is known to have early and late side effects.

Comments

1 In this case, a longitudinal design was justified as the authors wanted to capture the effects of radiotherapy on quality of life over a 1-year period. The aim was to find out if, and how, quality of life varied over this period and also whether the immediate decrease in quality of life, reported in the literature, would persist at 1 year after treatment.

2 This study is prospective because it starts collecting data in the present and continues up to 1 year thereafter.

3 One of the problems with longitudinal studies is the loss of participants (attri-

tion), especially during the later phase of the study. Therefore, the projected number of participants who may not continue with the study should be taken into account when calculating the sample size. In this study, the authors' projection was that there would be 10 per cent attrition at 4–6 weeks, 20 per cent at 6 months and 40 per cent at 1 year. However, the actual response rates (97 per cent, 90 per cent and 93 per cent at the three respective time-points showed that this was an over-estimation.

4 The results showed that most of the participants experienced a significant decline in their quality of life at 4–6 weeks after radiotherapy but that this improved at 6 months post treatment. However, a minority of them continued to experience a lower quality of life at 1 year than before radiotherapy.

Most research has the potential to influence the subsequent behaviour of the respondents, although the extent to which this happens depends on the methods the researcher uses and the nature of the research. The effect of the observer on the observed is well documented (see Chapter 18). Surveys also can raise issues and trigger reactions among respondents. Longitudinal studies, because of their prolonged nature, are potentially likely to raise respondents' awareness and give them time to change their attitudes and behaviours, thereby preventing researchers from studying behaviours as they would have been if there had been no research interference. While studying 'the changing situations of a panel of family caregivers of elderly relatives in the home' using a longitudinal design, Collins et al. (1989)

became 'increasingly aware of the unintended effects that study participation has had on the family caregiver'. They concluded from their study that:

> through the research process researchers actively influenced the experiences of many of the family caregivers in the study. Caregivers seem to have been stimulated to evaluate and change their appraisals of their care-giving situations and, at times, their use of external resources and patient management strategies.

Another problem with longitudinal studies is that they take time and are costly as they may span a number of years. To get round these problems to some extent, it is sometimes possible to survey a cross-section of respondents, who can provide data to describe the changing nature of the phenomenon. For example, instead of interviewing a group of people experiencing bereavement at 6-monthly intervals, the researcher can choose to collect data from people who are at different stages of bereavement. She will interview a group at 1 month after the loss, a group who are bereaving at 6 months and another group who are at the 1-year stage. All these data will be gathered only once from each group and together will provide an insight into the process of bereavement.

Most surveys are, however, cross-sectional because this design allows researchers to access a cross-section of the population (Research Example 17). A cross-sectional design is one in which data are collected from different groups of people who are at different stages in their experience of the phenomenon. Carlson and Morrison (2009) used a cross-sectional study design to identify the specific palliative services provided to patients who enrolled with a hospice and the extent to which services varied across hospices. They found that 'the cross-sectional study design was an efficient way to evaluate a large sample of patients receiving hospice [care], to understand the prevalence of specific services, and to generate hypotheses regarding why service delivery might vary across hospices'.

A cross-sectional design

Determinants of cigarette smoking among school adolescents in eastern Ethiopia
Reda et al. (2012)

The aim of the study was to assess the prevalence of cigarette use and its determinant factors among high-school students in eastern Ethiopia. A cross-section of 1,890 adolescents from seven secondary schools and two high schools were administered a questionnaire.

Comments

1 As the aim was to assess smoking prevalence at the time of the study, a cross-sectional design is appropriate. It gives a 'snapshot' of the smoking behaviour and patterns of smoking in this cohort of adolescents.

2 The sample was a cross-section of young people in terms of gender, ethnicity, religion and education, among other factors.

3 If the aim had been to investigate whether the smoking behaviour of these (same) adolescents would change over time (for example, from adolescence to adulthood), a longitudinal study would have been the design of choice.

Research example 17

The strength of a cross-sectional design is that researchers get instant answers to some of their questions. For example, if a researcher wanted to know whether people became more resilient as they grew old (hypothesis), she could measure resilience in a group of young people and a group of older people. In this 'snapshot' survey, the data would show whether or not the hypothesis was supported. Therefore the researcher could get the answer in a matter of days or weeks. However, a more valid result would be to measure resilience in a group of young people and repeat the measurement, say every 10 years, until they were old to know whether or not their resilience was increasing. Therefore the limitations of the cross-sectional approach lie mainly in the fact that the same group is not studied over time and that the various groups may not have similar characteristics.

Retrospective and prospective studies

Phenomena that have already occurred have their explanations in the past. Researchers have to 'work backwards' and search for variables or factors to account for them. A wealth of valuable information resides in people and documents, which can help to shed some light on many current concerns. Records are kept for the purpose of describing, and accounting for, what people do. For example, community nurses' diaries contain information that can help towards understanding what they do. Patients' notes give information on the treatment and progress of their illnesses, as well as a considerable number of demographic and other personal details. These were not collected for the purpose of research, but they can be used retrospectively to explain and inform current phenomena.

A retrospective design is one in which researchers study a current phenomenon by seeking information from the past. For example, to inform the policy of managing unscheduled presentations of cancer outpatients (a current problem or issue), Aprile et al. (2013) reviewed records of patients over a 2-year period and extracted data relating to demographics, clinical variables and reason(s) for presentation. This study was mainly descriptive. However, a study can also be correlational, as when the researcher investigates a condition or illness that has already occurred and searches for variables in records or personal accounts that may be associated with it. For example, researchers have looked at upbringing, lifestyles and life events (information from the past) in an attempt to find causes that may be related to patients currently suffering from schizophrenia (that is, something that has already occurred). For an example of a retrospective study, see Research Example 18.

Retrospective studies must be differentiated from historical studies. If one takes the view that everything that has gone before us is history, all retrospective studies can be termed historical. The crucial difference between the two, in research terms, is that retrospective studies aim to describe or explain a current phenomenon by examining factors that are associated with it or gave rise to it. A historical study, however, does not need to have a 'foot in the present'. It seeks to understand phenomena as embedded in that particular period in history. For example, a nurse historian may carry out a study of leadership styles of matrons in the nineteenth century or describe moral treatments that psychiatric patients received in asylums.

A retrospective design

Aromatherapy and massage intrapartum service impact on use of analgesia and anaesthesia in women in labour: a retrospective case note analysis *Dhany et al. (2012)*

Dhany et al. (2012) carried out a study to find out if an intrapartum aromatherapy and massage service reduced the need for analgesia during labour in a general maternity unit. They used clinical data that had already been collected (since 2007) to compare those who received the service with those who did not.

Comments

1 The reason for using a retrospective design was because it was not feasible to conduct a randomised, controlled trial to compare the two groups.

2 The authors explained that every woman who gave birth in the unit had comprehensive pregnancy, labour and delivery records entered into the computer system.

3 Extracting data from existing records requires ethical approval. In this study, data extracted from the case notes were anonymised prior to entry in the SPSS software.

Although some comparisons can be made with current leadership styles or psychiatric treatments, the aim of these studies is to focus on these events only as they happened at the time, with or without relevance or reference to what happens now. Here are some examples of historical research:

● the historical context of addiction in the nursing profession, 1850–1982 (Heise, 2003);
● a review of learning disability nursing research, 1995–2003 (Northway et al., 2006);
● trends in hospitalisation rates and severity of injuries from abuse in young children, 1997–2009 (Farst et al., 2013).

One of the main drawbacks of retrospective designs is that the researcher relies on existing data that were, most probably, not collected for research purposes and therefore lack the rigour with which research is carried out. Descriptions of past behaviour may be highly subjective. Records may be incomplete, or difficult to make sense of or even to decipher. Relying on respondents' memory also has its limitations. Apart from forgetting important details, respondents can be selective in how they view the past. Despite these shortcomings, retrospective studies have been useful in, for example, making links between lung cancer and smoking, and heart disease and fat intake.

A prospective design is one in which researchers study a current phenomenon by seeking information from the future (see Research Example 16, above). Nurses may want to know the effects of their practices on patients' behaviour over time, or how the diagnosis of a condition such as breast cancer subsequently affects the lifestyle of its sufferers. Researchers using a prospective design can have some control over whom they want to include in their study and how data are collected. To ensure that the lifestyle of the newly diagnosed cancer patients would not have changed anyway, another group of people without breast cancer can be studied at the same time. With this design, data are collected at one or more points in the future, as is the case in longitudinal studies. In fact, the two designs have a lot in common. The main difference between them is that longitudinal studies can be both prospective and retrospective.

Williams et al. (1994) used a prospective design to study 'early outcomes after hip fracture among women'. Outcomes were compared in three groups of formerly community-living women: 'those discharged home from the hospital, those discharged to a nursing home and staying there for more than 1 month, and those staying for less than 1 month'. For an example of a prospective study see McCaughan et al. (2013) in Research Example 16.

Evaluative studies

In the era of evidence-based practice and client-centred care, evaluative studies assume great importance. Practitioners can evaluate their practice by reflecting on what they do. The difference between this and an evaluative study is that the latter is a systematic appraisal using research methods. Evaluative studies tend to focus on a particular practice, policy or event. They are normally carried out when the researcher wants to find out if, how and to what extent the objectives of particular activities have been or are being met. These activities could be the provision of a service, a teaching programme or a series of therapeutic sessions. By focusing on these specific, well-defined activities, evaluative studies tend to take the form of case studies. In Baker et al.'s (2012) 'evaluation of the impact of the Chief Nursing Officer's review of mental health nursing in mental health trusts in England', the aim was to find out the progress made with regards to the 17 key recommendations made in the original review.

Researchers may also decide to select aspects they want to evaluate no matter what the original objectives were. However, if the purpose of the evaluation is to improve that particular activity or to learn from the experience, it makes sense that the aims and objectives should provide the benchmark against which the success of the programme or activity can be measured.

In evaluative studies, researchers can use quantitative and/or qualitative methods. Frank et al. (2011) evaluated 'patient participation in an emergency department' by means of the Patient Participation Emergency Department Questionnaire. On the other hand, Crilly et al. (2012) used semi-structured interviews in their qualitative evaluation of 'an Australian hospital avoidance admission programme for aged care facility residents'. For examples of mixed methods evaluative studies, see Hesselink and Harting (2011) and Higgins et al. (2012). The main limitation of evaluation studies lies in the fact that they are aimed at understanding specific practices and policies. Their contribution to knowledge in general, and research methodology in particular, remains a secondary objective.

There are many similarities and differences between audit and research (Closs and Cheater, 1996; Blood and Transplant, 2012). Evaluative studies seem to resemble audit mainly because both tend to address issues in specific settings. Both audit and evaluation research must use rigorous methods to collect and analyse data. Finally, the contribution of audit and evaluative studies to the development of theory is rather limited.

The main difference between them is that the research evaluation of a project can sometimes be an afterthought, although the original aims and objectives can be used as benchmarks. Audit, on the other hand, is a cycle that 'involves setting standards for practice, monitoring that practice, comparing actual practice with the standards set, if necessary making changes to practice and then remonitoring practice to see if the agreed standard is attained' (Closs and Cheater, 1996). This important practice element is not usually present in evaluative studies. Research Example 19 gives an account of an evaluative study.

An evaluative study

Evaluation of the implementation of assistant in nursing workforce in haemodialysis units *Chow and Miguel (2010)*

Chow and Miguel (2010) evaluated the impact of a new skill-mix model involving the introduction of assistants in nursing to the five haemodialysis units at a major tertiary area health service in Sydney, Australia. The nurses' attitudes and their satisfaction with the organisation of care delivery in their dialysis units prior to, and 6 months after, the introduction of the change were measured. The impact on patient care in terms of nosocomial infections, falls, medication and patient complaints, as well as nurse work-related injuries including needlestick injuries, were investigated.

A quantitative approach was adopted in this study. The Revised Nursing Work Index Data Questionnaire and a demographic questionnaire were used to collect data.

Other sources of data included the area health service's workforce database to compare staffing levels at baseline and 6 months after. Data from the Incident Information Management System in New South Wales were also accessed to evaluate changes in rates of reported clinical incidents.

Comments

1 In this evaluation, key outcomes for nurses and patients were measured and compared before and after the introduction of the new model.

2 Apart from collecting data specifically for this study (that is, through the administration of questionnaires), the researchers made use of existing databases; this is a common practice in evaluation study.

Research example 19

Comparative studies

Many research designs involve some form of comparison. Experimental studies compare the results of experimental and control groups. Surveys collect data that allow comparisons according to demographic factors such as age, gender or class. The difference between these and comparative studies is that the purpose of the latter, at the outset, is to compare – whether it is people's characteristics, policies, practices or events.

As the main purpose of comparative studies is to compare, the rationale for this must be provided. The reasons given by Tiwari et al. (2003) in their study of 'critical thinking disposition of Hong Kong Chinese and Australian nursing students' include a lack of understanding of how critical thinking may vary across cultures.

Comparative studies can be quantitative, qualitative or both. Research Example 20 describes a comparative study in which a quantitative approach is used. McCaughan et al. (2011), on the other hand, used qualitative methods (semi-structured interviews) to explore and compare the experience and coping behaviour of men and women with colorectal cancer at diagnosis and during surgery. Comparative studies are a useful way of learning about people and practices. In healthcare, it is well known that there are different treatments for the same condition. While evaluation studies provide data on the effectiveness of particular treatments, comparative studies make it possible to compare different treatments.

Research example 20

A comparative study

A comparison of the hand hygiene knowledge, beliefs and practices of Italian nursing and medical students *van De Mortel et al. (2012)*

The review of the literature for this study showed that there was ample evidence of a higher rate of compliance with hand hygiene guidelines among registered nurses when compared with doctors. The difference persisted even after hand hygiene compliance interventions. The authors wanted to know if these differences were apparent during nurses' and doctors' training and whether they were related to their hand hygiene knowledge and beliefs.

A quantitative approach was used in this study. The practices, knowledge and beliefs of 117 nursing students and 119 medical students were measured and compared by means of a questionnaire.

The results showed that while their beliefs were similar, nursing students had a higher level of knowledge and self-reported compliance than doctors.

The Delphi technique

Another form of research, which is a variation of the survey design, is the Delphi technique. This consists of gathering the views of experts on a particular issue with the added agenda of seeking an agreement or consensus on the issue. This necessarily entails 'going back' to the experts until a consensus is reached. There are many issues in nursing that some researchers believe can be enlightened by experts. This type of design is particularly useful when setting priorities, clarifying roles, defining concepts and identifying competencies.

The Delphi technique consists mainly of seeking the views of a panel of experts on a particular issue, usually by means of a questionnaire. After analysis of the data, the same experts are given feedback from the findings and asked to reconsider their views with a view to reaching consensus. This exercise is repeated until the researcher is satisfied that the study has achieved its aims. Examples of Delphi studies include:

'Benchmarks for effective primary care-based nursing services for adults with depression' (McIlrath et. al., 2010), 'Developing a guideline for clinical trial protocol content' (Tetzlaff et al., 2012) and 'Research priorities of midwives' (Jordan et al., 2013).

There are different versions of the Delphi technique, although the core principles should include a panel of experts, more than one round of questionnaires, an attempt to reach consensus of opinion through feedback and the assurance of anonymity (between experts) throughout the process (Beretta, 1996). The Delphi technique has the advantage of collating the views of experts using questionnaires without incurring the cost of getting the experts together. The fact that these people do not meet and are not aware of who the others are means that they do not have the opportunity to influence one another, therefore allowing diverse opinions to be expressed. The disadvantages include the subjective bias in the researcher's choice of 'experts' and the pressure on the respondents to agree, thereby introducing the possibility of hasty decisions being taken. There is also the problem of low response rates, especially in the later rounds of the questionnaire, which casts doubt on the 'consensus' reached. Could it be that those who drop out do so because they do not want to change their initial views?

According to Powell (2003), the findings of a Delphi study 'represent expert opinion rather than indisputable fact', and 'further inquiry to validate the findings may be important'. For a review of Delphi studies and further discussion of the technique, see Keeney et al. (2006). The opportunities for interaction and communication between experts that the internet affords, at very little cost, suit the Delphi approach. Cole et al. (2013) offer a useful discussion on internet-based Delphi research. See Research Example 21 for a Delphi study.

A Delphi study

Competencies for practice in renal case: a national Delphi study *Lindberg et al. (2012)*

The purpose of this Delphi study was to identify the essential competencies for professional renal nursing in Sweden. According to the authors, this (Delphi) design was selected because a consensus about the core competencies for renal nursing care was required.

A literature review and a workshop with key stakeholders were conducted to generate an initial and provisional list of 56 competencies. This list was sent to a panel of 25 registered nurses in renal nursing care.

Comments

1 One of the difficulties with the Delphi technique relates to the definition and recruitment of experts. In this study, the criteria for selecting panel members were that they needed to be registered nurses working in a renal department with a minimum of 12 months' experience who rated themselves as 'experts' in renal nursing. They were recruited through the Swedish Nephrology Nurses Association.

2 The number of 'rounds' of questionnaires can vary in Delphi studies. In this case, there were four rounds. In the first two rounds, panel members reworded, deleted or added items. In the third and fourth rounds, no competencies were discarded.

3 The final list of competencies was reduced from 56 to 43.

4 The authors concluded that this national description of competencies could be used to inform the development of education and training curricula in this field of nursing.

Research example 21

Action research

Action research, as the term suggests, has two main components – action and research. The purpose of conventional research is mainly to contribute to the body of knowledge. Some of this knowledge could eventually, but not necessarily, be used in practice. With action research, the emphasis is on 'action', and research methods are used to inform this action. Defining action research is problematic since there are a number of models (see, for example, Hart and Bond, 1995). In essence, it involves a collaboration between researcher and practitioner in:

● identifying a practice problem;
● using research methods to assess this problem;
● planning and implementing the change;
● evaluating the outcome.

And so the cycle continues. The number of steps depends on whose model one uses.

In its conventional form, research is normally carried out by outside researchers on practitioners and their practice to advance the researchers' cause. They use the practice setting to collect data and rely on the goodwill of practitioners but give little back. In action research, there is more 'give and take' in the relationship between these two protagonists. With conventional research, findings are often couched in research terminologies that can remain incomprehensible to practitioners. The researcher's interpretation of practice phenomena often does not coincide with the practitioner's perception of the same. Action research has the advantage that researcher and practitioner can enter into a dialogue, discuss their different interpretations and produce more valid findings by drawing from each other's special knowledge and experience. Research findings in conventional research can take up to 2 years before they are published. In action research, the emphasis is on the 'here and now'. Solutions to problems are immediately implemented and evaluated.

Action research is not possible without the collaboration of all those involved in, or affected by, the introduction and implementation of change. This has led to the belief that all action research involves participation. Participatory action research (PAR) is a form of action research that involves empowering and emancipating participants (for example, practitioners or carers) to have control over what they want to change and how this should happen (Fals-Borda and Rahman, 1991; Baum et al., 2006). According to Baum et al. (2006):

> PAR seeks to understand and improve the world by changing it. At its heart is collective, self reflective inquiry that researchers and participants undertake, so they can understand and improve upon the practices in which they participate and the situations in which they find themselves. The reflective process is directly linked to action, influenced by understanding of history, culture, and local context and embedded in social relationships.

In reality, the degree of real participation in action research varies according to the aims of individual projects. Participation ranges from token, minimal and moderate to full. There is increasingly a recognition that change is more difficult when it comes 'from above'. By listening, and understanding people's needs, motives and circumstances, it is possible to develop interventions or programmes that suit them best. This is why action research is also associated more with qualitative than quantitative approaches, although both can be useful.

Action research has a number of limitations, including difficulties in getting all those involved to be motivated enough to see the project to its successful completion. It is time-consuming as, unlike conventional research, it involves an (or several) implementation stage. When action research is carried out in a particular clinical setting, there may be little choice for some staff to 'opt out', as the project may have to involve all of them. 'Reluctant' participants may feel pressurised to conform. In conventional research, the decision to participate or not is up to the individual. Action research is about change, and change has political dimensions and implications. The potential for conflict of interest between researchers (often seen as outsiders) and practitioners, as well as between practitioners themselves, is real.

Drawing on their experience of an action research study in Australia, Nugus et al. (2012) offer useful insights into the tension between organisational politics and conducting action research. For example, they found that some managers' enthusiastic support of the project at the start changed to resistance once the findings were presented. They also reported that 'many frontline staff were less supportive, some were suspicious of or hostile towards management-led processes to improve and evaluate care'. For more discussion on the political and ethical aspects of action research, see Williamson and Prosser (2002) and Nugus et al. (2012). Despite these limitations, action research is gaining popularity in health and nursing at a time when the impact of research on practice is being questioned more and more.

Examples of action research studies include 'Developing the practice context to enable more effective pain management with older people' (Brown and McCormack, 2011), 'Development and implementation of a critical pathway for patients with chest pain' (Siebens et al., 2012) and 'Developing, testing, and sustaining rehabilitation interventions' (Ehde et al., 2013). In Research Example 22, Nilvarangkul et al. (2006, 2013) describe the aims, process and benefits of an action research study.

An action research study

Strengthening self-care among women weavers in North-East Thailand *Nilvarangkul et al. (2006, 2013)*

The aim of this action research study was to improve self-care and work safety practices among women weavers. The design consisted of the following phases: fact-finding, problem prioritisation, planning for action, implementation and evaluation. According to the authors, the principles of PAR were used to empower this group of women and their communities to care for themselves and to be able to address their problems.

Research example 22

After the initial assessment/fact-finding stage, the researchers and these women reflected on their findings. The women then prioritised their needs and developed a five-point plan focusing on health promotion, illness prevention, social welfare and self-care education to address their problems.

The authors concluded that this action research study benefitted the women as well as the researchers as it provided them with 'a greater understanding and a valuable experience concerning the actual situations'. It also demonstrated 'the value of action research processes for empowering local communities to gain greater understanding and ownership of their own health issues, and for developing local strategies for addressing them'.

Qualitative research approaches

Qualitative researchers, in general, do not use the terms mentioned above to describe their study design; instead they describe their approach as ethnography, phenomenology, grounded theory or discourse analysis, and then go on to explain what they do. The phenomenological, grounded theory and ethnographic approaches to research are described in Chapters 12, 13 and 14, respectively. A brief account of discourse analysis is given below. These are the four most often used qualitative approaches in nursing research, although there are more qualitative designs that can be described here.

Discourse analysis

In discourse analysis, the focus of study is discourse through words, phrases or sentences and the manner and context in which they are expressed. As explained in Chapter 4, language is not just a medium of conveying what we mean; it is a way of constructing social reality. By learning language, we learn values, beliefs and social norms from the particular culture or sub-culture in which it is embedded. Through language, we also transmit our view of the world and seek to shape it according to our beliefs.

Sources of data in discourse analysis are texts in the forms of transcribed interviews, recorded conversations, diary entries, letters, books, songs and other similar media. The frameworks that discourse analysts use to analyse data vary according to the preference of researchers. Conversation analysis is often based on the work of Potter and Wetherell (1987). Foucault (1972) is popular with critical analysts, in particular those who want to explore the power relationships between participants.

Discourse analysis, as an approach, has been used to study a number of topics in health and nursing including: 'How nurses understand and care for older people with delirium in the acute hospital' (Schofield et al., 2012), 'How is stroke thrombolysis portrayed in UK national and London local newspapers?' (Cluckie et al., 2012) and 'comparing Danish textbooks for nursing and medical students between 1870 and 1956' (Frederiksen, 2010). White (2004), Stevenson (2004) and Campbell and Arnold (2004) also offer useful insights into the use of discourse analysis in nursing research. Research Example 23 is a description of a study based on discourse analysis.

A study using discourse analysis

Masculinities, 'guy talk' and 'manning up': a discourse analysis of how young men talk about sexual health *Knight et al. (2012)*

Knight et al. (2012) interviewed 32 young men to explore men's discourses about sexual health. They were asked to describe situations in which they engaged in conversation or discussion, with their peers and sex partners, about sexual health. They also had to describe the social contexts in which these conversations took place.

The authors explain that they drew on methods from critical discourse analysis to explore the social processes that (re)produce and reflect knowledge and power relations through discourses. The purpose of using discourse analysis was to explore 'power distributions between and across socially dominant and subordinate groups (for example, within the social hierarchy of men)'.

Research example 23

In this chapter, some of the common terminologies used to describe research designs have been explained. Different levels and types of research designs in quantitative research have been described.

To facilitate understanding, it was felt necessary to present each one as distinct and separate from the others, but in practice there is a considerable overlap between, for example, descriptive and correlational studies. Experiments can be prospective, and a comparative study can be both descriptive and retrospective. What is important, however, is not what terminology is used but that the most appropriate design is selected and described in enough detail to make sense of what was done and to assess the reasons for, and implications of, such actions.

Summary

References

Aprile G, Pisa F E, Follador A et al. (2013) Unplanned presentations of cancer outpatients: a retrospective cohort study. *Supportive Care in Cancer*, **21**, 2:397–404.

Baker J, Swarbrick C, Campbell M, Playle J and Lovell K (2012) A follow-up evaluation of the impact of the Chief Nursing Officer's review of mental health nursing in mental health trusts and universities in England: comparisons of two e-surveys. *Journal of Advanced Nursing*, **68**, 3:625–35.

Baum F, MacDougall C and Smith D (2006) Participatory action research. *Journal of Epidemiology and Community Health*, **60**, 10:854–7.

Beretta R (1996) A critical review of the Delphi technique. *Nurse Researcher*, **3**:79–89.

Blood and Transplant (2012) The difference between clinical audit & research. Retrieved from http://hospital.blood.co.uk/library/pdf/INF451.pdf (accessed 21 August 2013).

Brown D and McCormack B G (2011) Developing the practice context to enable more effective pain management with older people: an action research approach. *Implementation Science*, **6**:9.

Campbell J and Arnold S (2004) Application of discourse analysis to nursing inquiry. *Nurse Researcher*, **12**, 2:30–41.

Carlson M D A and Morrison R S (2009) Study design, precision, and validity in observational studies. *Journal of Palliative Care Medicine*, **12**,1: 77–82.

Castles M R (1987) *Primer of Nursing Research* (Philadelphia: W B Saunders).

Chow J and Miguel S S (2010) Evaluation of the implementation of assistant in nursing workforce in haemodialysis units. *International Journal of Nursing Practice*, **16**: 484–91.

Closs S J and Cheater F M (1996) Audit or research – what is the difference? *Journal of Clinical Nursing*, **5**:249–56.

Cluckie G, Rudd A G and McKevitt C (2012) How is stroke thrombolysis portrayed in UK national and London local newspapers? A review and critical discourse analysis. *Age and Ageing*, **41**, 3:291–8.

Cole Z D, Donohoe H M and Stellefson M L (2013) Internet-based Delphi research: case based discussion. *Environmental Management*, **51**, 3:511–23.

Collins C, Given B and Berry D (1989) Longitudinal studies as intervention. *Nursing Research*, **38**, 4:251–3.

Creswell J W (1994) *Research Design: Qualitative and Quantitative Approaches* (Newbury Park, CA: Sage).

Cresswell K, Howe A, Steven A et al. (2013) Patient safety in healthcare preregistration educational curricula: multiple case study-based investigations of eight medicine, nursing, pharmacy and physiotherapy university courses. *British Medical Journal Quality and Safety* **22**:843–54.

Crilly J, Chaboyer W and Wallis M (2012) A structure and process evaluation of an Australian hospital admission avoidance programme for aged care facility residents. *Journal of Advanced Nursing*, **68**, 2:322–34.

Dhany A L, Mitchell T and Foy C (2012) Aromatherapy and massage intrapartum service impact on use of analgesia and anesthesia in women in labour: a retrospective case note analysis. *Journal of Alternative and Complementary Medicine*, **18**, 10:932–8.

Ehde D M, Wegener S T, Williams R M et al. (2013) Developing, testing, and sustaining rehabilitation interventions via participatory action research. *Archives of Physical Medicine and Rehabilitation*, **94**, 1 (Suppl):S30–42.

Fals-Borda O and Rahman M A (1991) *Action and Knowledge: Breaking the Monopoly with Participatory Action Research* (London: Intermediate Technology Publications).

Farst K, Ambadwar P B, King A J, Bird T M and Robbins J M (2013) Trends in hospitalization rates and severity of injuries from abuse in young children, 1997–2009. *Pediatrics* 2013; **131**:6 e1796-802.

Foucault M (1972) *The Archaeology of Knowledge* (London: Routledge).

Frank C, Fridlund B, Baigi A and Asp M (2011) Patient participation in the emergency department: an evaluation using a specific instrument to measure patient participation (PPED). *Journal of Advanced Nursing*, **67**, 4:728–35.

Frederiksen K (2010) A discourse analysis comparing Danish textbooks for nursing and medical students between 1870 and 1956. *Nursing Inquiry*, **17**, 2:151–64.

Hart E and Bond M (1995) *Action Research: A Guide to Practice* (Buckingham: Open University Press).

Heise B (2003) The historical context of addiction in the nursing profession: 1850–1982. *Journal of Advanced Nursing*, **14**, 3:117–24.

Hesselink A E and Harting J (2011) Process evaluation of a multiple risk factor perinatal programme for a hard-to-reach minority group. *Journal of Advanced Nursing*, **67**, 9:2026–37.

Higgins A, Sharek D, Nolan M et al. (2012) Mixed methods evaluation of an interdisciplinary sexuality education programme for staff working with people who have an acquired physical disability. *Journal of Advanced Nursing*, **68**, 11:2559–69.

Huang H L, Shyu Y I, Huang H L et al. (2013) Factors associated with dementia care practices among community health nurses: results of a postal survey. *International Journal of Nursing Studies*, **50**, 9:1219–28.

Jordan K, Slavin V and Fenwick J (2013) Research priorities of midwives: a Delphi study. *Practising Midwife*, **16**, 3:26–8.

Keeney S, Hasson F and McKenna H (2006) Consulting the oracle: ten lessons from using the Delphi technique in nursing research. *Journal of Advanced Nursing*, **53**, 2:205–12.

Knight R, Shoveller J A, Oliffe J L, Gilbert M, Frank B and Ogilvie G (2012) Masculinities, 'guy talk' and 'manning up': a discourse analysis of how young men talk about sexual health. *Sociology of Health and Illness*, **34**, 8:1246–61.

Lin, S C, Tsai K W, Chen M W and Koo M (2013) Association between fatigue and internet addictions in female hospital nurses. *Journal of Advanced Nursing*, **69**, 2:374–83.

Lindberg M, Lundström-Landegren K, Johansson P, Lidén S and Holm U (2012) Competencies for practice in renal care: a national Delphi study. *Journal of Renal Care*, **38**, 2:69–75.

McCaughan E, Prue G, Parahoo K, McIlfatrick S and McKenna H (2011) Exploring and comparing the experience and coping behaviour of men and women with colorectal cancer at diagnosis and during surgery. *Journal of Advanced Nursing*, **67**, 7:1591–600.

McCaughan E, McSorley O, Prue G, Parahoo K, Bunting B, O'Sullivan J and McKenna H (2013) Quality of life in men receiving radiotherapy and neo-adjuvant androgen deprivation for prostate cancer: results from a prospective longitudinal study. *Journal of Advanced Nursing*, **69**, 1:53–65.

McIlrath C, Keeney S, McKenna H and McLaughlin D (2010) Benchmarks for effective primary care-based nursing services for adults with depression: a Delphi study. *Journal of Advanced Nursing*, **66**, 2:269–81.

Modiba L M, Baliki O, Mmalasa R, Reineke P and Nsiki C (2011) Pilot survey of domestic abuse amongst pregnant women attending an antenatal clinic in a public hospital in Gauteng Province in South Africa. *Midwifery*, **27**, 6:872–9.

Nilvarangkul K, Wongprom J, Tumnong C, Supornpun A, Surit P and Srithongchai N (2006) Strengthening the self-care of women working in the informal sector: local fabric weaving in Khon Kaen, Thailand (Phase I). *Industrial Health*, **44**, 1:101–7.

Nilvarangkul K, Srithongchai N, Saensom D, Smith J F, Supornpan A and Tumnong C (2013) Action research to strengthen women weavers' self-care in North-East Thailand. *Public Health Nursing*, **30**, 3:213–20.

Northway R, Mitchell D and Kaur-Mann K (2006) *Review of Learning Disability Nursing Research 1995–2003* (Pontypridd: University of Glamorgan).

Nugus P, Greenfield D, Travaglia J and Braithwaite J (2012) The politics of action research: 'if you don't like the way things are going, get off the bus'. *Social Science and Medicine*, **75**, 11:1946–53.

Potter J and Wetherell M (1987) *Discourse and Social Psychology* (London: Sage).

Powell C (2003) The Delphi technique: myths and realities. *Journal of Advanced Nursing*, **41**, 4:376–82.

Reda A A, Moges A, Yazew B and Biadgilign S (2012) Determinants of cigarette smoking among school adolescents in eastern Ethiopia: a cross-sectional study. *Harm Reduction Journal*, **9**:39.

Sangster-Gormley E (2013) How case-study research can help to explain implementation of the nurse practitioner role. *Nurse Researcher*, **20**, 4:6–11.

Schofield I, Tolson D and Fleming V (2012) How nurses understand and care for older people with delirium in the acute hospital: a critical discourse analysis. *Nursing Inquiry*, **19**, 2:165–76.

Siebens K, Miljoen H, De Geest S, Drew B and Vrints C (2012) Development and implementation of a critical pathway for patients with chest pain through action research. *European Journal of Cardiovascular Nursing*, **11**, 4:466–71.

Stevenson C (2004) Theoretical and methodological approaches in discourse analysis. *Nurse Researcher*, **12**, 2:17–29.

Taylor R (2013) Case-study research in context. *Nurse Researcher*, **20**, 4:4–5.

Tetzlaff J M, Moher D and Chan A W (2012) Developing a guideline for clinical trial protocol content: Delphi consensus survey. *Trials* [Electronic Resource], **13**:176.

Tiwari A, Avery A and Lai P (2003) Critical thinking of disposition of Hong Kong Chinese and Australian nursing students. *Journal of Advanced Nursing*, **44**, 3:298–307.

van De Mortel T F, Kermode S, Progano T and Sansoni J (2012) A comparison of the hand hygiene knowledge, beliefs and practices of Italian nursing and medical students. *Journal of Advanced Nursing* **68**, 3:569–79.

White B (2004) Discourse analysis and social constructionism. *Nurse Researcher*, **12**, 2:7–16.

Williams M A, Obserst M T and Bjorklund B C (1994) Early outcomes after hip fracture among women discharged home and to nursing homes. *Research in Nursing and Health*, **17**:175–83.

Williamson G R and Prosser S (2002) Action research: politics, ethics and participation. *Journal of Advanced Nursing*, **40**, 5:587–93.

11

Experiments

Opening thought   The true method of knowledge is experiment.

William Blake

Introduction

In the previous chapter, we identified three levels of research in quantitative studies: descriptive studies, correlational studies and causal studies. The experiment as a research design corresponds to the third level. Its aim is to establish causal links between variables. It is the principal method in the natural sciences for testing hypotheses and theories, and it uses the deductive approach to data collection (hence the label 'hypothetico-deductive').

In this chapter, we will explore the meaning and purpose of experiments, the difficulties and limitations of using the experimental design in social and health research, the strategies that researchers use to enhance the validity and generalisability of their findings, the ethical implications of experiments involving humans as 'subjects' or participants, and the use and value of experiments in the study of nursing phenomena.

The current emphasis on systematic reviews of randomised controlled trials (RCTs) in itself warrants a closer examination of the experiment as a viable design in nursing research; this is why it is given a lengthy treatment here.

The meaning and purpose of experiments

The term 'experiment' conjures up images of scientists mixing chemicals in a laboratory or observing the behaviour of rats in conditions induced by a researcher. Television adverts often show a man or woman in a white coat making such statements as 'test after test proves' a particular brand of detergent or cat food is better than others.

In everyday life, too, we 'experiment'. A spice may be added to our usual recipe to find out whether it makes it taste better. Painkillers are taken to relieve headaches or sleeping tablets to induce sleep. The aim in each case is to attempt to produce a change (improve taste, relieve pain or induce sleep) by doing something (adding a spice, or taking painkillers or sleeping tablets). Whether or not we know it, we unwittingly carry out experiments, more often on ourselves, with the aim of making our lives more comfortable.

Most people are particular about the type of tablets they take for a headache. They have probably arrived at this choice by 'trying out' several brands. Some people with back pain will 'try' different forms of treatment, such as medication prescribed by a general practitioner, herbal medicine or the services of an osteopath. They know how they felt before and after each of these treatments and are thus able to make up their minds about its effectiveness. In 'trying out' these drugs or treatments, people have in fact engaged in a 'trial' or experiment.

Professionals, too, experiment during the course of their work. To enhance learning, teachers may 'experiment' with seminars, group discussions or lectures. Nurses may try a different type of dressing or introduce a different approach to the organisation of patient care, such as primary nursing or team nursing. If these do not produce the desired effect, they may try other approaches. By basing their practice on 'trial and error', some nurses unwittingly 'experiment' on their clients, and the negative implications of this can sometimes be serious.

In Chapter 2 it was explained that people need to know why things happen. A headache is explained by pressure at work, a hot summer may be attributed to global warming, and an increase in child violence is often blamed on the types of television programme children watch. Even when we cannot explain a phenomenon such as winning a lottery, we put it down to 'lady luck'. In fact, we are constantly preoccupied with 'cause and effect'. The relationship between cause and effect is the essence of an experiment.

Clinical trials

The difference between the types of experiment that lay people and practitioners unwittingly carry out and 'research experiments' is that, in the latter, the researcher systematically and rigorously studies cause-and-effect relationships between variables, by taking steps to ensure that the results obtained (the effect) can only be attributed to the intervention (the cause).

In healthcare, experiments are normally referred to as clinical trials. They are carried out mainly to study the effects of interventions (including drugs, psychosocial therapies, educational programmes, services and diagnostic tests). Trials of healthcare interventions are often described as either explanatory or pragmatic (Roland and Torgerson, 1998). Explanatory trials study the efficacy of interventions. They seek to understand why and how an intervention works so that we can gain a scientific (biological, physiological or psychosocial) understanding of the intervention. These types of trial are normally carried out under ideal circumstances. Participants are carefully selected according to narrow sets of criteria. While the results may show how and why an intervention works, they may not have wide generalisability.

In normal everyday practice, some patients with a certain condition such as rheumatism may differ in their characteristics, attributes and background from others. They frequently have multiple concurrent illness conditions. Clinicians are interested to know whether their interventions can work with the types of patient they encounter in their daily work. Pragmatic trials investigate the effectiveness of interventions in real-life situations. This means that few patients are excluded (only those for whom the intervention may be inappropriate). In Austvoll-Dahlgren et al.'s (2012) study, of a 'web portal for improving public access to evidence-based health information and health literacy skills', the reason given by the authors for selecting a pragmatic design was to include typical users for the web portal in the participant sample. While the results of pragmatic trials may be questionable because researchers have little control over the conditions in which the intervention is administered and evaluated, the results have wider applicability. In pragmatic trials the intervention is made to suit the patient's condition, while in explanatory trials the patient is selected to suit the intervention.

Effectiveness, in pragmatic trials, is often patient-centred and includes, for example, an evaluation of safety, comfort or side-effects as well as symptom reduction, healing and cure. Research Example 24 is an example of a pragmatic trial. For a comparison of explanatory and pragmatic trials, see Roland and Torgerson (1998).

Research example 24

A pragmatic and parallel design

A randomized controlled trial of nurses vs. doctors in the resolution of acute disease of low complexity in primary care *Iglesias et al. (2013)*

The aim of this study was to compare the effectiveness of care delivered by nurses with the usual care delivered by general practitioners, in adult patients in primary care practices in one region in Spain.

The competing demands on the time of general practitioners makes it difficult for them to see everyone who seeks their services. The authors decided to test an intervention designed to find out whether nurses could relieve some of the general practitioners' burden. Patients were allocated either to trained nurses (the intervention group) or general practitioners (the control group).

Comments

1   A randomised controlled trial was selected because it is the best design for providing evidence of effectiveness.

2   Two groups were receiving care at the same time, making it a 'parallel' design trial.

3   According to the authors, it was also a 'pragmatic' clinical trial conducted in clinical practice with real clinical situations.

The logic of experiments

Suppose a nurse observes that constipation is rife among patients on her ward. Having read in the literature that lack of fibre may be responsible for constipation, she decides to put this to the 'test'. After finding out that the amount of fibre in her patients' current diet is in fact low, she increases it and observes whether there is a reduction in the incidence of constipation. However, a colleague may be sceptical and say that these results would have been obtained with or without an increase in fibre and that other factors, such as medication, mobility, age or nursing care, may be implicated.

To rule out the possibility that the reduction in constipation would have happened anyway, the nurse can decide to have two groups of patients: one receiving the current diet, and the other the new diet. Additionally, she may account for or 'control' the other factors by making sure that patients in both groups are, in general, similar in the amount and type of medication they take, in their degree of mobility and in their age, and that they are nursed by the same team of nurses. To avoid the possibility of bias in the selection of patients, the researcher can randomly assign them to either group. In so doing, she has carried out a research experiment. She has:

- put a hypothesis to the test (that a high-fibre diet reduces constipation);
- introduced an intervention (a new high-fibre diet) and measured the outcome (a reduction in constipation);
- compared the pre-test scores (the level of constipation before the experiment) with the post-test scores (the level of constipation after the experiment);
- compared the scores of the group of patients on whom she has experimented (experimental group) with those of the group receiving the usual diet (control group);
- controlled other factors that may work for or against a reduction in constipation (by making sure that one group does not receive more laxatives than the other);
- randomly allocated patients to the two groups (to ensure that both groups are similar (equivalent) in relevant factors except in the amount of fibre in their diets).

Our nurse has in effect met the three requirements of a true experiment: intervention, control and randomisation.

Intervention

Without intervention, there is no experiment. A researcher has to do something to produce an effect or outcome. In the above example, the intervention is the introduction of a new diet, and the outcome is a reduction in constipation. In a correlational study, the researcher would not actively have intervened by introducing the new diet but instead could have, for example, carried out a survey of the fibre content of patients' diets and their bowel habits to find out whether or not there was a link between these two variables. Stulz et al.'s (2013) study of the 'relationship between attention deficit/hyperactivity disorders (ADHD) and eating disorders' is an example a correlational design. They did not introduce an intervention but instead obtained data from a clinical interview with, and self reports of, 32 women with eating disorders. The findings suggest a weak link between the severity of

ADHD key features and the severity of single eating disorder symptoms in female patients with eating disorders.

In experimental studies the researcher attempts to make things happen, while in correlational ones she studies phenomena as they are. In health research, the term 'treatment' is often used instead of 'intervention'.

The experiment is the design of choice to test hypotheses and theories. In Chapter 9, a hypothesis was defined as a 'statement in one sentence, about the expected relationship, if any, between two or more variables'. In its simplest form, the hypothesis has two variables: independent and dependent. Moore (2001) carried out an experiment to test the following null hypothesis: topical amethocaine will have no effect in reducing behavioural and physiological responses in neonates. The independent variable was treatment with amethocaine gel, and the dependent variables were the behavioural and physiological responses to intravenous cannulation.

The purpose of an experiment is to collect data to support or reject the null hypothesis. Although experiments should have a formal hypothesis, you will find when reading research articles that many of them express the purpose of their studies in the form of questions. For example, Pearson and Hutton (2002), in their study comparing the ability of foam swabs and toothbrushes to remove dental plaque, used an experimental design to answer the following questions:

- Is there a difference between the ability of foam swabs and a toothbrush to remove dental plaque from approximal and crevice surfaces?

And, if there is a difference:

- What is the magnitude of the difference between the ability of foam swabs and a toothbrush to remove dental plaque from approximal and crevice surfaces?

On the other hand, Robbins et al. (2003), in their study evaluating the effectiveness of a home visit and booklet in providing education to parents about infant illnesses, formulated their research questions in the form of objectives. As they explain, the objectives of the study were to evaluate the effects of the intervention on:

- the use of health services;
- parental feelings of confidence and knowledge of common childhood illnesses;
- parents' intention of carrying out home care activities for their child's symptoms;
- parents' intention of seeking professional advice.

One can see that the above questions and objectives have the potential of being translated into hypotheses such as 'foam swabs are more effective in removing dental plaque than toothbrushes' or 'A visit and a booklet will increase the use of health services by parents'. See how many hypotheses you can develop from the above questions and objectives.

Control

Experimental and control groups

To make sure that the intervention she has introduced is the only variable responsible for the outcome, the researcher can devise strategies to control extraneous variables. These are variables other than the experimental intervention that may also affect the outcome.

Suppose that a researcher uses an experimental design to test the effectiveness of counselling in the treatment of a group of depressed patients. She may find that after a series of counselling sessions, their conditions have improved. She cannot be certain, however, that they would not have got better anyway 'with the passing of time', or that other factors such as the drug treatment they were also receiving or their nursing care did not contribute to their improvement. To find out whether the counselling sessions were indeed the only contributing factor, she could have compared her group of patients with another group receiving no treatment. However, in healthcare settings it is likely that patients are receiving some form of treatment. She can, therefore, compare the group of patients receiving the counselling sessions with another group receiving the usual treatment. The group that is receiving the new intervention is called the *experimental group*, and the group with which the comparison is made is called the *control group*.

Because there is a possibility that some of the patients in one group may be more acutely ill or one group may comprise more women than men, for example, the researcher has to make sure that the two groups are similar in the main relevant characteristics, such as age, gender, social class, type and duration of depression, that may affect the recovery from depression. In this way, she will have more confidence that her results are unaffected by these variables. She has, therefore, exerted control over these extraneous variables. The main types of design that researchers used in their trial to control extraneous variables are between-subject (or parallel groups), crossover and single subject.

Between-subject or parallel groups design

By allocating subjects to either the experimental or the control group, the researcher is making a comparison between the two parallel groups of subjects. This type of control is known as between-subject or parallel groups design. It is the most common design in randomised controlled trials. In Robbins et al.'s (2003) study of 'minor illness education for parents of young children', the parents in the experimental group received a visit and booklet from the research nurse. The parents in the control group received only the service offered routinely by the health visitor.

Between-subject designs can have more than two groups. The number of groups depends on the purpose of the experiment. For example, in a study of the effects of relaxation, music and the combination of music and relaxation on postoperative pain, Good et al. (2001) allocated participants to one of the following four groups: group 1 – relaxation; group 2 – music; group 3 – music and relaxation; and group 4 – control.

The most important consideration in parallel groups trials is ensuring that the groups are similar in their key characteristics. If there were differences in, for example, age, gender or illness conditions in the profile of the groups, it would be difficult to attribute the results only to the intervention. One way to achieve an equalisation of groups is to randomly allocate the participants. Randomisation is the objective process of allocating participants to groups and is explained further in the next section. For an example of parallel design, see Research Example 24 above.

Within-subject or crossover design

Despite the efforts of researchers to select subjects with similar characteristics for the experimental and control groups, the fact remains that they are different groups of individuals and we can never be sure whether or not some of their differences, however negligible, account for differences, if any, in the outcome. To overcome this problem, the same group of people can sometimes serve as both the control and the experimental group. For example, if a researcher wants to find out whether aromatherapy can induce sleep in patients with sleeping problems, she can select a group of 20 patients, administer aromatherapy to 10 patients and give the other 10 their usual sedatives for a period of three weeks. She can then change this over, giving the first group their usual sedatives and the other group the aromatherapy. By comparing the results for each patient, the researcher can assess the effects of the new intervention. This type of allocation is called a crossover or within-subject design as it involves the same subjects 'crossing over' to the new intervention after receiving their usual treatment and vice versa.

Pearson and Hutton (2002) used a crossover design in their study on the effectiveness of foam swabs to remove dental plaque. They explain that participants were allocated to one of two groups (foam swabs or toothbrushes) for 1 week. In the second week, the treatments were reversed. This was done to 'ensure that any learning effect resulting from the order of treatment (tooth brushing or using foam swabs) could be assessed'. This design minimised the possibility of differences between groups as 'each person acted as their own control' (Pearson and Hutton, 2002).

The advantage of this type of design is that subjects are paired with themselves and therefore the patient characteristics are the same in both groups (Mills et al., 2009). Additionally, each participant counts as two because they receive both the intervention and the usual treatment. One of the main problems with the crossover design is related to the carry-over effect, which happens when the effect of the first treatment continues into the second treatment period. In the above example of aromatherapy and sleeping problems, it could happen that the aromatherapy the first group of patients received was so effective in relaxing them that its effects continued for a while even after the therapy had been discontinued. If this group were to have their usual sleeping tablets immediately after the aromatherapy was stopped, it would be difficult to assess whether their sleep was helped by their usual drug therapy or by the carry-over effects of aromatherapy. Researchers must pay particular attention to this problem and often leave a time gap between the two interventions.

Crossover trials are most popular for the study of new and developmental drugs and are best suited to trials related to symptomatic but chronic conditions or diseases (Mills et al., 2009). In Research Example 25, Shaygannejad et al. (2012) showed how they used a crossover design in their study of fatigue in people with multiple sclerosis.

A crossover trial

Comparison of the effect of aspirin and amantadine for the treatment of fatigue in multiple sclerosis *Shaygannejad et al. (2012)*

In this study, the authors compared the effects of two drugs (aspirin and amantadine) in a group of 52 patients with multiple sclerosis. These were divided into two groups. The first group received aspirin for 4 weeks, while the second received amantadine for the same period. After a 2-week washout period, they crossed over to receive the alternative treatment.

Comments

1 In this study, the authors allowed for a 2-week washout period to control for the possibility of the effects of the drugs lasting after the drugs had been administered.

2 As the same participants received the two treatments, the sample size is double what it would be if the usual control versus experimental group design had been used.

Research example 25

Single-subject design

One of the problems of experiments involving people in healthcare settings is finding large samples. Even when this is possible, it is difficult to allocate them into groups that are identical in relation to the relevant variables. The problem is further exacerbated when subjects, for various reasons, drop out of the experiments.

A single-subject or single-case design, on the other hand, minimises these logistical problems since it involves only one participant at a time (although obviously if the one participant drops out, the experiment has to be scrapped). In its simplest form, it involves a pre-test followed by an intervention and a post-test. For example, a single-subject design could be used in an experiment to find out the effect of relaxation therapy on stress in one particular patient. Baseline measurements can be taken to find out how stressed the patient is before receiving relaxation therapy. A post-test measurement will then determine whether or not the therapy has been effective. Such a design is known as the AB design, where A is the pre-test, B the post-test and the intervention the middle. It will, however, take more than just one intervention for a firm conclusion on the effect of relaxation therapy to be drawn. This will have to be repeated many times, especially on different days and if possible in different circumstances, to avoid other influences.

Single-case designs give researchers the opportunity to focus on an individual and therefore pay more attention to details. It is particularly suited to the principle of patient-centred care, since the interaction between the individual and the treatment is unique, although lessons learnt can be applied to other cases as well. This type of design is useful when little is known about the effectiveness of interventions coupled with difficulties in undertaking a large-scale conventional experiment. Much of child psychology developed from the work of Piaget, who based many of his theories on observations of his own children. In the field of learning, Skinner, Pavlov and Thorndike emphasised the importance of the intensive study of an individual in deriving an understanding of conditioning.

One of the major limitations of single-case designs is that their findings cannot be generalised to similar populations, since they are individual cases. Some single-design studies have more than one participant to increase the generalisability value of the findings. However, a conventional RCT with at least two groups and an adequate sample size would be required before the findings could be generalised to other similar populations. For an overview of the methodology, strengths, limitations and possible clinical applications of single-subject designs, see Janosky (2005). In Research Example 26, Sil et al. (2013) show the use of a single-subject design.

Research example 26

A single-subject design

Videogame distraction reduces behavioral distress in a preschool-aged child undergoing repeated burn dressing changes *Sil et al. (2013)*

In this study, a 4-year-old girl undergoing changes in burn dressing was recruited to test and compare the effectiveness of two interventions: passive versus interactive videogame distraction. In the interactive intervention the participant played a video game, and in the passive one, she watched a pre-recorded tape of the same game played by someone else. The outcome measured was the level of behavioural distress.

Baseline measurements (before the interventions were introduced) were taken three times. Each intervention was administered five times (in random sequence) and post-interventions measurements were taken after each of them.

Comments

1 Single-case designs resemble case studies since they tend to focus on one or a few cases. In fact, the authors of this study used the terms 'case study' and 'single-subject design' to describe their trial. Qualitative interviews were also undertaken with nurses, parents and the participant.

2 The single-subject design was appropriate as it would have been difficult to obtain the required sample size for a conventional two-group design.

3 The authors recognised the limited generalisability of the findings of their study and recommended a trial with larger sample.

Quasi-experiments

For a number of reasons, ethical and practical, it may sometimes not be possible to carry out true experiments in nursing and midwifery. For example, if a researcher introduces a new model of nursing in a ward, it is not feasible to randomly allocate patients to two groups in the same ward or even to allocate them to different wards because of clinical, organisational and ethical considerations. The best she can do is to compare the ward introducing the new model with a similar ward in the same hospital. Although the researcher has a new intervention, she does not have a 'proper' control group but a comparison group, as she cannot randomise subjects to each group. She has only partly met the criteria of a true experiment. In effect, she has carried out a quasi-experiment, a design that must have a new intervention but not necessarily a control group, and has no randomisation.

This type of experiment is appropriate in cases where the researcher seeks to introduce minimum disruption in a natural setting. Because in quasi-experiments researchers do not have the high degree of control over extraneous variables that is seen in true experiments, it is not possible to state with confidence that any new intervention is actually responsible for the effects measured. Therefore quasi-experiments cannot establish cause-and-effect relationships with certainty, but they can establish links.

There are a variety of quasi-experimental designs. At the very least, the researcher can introduce a new intervention into a group and measure the outcome. For example, relaxation therapy may be introduced to a group of patients, and the researcher may want to find out whether they report a decrease in their level of anxiety. This is the weakest form of experiment since there are no baseline scores (pre-test) and no other groups with which to compare the final scores.

The next step up is when a researcher measures the anxiety level prior to and after the introduction of relaxation therapy. This time, there is more confidence that a change has happened (if it has), although it is still difficult to establish with certainty that relaxation therapy is the cause, because a number of other factors may be implicated. To be more certain, the researcher may decide to have two groups: one experimental and one comparison. She measures the anxiety level on the experimental ward before and after the intervention. She also carries out the same measurements at the same time with patients on a similar ward (the comparison group) who did not receive relaxation therapy. She can then begin to have more confidence in her results. This last design is called a non-equivalent groups design. It may be that the subjects in both groups are similar in many respects but that the researcher did not have enough control over their selection and allocation to ensure that they were in fact equivalent.

Examples of quasi-experimental studies in nursing include 'The effectiveness of a disaster training programme for healthcare workers in Greece' (Bistaraki et al., 2011), 'Preventing belt restraint use in newly admitted residents in nursing homes' (Gulpers et al., 2012) and 'New media simulation stories in nursing education' (Webb-Corbett et al., 2013). See Research Example 27 for a study using a quasi-experimental approach.

A quasi-experimental study

Improvement of Iranian nurses' competence through professional portfolio *Bahreini et al. (2013)*

The aim of this study was to find out whether a 'portfolio-based professional development programme' had an effect on nurses' competence in a hospital in Iran. A pre-test/post-test, quasi-experimental design was used in which two wards were randomly allocated to the experimental group and two wards to the control group. Nurses in the experimental group participated in the portfolio programme, while those in the control group received routine professional development programmes.

Comments

1 This design is quasi-experimental because it meets two out of three criteria for an RCT: it has an intervention and a control group. However, the nurses themselves were not individually randomised to either the control or the experimental group.

2 The reason why nurses in this study could not be randomised is probably because it would have caused significant disruption to the clinical areas where this study was carried out. In such situations, randomisation of participants is not feasible.

Factorial designs

A factorial design is one in which the effect of two or more independent variables on one or more dependent variables can be tested in the same study. The term 'factor' in factorial designs refers to 'variables'. Factorial designs are particularly suited to the study of interactions between variables and of the 'added' value of using a combination of interventions. This type of design also allows for treatments (for example, drugs or psychosocial interventions) to be varied. The strength of the approach is that it can all be done in one study. For an example of a factorial design, see Research Example 28.

A factorial design in a randomised trial

The effect of two lottery-style incentives on response rates to postal questionnaires in a prospective cohort study in pre-school children at high risk of asthma: a randomised trial *van der Mark et al. (2012)*

The aim of this study was to find out if any of three lottery-style strategies would be effective in increasing response rates and retention in a study of asthma in pre-school children.

There were three intervention groups and a control group. The first intervention group had a chance to win, in a lottery style, a gift voucher only, the second a gift voucher and a day trip, and the third a day trip and no gift voucher; the fourth (control group) received neither a gift voucher nor a day trip. They were eligible to participate in the lottery or raffle only if they returned all the questionnaires at the end of the study.

Comments

1 The rationale for the factorial design trial was the lack of conclusive evidence on the effects of non-cash incentives in increasing response rates and promoting retention in research studies.

2 In this study, none of the lottery-style incentives reduced the loss to follow-up or the need for reminders, or increased response rates.

Randomisation

In experimental terms, randomisation means using an objective method or strategy to randomly allocate subjects to groups. There are different ways in which randomisation can be carried out. Some of the common types of randomisation are simple, matched pairs, cluster and block.

Simple randomisation

If a researcher decides to allocate participants to group A or group B, she can flip a coin or allocate participants alternatively to each group as they enter the study. This type of randomisation has an objective element (the chance of a head or tail) and a subjective element (the researcher may decide to flip the coin again if he does not want a particular participant to be in the group allocated by the coin). A more objective way is to use sealed, opaque envelopes with the letter A or B inside. These envelopes would be used by another person who is 'blind' to the trial to allocate subjects to groups. If a list of potential of participants is available, the allocation can be made by using numbers randomly allocated by computers or a table of random numbers freely available on the internet). Fincher et al. (2012), in their study of 'The effectiveness of a standardised preoperative preparation in reducing child and parent anxiety', used computer-generated random numbers for allocation to the intervention and control groups.

Matched pairs

One strategy that has been useful in ensuring that the subjects in the two groups are similar in the relevant characteristics is 'matching'. If a researcher requires an equal distribution of the following characteristics – women aged between 48 and 50, middle class and newly diagnosed with breast cancer – in her experimental and control groups, she will look for two women who meet these criteria and allocate one to each group until the required sample size is reached. This matched-pairs allocation technique is usually appropriate when the researcher knows in advance which variables to control. Also, as Dane (1990) points out, 'there is no end to the number of potential variables that may require matching, and therefore you can never be sure you have matched participants on all relevant characteristics'. Another limitation of this approach is that it can take a long time to find enough matched pairs for an adequate sample size. To partly overcome this problem, the researcher may try to match groups instead of pairs. For an example of matched pairs randomisation, see Vieira et al.'s (2012) study of reducing falls among older patients undergoing rehabilitation.

Cluster randomisation

Instead of randomising and allocating individuals to groups, researchers increasingly randomise clusters (for example, hospitals or schools) instead of individuals. For example, in Meyer et al.'s (2003) study of the effect on hip fractures of an increased use of hip protectors in nursing homes, a cluster was defined 'as a nursing home in itself or an independently working ward of a large nursing home'. Forty-nine clusters agreed to take part and, by randomisation, 25 clusters (with 459 residents) were allocated to the intervention group, with 24 clusters (483 residents) constituting the control group (Meyer et al., 2003). The Medical Research Council (2002) gives several reasons to explain when cluster randomisation is appropriate, including the following:

- The intervention to be studied is itself delivered to and affects groups of people rather than individuals. Examples include changes in general practice organisation and the use of local radio for health promotion.
- The intervention is targeted at health professionals with the aim of studying its impact on patient outcomes. An example would be education about guidelines for a particular medical condition; it would be difficult for professionals receiving such education not to let this affect the management of all of their patients.
- The intervention is given to individuals but might affect others within that cluster – that is, there might be contamination. For example, the recipients of a behavioural intervention to promote weight loss or reduce smoking might share their information with others attending the same clinic.
- If the intervention involves supplying equipment or staff to an administrative unit, the randomisation of these units rather than individuals would mean that only a subset of the units would receive the equipment or staff. This might be cheaper or administratively more convenient.

The unit of analysis can be the clusters or individuals. If analysis is at the level of individuals, the sample size has to be increased in order to compensate for the differences between clusters. Informed consent could be a problem, but the need for individual informed consent should not be ignored in cluster randomisation.

There has been a large increase in the numbers of trials using cluster randomisation. For bibliometric surveys on cluster randomisation trials, see Bland (2004).

Random block design

Conventional randomisation may produce groups that have similar profiles. For example, after randomisation, the average age of participants in the control group and experimental group may be similar. However, the age distribution may not be similar. Therefore, although it looks as if the groups are similar in 'average' age, in fact one group may comprise mainly middle-aged people and the other, half younger and half older people (Ross, 1999).

The randomised block design may offset this weakness in conventional randomisation by grouping participants who share the same characteristics (for example, age, gender, condition or behaviour) so that 'like' can be compared with 'like'. Participants are matched and put into groups. The groups are then randomly selected to be either control or experimental. The number of groups depends on the purpose of the study. One of the limitations of this design is the difficulty involved in managing a large number of groups and in getting adequate sample sizes for each. Wu et al. (2004) reported that they used 'the variables of age, sex, pulmonary function, smoking, and steroid use to match (block)' the participants in their study of 'acupressure in improving dyspnoea in chronic obstructive pulmonary disease'.

Placebos and blind techniques

Two other strategies to control extraneous variables are the use of placebos and blind techniques in experimental designs.

Placebos

The idea of receiving a new form of treatment can itself make some people feel better. If some subjects in an experiment have high expectations of a new drug or other form of treatment being tested, this can affect the results of the study. To overcome the possible suggestive effect of the new intervention, a placebo – a substance that has no pharmacological or therapeutic property – can be administered to one group for comparison purposes. It is made, as much as possible, to resemble the new drug or treatment.

Kleijnen et al. (1994) point out that in any medical intervention there is some degree of placebo effect, which includes the perception of the therapist by the patient, the effect of the therapeutic setting and the credibility of the medication itself (size, shape, colour, taste). In a study comparing the effectiveness of oral vitamin B12 and placebos for patients suspected of subtle cobalamin deficiency, Favrat et al. (2011) explained that both the vitamin and placebo pills were similar in appearance and taste and were given in a similar container. For another example of the use of placebos in an experiment, see Moore's (2001) study comparing the effectiveness of amethocaine gel with a placebo in the management of procedural pain in neonates.

It is often not possible to devise a placebo to match a psychosocial intervention, such as counselling. For this reason, the use of a placebo is uncommon. Most clinical trials test the best known (usual) treatment against the new treatment.

Single-blind and double-blind techniques

Being aware of which interventions the control and experimental groups are receiving may introduce bias on the part of the subjects and researchers. Patients may have a preference for a particular drug with which they are familiar, or may have high expectations of the new therapy being tested. These may influence their assessment of the interventions. Researchers, too, may be biased in favour of the intervention being tested, and this may affect their observations and recording of data. To avoid these types of influence, it is possible, especially when two 'drugs' look and taste similar, as when placebos are used, not to let the subjects and the health professional know whether they are in the experimental or the control group. For ethical reasons, their informed consent for taking part in the experiment must be obtained. 'Blinding' or 'masking' is the term used to indicate that those taking part in the trial are not aware of who are allocated in what groups.

A single-blind trial is one in which either the participants or the researchers are unaware of the allocation to groups. In a single-blind RCT of the effectiveness of telephone counselling in improving breastfeeding practices (Tahir and Al-Sadat, 2013), only the researcher collecting outcome data was blinded to the group allocation. This is because the women were aware of what they were receiving and the counsellors were aware of which group was receiving the intervention. With psychosocial interventions, it is difficult to conceal group allocation from the participants and the persons giving the treatment.

A design in which both the subjects and the therapists are unaware of which drug each group is receiving is called a double-blind trial. A triple-blind design is one in which those who collect and analyse the data (researchers) are also not aware of the group allocation. For an example of a double-blind, placebo-controlled, parallel group (one control and one intervention) RCT, see Fagerström et al. (2010).

Internal and external validity

An RCT is an experiment in which subjects are randomly allocated to one or more control groups and to one or more experimental groups, depending on the number of interventions. It is a popular type of experiment for testing the effectiveness of drugs and other forms of therapies, and is increasingly being used to assess the effectiveness and cost-efficiency of other types of interventions, services and policies as well. The uses and limitations of RCTs are discussed later in this chapter.

The purpose of experiments in nursing and healthcare in general is ultimately to contribute to better treatment, care and other services. The usefulness of their findings, however, depends on their internal and external validity. Internal validity is the extent to which changes, if any, in the dependent variable can be said to have been caused by the independent variable alone. External validity is the extent to which the findings of an experiment can be applied or generalised to other similar populations and settings.

Internal validity

A number of unwanted factors internal to the study can, on their own or combined, interfere with the experiment and make it difficult to conclude with confidence that the findings reflect the true relationship between the two variables being investigated and nothing else. The purpose of control is precisely to eliminate or minimise these unwanted effects. Brennan and Croft (1994) ask two questions that can be used to assess the internal validity of an experiment:

1   To what extent might flaws in the study design have biased the study result?
2   If the result is thought to be free from bias, to what extent might other causes have confounded the observed association?

From these questions emerge two terms central to the understanding of internal validity: biases and confounders. Biases can be present at every stage of an experiment, from the admission of subjects to the experiment to the interpretation and reporting of findings. On the other hand, some factors in the study may work in the same or opposite direction to the independent variable and therefore affect the dependent variable. These factors or variables are known as confounders or confounding variables. The following hypothetical experiment gives an example of confounders.

A teacher carries out an experiment to investigate the effectiveness of a new study method: self-directed learning. She allocates 20 students to the experimental (self-directed learning) group and 20 students to the control group, the latter being exposed to their usual teaching method (lectures). The teacher then compares the students' knowledge at the end of the module and finds that those receiving lectures have a higher knowledge score than do the self-directed learning students. She had 'controlled' other variables such as age, gender and educational level to prevent these from influencing the results by making sure that, on average, both groups had students of the same age and educational level and had an equal number of males and females.

However, one variable of which she may have been aware but which she found difficult to control was the 'learning ability' of each student. It could be that the learning ability of those receiving lectures was higher than that of the other group. The researcher cannot state with confidence that the lecture is the better method of imparting knowledge, nor can she know whether the difference in the two groups' learning abilities is responsible for the difference in knowledge scores. In this experiment, 'learning ability' may be a confounding variable as it may be confounding, or confusing, the results. On the other hand, the researcher may also find that some members of the lecture group have also been exposed to a television programme on their module topic during the course of the experiment. She was powerless to do anything to prevent this as she learnt about it after the experiment had been completed. Therefore, 'exposure to the TV programme' is a confounding variable. Researchers may be aware of such variables and be unable to control them, or may be unaware of them. Their task is to speculate on the effects of all possible confounders as they are more familiar with their study than are those reading the report.

The random allocation of subjects should remove possible confounders by making the groups more or less similar in their relevant characteristics, but it does not always do so. It may happen, for example, that by randomly allocating patients with the same type of illness to two groups, one group ends up with some patients who are more acutely ill than the other group. The severity or acuteness of the illness can therefore constitute a confounding variable. This has the potential to affect the results, especially if a drug or therapy is the subject of an experiment. It is sometimes possible to make an allowance for such effects when the data are analysed and interpreted. However, such undesirable interference from confounding variables can and must be avoided where possible.

Biases and confounders threaten the internal validity of experiments, hence the term 'threats to internal validity'. Cook and Campbell (1979) have identified a number of factors that can affect study findings. Some of these will be used here to assess the internal validity of experiments. These are history, maturation, testing, instrumentation, selection, mortality and statistical regression.

History effects

A history effect is produced whenever some uncontrolled event alters the participants' responses (Dane, 1990). In the above experiment on teaching methods, the uncontrolled event is the television programme that was shown during the time the experiment took place. An example of a historical effect comes from a study by Berg et al. (1994) on 'nurses' creativity, tedium and burnout', in which the authors speculate that the 'results may have been affected by factors of an individual or social type'. They explained that 'there was a large organisational change in the public sector during the intervention which meant that both wards were completely reorganized from the county council to the community and also Sweden, in general, was facing increasing unemployment'.

Maturation effects

Some changes in people's behaviour and attitudes can happen over time with or without a specific intervention. For example, an intervention designed to reduce the anxiety of patients newly admitted to hospital may account for a reduction in anxiety when the pre-test scores and the post-test scores are compared. However, it could be that patients were less anxious with the passing of time because they were becoming more familiar with their surroundings and with staff. This type of effect is known as maturation. It is a threat to internal validity 'due to the respondent's growing older, wiser, stronger, more experienced, and the like between pretest and posttest' (Cook and Campbell, 1979).

Testing effects

The process of repeated testing can itself affect performance. People can alter their answers in the post-test if they obtained low scores in the pre-test. They may also have thought about their performance in between tests or become more familiar with the test format. Differences in scores may be only partly due to the intervention. Therefore testing is a threat to internal validity if it is not 'controlled' as part of the experiment.

Instrumentation effects

The measuring process itself can be biased. The choice of data collection methods may also reflect the researcher's preference and may not be the most appropriate for the study. For example, Allen et al. (1992), in their study of the 'effectiveness of a preoperative teaching programme for cataract patients', admitted that the questionnaire they had developed had some limitations. They explained:

> the areas of knowledge tested may not be the most important ones despite a content review by ophthalmic nurses and ophthalmologists. A true–false format was perceived by the researchers to be the most appropriate for elderly subjects. Although subjects did not have difficulty in answering this kind of question, it may be that another format would be more appropriate. A common problem with measuring tools is that they are sometimes not sensitive enough to measure the small differences between experimental and control group scores.

Selection effects

There are at least two points in the selection of participants at which bias can 'creep in'. Although the experimenter can set inclusion criteria (such as patients of a certain age group who are not seriously ill), she still has to make a judgement about whom to include or exclude. Assessing the severity of illnesses is not as straightforward as it seems: it involves a degree of subjectivity. The allocation of subjects to groups can also give rise to bias. The more objective the allocation of subjects, the less likely it is to be biased.

Mortality effects

Researchers take care in allocating subjects so that groups are as far as possible similar in all the important characteristics. When subjects drop out, either because they die, cannot tolerate treatment or simply want to stop taking part, it can create an imbalance between the groups. The loss of participants to a study is known as mortality or attrition. Not only do the groups become smaller in size, but they may also become dissimilar in the relevant characteristics. In fact, the benefits of randomisation can be undermined by mortality, especially in cases where the number of drop-outs is not even between groups. The reasons why subjects fail to complete the experiment must be made clear and must be taken into account in the analysis of data.

Internal validity is the crucial test that every experiment should pass. As Cook and Campbell (1979) explain:

Estimating the internal validity of a relationship is a deductive process in which the investigator has to systematically think through how each of the internal validity threats may have influenced the data. Then, the investigator has to examine the data to test which relevant threats can be ruled out. In all of this process, the researcher has to be his or her own best critic, trenchantly examining all of the threats he or she can imagine.

Your task as a reader is to assess the extent to which the researcher does this and to think of possible biases and confounders that may have been overlooked but which may have affected the findings.

Internal validity is not an all-or-nothing issue. It is more a question of the extent to which an experiment has internal validity, as it is not possible to be aware of, or eliminate the effects of, all biases and confounders. The validity of the findings is determined by checks on biases and extraneous variables. The list of all possible confounders must be exhausted before a causal relationship between the variables under study can be established.

Statistical regression

Statistical regression, also known as regression to the mean, has been used to explain differences between pre-test and post-test scores. It is a statistical phenomenon that can make natural variations in repeated data look like real change (Barnett et al., 2005). Statistical regression is the tendency of high or low scores (outliers) to come closer to the mean (regression) when measured for the second time. This is because it is believed that very high scores and very low scores occur by chance, and the chance of this happening is lower than for scores that reflect the mean or average. This can be illustrated by an example from the television card game show *Play Your Cards Right*. Participants are asked to guess whether the next card is higher or lower than the previous one. Inevitably when, for example, a 10 of hearts is shown, the next card is predicted to be lower. Participants seem to estimate that the chance of a lower number coming up is greater than that of a higher number (as there are fewer cards above than under 10).

In research, statistical regression can be a threat to validity, in particular in single-group trials. The absence of a control group makes it difficult to ascertain whether the difference in pre-test and post-test scores is due to the intervention or to chance. As very high or very low scores have a tendency to regress to the mean, one should be careful in interpreting the results of trials when the pre-test scores are unusually much higher than the mean.

External validity

The internal validity of a study is a necessary but not sufficient condition for its findings to be generalisable to other similar populations and settings; it must also have external validity. An experiment takes place in a particular setting with a specific group of people at a particular time. Together, these factors contribute to make the experiment a unique happening. The question to ask is, 'Can its findings apply readily to similar populations in different settings?' For this to be possible, the population and setting of the experiment must closely approximate the population and setting where the findings are to be used. For example, if a study shows that giving relevant information prior to surgery relieves postoperative stress, does this mean that giving information to preoperative surgical patients in hospitals other than where the experiment was carried out would also relieve their postoperative stress? Does information-giving have the same effect in a ward where the atmosphere is relaxed and nurses are attentive to patients' concerns as in another ward where the atmosphere is tense and the nurse–patient relationship leaves a lot to be desired?

The main threat to external validity comes from the selection and allocation of subjects. Randomisation in experiments means the random allocation of available subjects to groups. It does not mean that the samples are representative of the target populations (see Chapter 15). Subjects in experiments are typically recruited at the time of diagnosis or admission to hospital. These can be described as accidental samples and are convenient, since the potential subjects happen to present themselves at the time of recruitment. Seldom are sample frames available from which representative samples can be drawn. RCTs also recruit volunteers, who are then randomly allocated to groups. It may be that by taking subjects who are available or who volunteer, most of those who come forward are from an educated and middle-class background, and see the experiment as an opportunity to do something about their health. What randomisation does is simply to allocate randomly those who come forward, for the purpose of having equal groups.

Not all those who are available or who volunteer are recruited to an experimental study. The researcher normally selects a sample by specifying inclusion or exclusion criteria. Those who are physically or mentally incapacitated and those who cannot speak the country's language are often excluded. In this way, the sample is 'sanitised'.

When evaluating an experiment, you can use the different aspects of internal and external validity discussed here as a 'checklist'. You will find that not all authors provide enough information on their experiments for you to carry out an evaluation effectively. One of the common omissions is information related to the intervention received by the control group. While a detailed description of the new intervention may be provided, the control group's intervention is simply described as the 'usual treatment'. Some researchers forget that while they may be familiar with the 'usual treatment', many readers are not.

For example, in one study on the effect of an educational programme on the knowledge and attitude of patients to a particular topic, the teaching methods, the content and the duration of the programme that the experimental group received were described in detail. No such information was available about the control group. When no significant difference in knowledge and attitude was found, the researcher was at pains to explain why this was so. Attempts were made to explain what the control group 'would have received' rather than what they 'actually' received. It was not clear how much attention the researcher gave to finding out what the control group was exposed to. It is difficult to assess the internal validity of an experiment that sets out to compare two interventions when information on one intervention is not adequate.

Information about randomisation is sometimes lacking. Readers must be made aware of the precise method of random allocation and its implication for the internal or external validity of the findings.

Ethics of experiments

A number of ethical issues raised here apply equally to non-experimental research. Because experiments involve interventions by the researcher, they have more potential for causing physical and mental harm. There is an unequal distribution of power between the experimenter and the subject, more power resting with the former. The researcher also has power over whom to enter into the experiment and who should receive the current or the new treatment, except where randomisation is used. This unequal power relationship is evident in the fact that researchers possess information about the experiment and its implications, and control how much is given to participants. Participants sometimes actively seek to be included in clinical trials if they perceive that they will receive better treatment.

There are, however, rules of ethical conduct which, if followed, can to some extent prevent abuse on the part of researchers. Ethical research committees exist for the purpose of ensuring that participants' rights and well-being are protected. Clinicians and managers can and should also act as gatekeepers in order to protect patients' interests.

When ethical issues of research are discussed in articles and reports, the main aspects dealt with are often anonymity and confidentiality. While these are undoubtedly important, researchers must also be concerned with the physical and mental harm that can be done to participants in experiments. Causing them to worry is stressful enough. As regards clinical trials, Fetter et al. (1989) ask 'three central questions': 'Is experimentation with human subjects justified?', 'Do the possible benefits of conducting the study outweigh the potential risks?' and 'Has informed consent been respected?' Let us now look at each of these questions.

Is experimentation with human subjects justified?

Clinicians 'do things' to people all the time without being fully aware of their effectiveness. As explained earlier in this chapter, this form of trial and error is itself a form of 'back door' and uncontrolled 'experimentation'. At least research experiments are more in the open, with the result that participants' rights can be more protected. The purpose of clinical trials is to assess the effectiveness of particular treatments and to learn more about them for the benefit of more people than those included in the experiment.

Experiments should only be carried out when necessary. Just because patients are a captive population does not mean that they should be used by anyone wishing to 'prove' anything.

Do the possible benefits of conducting the study outweigh the potential risks?

If clinical trials are carried out to assess the effectiveness of particular drugs or other therapies, it stands to reason that in cases where this information is already available, there is no need for the experiment unless the evidence is inconclusive and the intention is to replicate the study. No experiment can be justified if patients are denied the best available treatment for the purpose of experimentation. When an experiment is carried out, researchers must ensure that control groups are given the best available treatment.

Has informed consent been respected?

Patients entering trials are often in a vulnerable position as well as being a captive population. They may be in a confused state, especially if they have just learnt that they have an illness. One can also ask whether or not they are in a position to refuse to take part in an experiment, especially in cases where the clinicians treating them are also the researchers involved in the study.

While researchers may believe that randomisation is a fairer way to allocate subjects to control or experimental groups, some patients want to have a choice of groups. It also shows that patients are not as 'passive' as one might think. However, there is no doubt that some may feel obliged to take part for one reason or another.

People approached to take part in a study should be fully informed of its implications, and of their right to refuse or withdraw at any time during the experiment. Their informed consent should be sought prior to the study, and this consent must be offered free from pressure of any kind. Researchers have a vested interest in recruiting participants to their study. Giving information on the negative implications of the experiment may lead to refusal to participate. Where the number of potential participants is large, this may not be an issue, but when participants are hard to recruit, it may create a tension between the obligation to provide 'balanced' information and the need to recruit.

In the case of single- or double-blind experiments, the question of telling patients which treatment is the placebo negates the purpose of blindness in the study. However, giving a tablet of no pharmacological property or an injection of sterile water in an attempt to deceive patients into thinking that they are real treatments is an infringement of their rights. Researchers must, however, tell patients that a placebo is used in the experiment and that they may or may not receive it. It is up to them to accept or refuse to take part.

Debriefing participants can help to bring them back to earth. However, one can still question the ethics of the intensive monitoring of patients during the period of the experiment, only to leave them alone feeling abandoned once the data have been collected. The security afforded during their interactions with researchers is suddenly removed at the end of the experiment. If the treatment has been beneficial, drug manufacturers sometimes make 'compassionate supplies' freely available to participants who leave a trial.

No experiment is more important than the right of individuals to privacy and safety. Researchers must examine their own conscience and motives when taking decisions that can affect the participants' well-being. The role of ethics committees, practitioners and managers as gatekeepers and advocates for patients and others who take part in experiments is of the utmost importance.

RCTs in nursing

Nursing, like all other health professions, needs to justify its practice on sound evidence. The RCT is generally considered to be the most appropriate study design for evaluating the effects of an intervention mainly because, when properly conducted, it limits the risk of bias (Centre for Reviews and Dissemination, 2009). The variation in nursing practice for the same condition is well documented in the literature (see Chapter 1). The RCT has the potential to compare existing practices or to evaluate new ones.

In a MEDLINE and hand search, Cullum (1997) found 522 'reports of RCTs' that evaluated aspects of nursing care between 1966 and 1994 (28 years). A quick search on the MEDLINE database (1946 to 27 August 2013) using a combination of the terms 'randomised controlled trial.mp.', 'randomized controlled trial. mp. or Randomized Controlled Trial/' and 'nursing.mp. or Nursing/' identified 5,433 items. A further similar search with the terms 'quasi-experiment.mp.', 'quasi-experimental.mp.' and 'nursing.mp. or Nursing/' showed 1,117 items. It seems that nurses have overcome much of the 'apparent antipathy to RCTs' reported by Shuldham and Hiley (1997). Some of the recent examples of RCTs in nursing include:

- tailored nursing interventions to improve enrolment in cardiac rehabilitation (Cossette et al., 2012);
- web-based nursing intervention for the self-management of pain after cardiac surgery (Martorella et al., 2012);
- cardiovascular risk management by practice nurses supported by self-monitoring in primary care (Tiessen et al., 2012);
- a 21-month randomised controlled trial of patient satisfaction with nursing consultations in a rheumatology outpatient clinic RCT for patients with inflammatory arthritides (Koksvik et al., 2013).

Evaluating experiments

When evaluating a research study, the first task is to make sense of the information provided in the article or report. In the case of experimental studies, it is vital to look for the hypothesis (or hypotheses) or objectives, and to identify the independent and dependent variables. The next step is to find out how they are operationally defined. If the experimental hypothesis is that 'the use of an information booklet will lead to an increase in knowledge', readers must be clear about what the 'information booklet' consists of, how the participants 'use' it and how 'knowledge' is measured. Does a list of questions adequately measure participants' knowledge? In health research, the criteria for measuring outcomes can reflect professional prejudices. For example, if the hypothesis is 'dressing A is more effective than dressing B in the treatment of leg ulcers', the 'effectiveness' outcome can be measured by the time each type of dressing takes to heal the wound. However, other criteria, such as the side effects of the dressing or the degree of comfort of patients with it should also be part of the outcomes to be assessed.

The population taking part in experiments must be clearly defined. Readers need to know what the inclusion criteria are, as this has implications for the generalisability of the findings. A description of subjects in each group with reference to the relevant variables must be given. It is not enough to say that the groups are similar in important characteristics such as age, gender or educational background. Figures must be provided to allow readers to decide for themselves whether this is the case. Not all crude data can or should be made available. However, data on the profile of subjects in each group are important because any of their characteristics could be a confounding variable. An important piece of information often withheld is the illness condition of the subjects in the two groups. Without knowing how similar or different the groups are, it is difficult to decide with certainty that severity of illness is not a confounding factor.

As explained earlier, researchers often omit to give adequate information about the treatment of control groups. Readers need to know whether both groups have received the same attention and care apart from the experimental drug or intervention. Could it be that in testing 'the effects of information giving on anxiety levels', the fact that those in the experimental group had someone to talk to was enough to reduce their anxiety? Did those in the control group receive the same amount of attention from the experimenters?

The allocation of subjects to the experimental and control groups can in itself be biased. Many reviewers would simply not bother to read about an experiment if it were not randomised. When subjects are randomised, the precise method of allocation must be described for readers to decide whether there is a possibility that bias may have crept in.

Researchers must also explain clearly who was 'blind' in the experiment and how this was achieved. The difficulty in maintaining blindness was discussed earlier. You must look for assurances from the researcher that adequate measures were taken to ensure blindness. For example, in a ward where some patients are given the experimental intervention and others the usual one, how can the experimenter be sure that the subjects did not talk to each other?

Those who have left or have been withdrawn from the experiment must also be accounted for: it could be that the new intervention did not work for them. In any case, subject 'mortality' must be taken into account in the analysis and interpretation of data and should not be ignored.

The precise method of data analysis must also be clearly described and the findings stated unambiguously. To evaluate the validity and reliability of the findings, the factors identified in the previous section, such as history, instrumentation, selection and mortality effects, must be considered. Researchers must identify the limitations of their study. In practice, it is rare that experimenters do not suspect confounding variables of having interfered with the experiment. Therefore those who do not discuss the possible effects of confounders run the risk of taking their findings at face value. Finally, you must assess whether the findings, if valid and reliable, are applicable to your own clinical situation.

Systematic reviews of RCTs have revealed a number of deficiencies in the reporting of trials. The Consolidated Standards of Reporting Trials (CONSORT) statement was developed to help authors improve their reporting by use of a checklist and flow diagram (Moher et al., 2001; Schulz et al., 2010). Checklists for evaluating and appraising RCTs are readily available on the internet. Helpful sites include the Scottish Intercollegiate Guidelines Network, Healthcare Improvement Scotland (http://www.sign.ac.uk/methodology/checklists.html) and the Cochrane Principles of Critical Appraisal (http://ph.cochrane.org/sites/ph.cochrane.org/files/uploads/Unit_Eight.pdf).

Summary

In this chapter, we have explained the meaning of 'experiment' and identified the main characteristics of a true experiment as intervention, control and randomisation. Different types of design, such as between-subject, within-subject and single-case, have been highlighted, as have the main differences between true and quasi-experiments.

We have shown that experiments have strengths and weaknesses, as do other approaches. The methodological problems and ethical implications can, to some extent, be managed. The number of experiments in nursing has increased in recent years, and there are numerous examples of nursing practice issues that have been explored with the use of the experimental design. Quasi-experiments, RCTs and other research designs can all contribute towards the pool of nursing and human knowledge.

References

Allen M, Knight C, Falk C and Strang V (1992) Effectiveness of a preoperative teaching programme for cataract patients. *Journal of Advanced Nursing*, **17**:303–9.

Austvoll-Dahlgren A, Bjørndal A, Odgaard-Jensen J and Helseth S (2012) Evaluation of a web portal for improving public access to evidence-based health information and health literacy skills: a pragmatic trial. *PLoS ONE*, **7**, 5:e37715.

Bahreini M, Moattari M, Shahamat S, Dobaradaran S and Ravanipour M (2013) Improvement of Iranian nurses' competence through professional portfolio: a quasi-experimental study. *Nursing and Health Sciences*, **15**, 1:51–7.

Barnett A G, van der Pols J C and Dobson A J (2005) Regression to the mean: what it is and how to deal with it. *International Journal of Epidemiology*, **34**, 1:215–20.

Berg A, Hansson U W and Hallberg I R (1994) Nurses' creativity, tedium and burnout during 1 year of clinical supervision and implementation of individually planned nursing care: comparison between a ward for severely demented patients and a similar control ward. *Journal of Advanced Nursing*, **20**:742–9.

Bistaraki A, Waddington K and Galanis P (2011) The effectiveness of a disaster training programme for healthcare workers in Greece. *International Nursing Review*, **58**, 3:341–6.

Bland J M (2004) Cluster randomised trials in the medical literature: two bibliometric surveys. *BMC Medical Research Methodology*, **4**:21–7.

Brennan P and Croft P (1994) Interpreting the results of observational research: chance is not such a fine thing. *British Medical Journal*, **309**:727–30.

Centre for Reviews and Dissemination (2009) *Systematic Reviews: CRD's Guidance for Undertaking Reviews in Health Care* (University of York: CRD).

Cook T D and Campbell D T (1979) *Quasi-experimentation: Design and Analysis Issues in Field Settings* (Boston, MA: Houghton Mifflin).

Cossette S, Frasure-Smith N, Dupuis J, Juneau M and Guertin M C (2012) Randomized controlled trial of tailored nursing interventions to improve cardiac rehabilitation enrollment. *Nursing Research* **61**, 2:111–20.

Cullum N (1997) Identification and analysis of randomised controlled trials in nursing: a preliminary study. *Quality in Health Care*, **6**, 1:2–6.

Dane F C (1990) *Research Methods* (Belmont, CA: Brooks/Cole).

Fagerström K, Gilljam H, Metcalfe M, Tonstad S and Messig M (2010) Stopping smokeless tobacco with varenicline: randomised double blind placebo controlled trial. *British Medical Journal*, **341**:c6549.

Favrat B, Vaucher P, Herzig L et al. (2011) Oral vitamin B12 for patients suspected of subtle cobalamin deficiency: a multicentre pragmatic randomised controlled trial. *BMC Family Practice*, **12**:2.

Fetter M S, Feetham S L, D'Apolito K et al. (1989) Randomized controlled trials: issues for researchers. *Nursing Research*, **38**, 2:117–20.

Fincher W, Shaw J and Ramelet A S (2012) The effectiveness of a standardised preoperative preparation in reducing child and parent anxiety: a single-blind randomised controlled trial. *Journal of Clinical Nursing*, **21**, 7–8:946–55.

Good M, Stanton-Hicks M, Grass J A et al. (2001) Relaxation and music to reduce post-surgical pain. *Journal of Advanced Nursing*, **33**,2: 208–15.

Gulpers M J, Bleijlevens M H, Capezuti E, van Rossum E, Ambergen T and Hamers J P (2012) Preventing belt restraint use in newly admitted residents in nursing homes. *International Journal of Nursing Studies*, **49**, 12:1473–9.

Iglesias B, Ramos F, Serrano B et al. (2013) A randomized controlled trial of nurses vs. doctors in the resolution of acute disease of low complexity in primary care. *Journal of Advanced Nursing*, **69**, 11: 2446–57.

Janosky J E (2005) Use of the single subject design for practice based primary care research. *Postgraduate Medical Journal*, **81**: 549–51.

Kleijnen J, de Craen J M, Van Everdingen J and Krol L (1994) Placebo effect in double-blind clinical trials: a review of interactions with medications. *Lancet*, **344**:1347–9.

Koksvik H S, Hagen K B, Rodevand E, Mowinckel P, Kvien T K and Zangi H A (2013) Patient satisfaction with nursing consultations in a rheumatology outpatient clinic: a 21-month randomised controlled trial in patients with inflammatory arthritides. *Annals of the Rheumatic Diseases*, **72**, 6:836–43.

Martorella G, Côté J, Racine M and Choinière M (2012) Web-based nursing intervention for self-management of pain after cardiac surgery: pilot randomized controlled trial. *Journal of Medical Internet Research*, **14**, 6:e177.

Medical Research Council (2002) *Cluster Randomized Trials: Methodological and Ethical Considerations*. MRC Clinical Trials Series (London: MRC).

Meyer G, Warnke A, Bender R and Mühlhauser I (2003) Effect on hip fractures of increased use of hip protectors in nursing homes: a cluster randomised controlled trial. *British Medical Journal*, **326**:76.

Mills E J, Chan A-N, Wu P, Vail A, Guyatt G H and Altman D G (2009) Design, analysis, and presentation of crossover trials. *Trials*, 10:27.

Moher D, Schulz K F and Altman D G (2001) The CONSORT statement: revised 6 recommendations for improving the quality of reports of parallel-group randomised trials. *Lancet*, **357**:1191–4.

Moore J (2001) No more tears: a randomized controlled double-blind trial of amethocaine gel vs. placebo in the management of procedural pain in neonates. *Journal of Advanced Nursing*, **34**, 4:475–82.

Pearson L S and Hutton J L (2002) A controlled trial to compare the ability of foam swabs and toothbrushes to remove dental plaque. *Journal of Advanced Nursing*, **39**, 5:480–9.

Robbins H, Hundley V and Osman L M (2003) Minor illness education for parents of young children. *Journal of Advanced Nursing*, **44**, 3:238–47.

Roland M and Togerson D J (1998) Understanding controlled trials. What are pragmatic trials? *British Medical Journal*, **316**:285.

Ross N (1999) Randomised block design is more powerful than minimisation. *British Medical Journal*, **318**:263.

Schulz K F, Altman D G, Moher D et al. (2010) CONSORT 2010 Statement: updated guidelines for reporting parallel group randomised trials. *British Medical Journal*, **340**:698–702.

Shaygannejad V, Janghorbani M, Ashtari F and Zakeri H (2012) Comparison of the effect of aspirin and amantadine for the treatment of fatigue in multiple sclerosis: a randomized, blinded, crossover study. *Neurological Research*, **34**, 9:854–8.

Shuldham C and Hiley C (1997) Randomised controlled trials in clinical practice: the continuing debate. *Nursing Times Research*, **2**, 2:128–34.

Sil S, Dahlquist L M and Burns A J (2013) Case study. Videogame distraction reduces behavioral distress in a preschool-aged child undergoing repeated burn dressing changes: a single-subject design. *Journal of Pediatric Psychology*, **38**, 3:330–41.

Stulz N, Hepp U, Gächter C, Martin-Soelch C, Spindler A and Milos G (2013) The severity of ADHD and eating disorder symptoms: a correlational study. *BMC Psychiatry*, 13:44 .

Tahir N M and Al-Sadat N (2013) Does telephone lactation counselling improve breastfeeding practices?: a randomised controlled trial. *International Journal of Nursing Studies*, **50**:16–25.

Tiessen A H, Smit A J, Broer J, Groenier K H and van der Meer K (2012) Randomized controlled trial on cardiovascular risk management by practice nurses supported by self-monitoring in primary care. *BMC Family Practice*, **13**:90.

van der Mark L B, van Wonderen K E, Mohrs J, Bindels P J E, Puhan M A and Ler Riet G (2012) The effect of two lottery-style incentives on response rates to postal questionnaires in a prospective cohort study in pre-school children at high risk of asthma: a randomised trial. *BMC Medical Research Methodology*, **12**:186.

Vieira E R, Berean C, Paches D et al. (2012) Reducing falls among geriatric rehabilitation patients: a controlled clinical trial. *Clinical Rehabilitation*, **27**, 4:325–35.

Webb-Corbett R, Schwartz M R, Green B, Sessoms A and Swanson M (2013) New media simulation stories in nursing education: a quasi-experimental study exploring learning outcomes. *Computers, Informatics, Nursing*, **31**, 4:198–203.

Wu H S, Wu S C, Lin J G and Lin L (2004) Effectiveness of acupressure in improving dyspnoea in chronic obstructive pulmonary disease. *Journal of Advanced Nursing*, **45**, 3:252–9.

Phenomenological Research

12

> Nothing ever becomes real till it is experienced.
>
> John Keats

Introduction

Phenomenology, as a research method, is one of the most popular approaches in nursing research. In this chapter, we will briefly trace the origin of phenomenology and describe the main ideas of the different versions of phenomenology. This is followed by an outline of three commonly used phenomenological research methods. The value and limitations of phenomenology to research will also be discussed.

Phenomenological research in nursing

Phenomenology is an established approach in nursing research. There is no doubt that one of the attractions of phenomenology is its focus on the experience of individuals. Nurses and other health professionals care for people with a wide range of experiences that impact on how they perceive, access and use services, and how they react to and cope with illness. Although there is a range of methodologies to study patient experience, qualitative approaches, in particular phenomenology, offer a unique 'entry' into the world of patients. Knowing what and how people experience illness and related issues can enable health professionals to help patients on their journey from diagnosis to recovery.

Yet the phenomenological method can be one of the most difficult qualitative approaches to put into practice in a research study. A recent systematic review, by Norlyk and Harder (2010), of 88 articles representing 41 journals revealed 'considerable variations ranging from brief to detailed descriptions of the stated phenomenological approach, and from inconsistencies to methodological clarity and rigor'. There were omissions relating to how the selected approach was implemented. These variations, inconsistencies and omissions make unclear the extent to which, if at all, some of these studies were indeed phenomenological.

One of the reasons why researchers find it challenging and confusing when undertaking a phenomenological study is because 'phenomenology' as a philosophy itself is difficult to understand, unless one is a philosophy scholar and/or fluent in the languages (German and French) in which the original texts were mainly written. While many of these texts have been translated into other languages, in particular English, the potential for meanings to be 'lost' in translation is considerable (see Paley, 1997,1998, 2005, for more on the misinterpretation of phenomenological texts).

Phenomenology is a philosophy that has been adapted, revised and changed over time by either the original philosophers themselves or by others after them. Therefore there is not 'one' phenomenology but many. Researchers can select from a range of phenomenological versions in their attempt to carry out their studies. Both the language barriers and the challenges involved in understanding dense philosophical concepts and principles sometimes lead to a reliance on secondary sources. Understanding the core ideas of the main and influential phenomenological philosophers is a starting point for those interested in this approach to research. Of necessity, an attempt will be made here to simplify what are, in fact, complex ideas and concepts. Those who wish to gain an in-depth of phenomenology should refer to the original texts.

The origins of phenomenology

Philosophers, scientists, theologians and others have, forever, grappled with the question of human existence and our relationship with the environment. How do we know we exist? Are you reading this book or are you dreaming you are reading this book? If you are not dreaming, how do you know?

Do physical things around us, such as chairs and tables, exist on their own, or do we have to be aware of them for them to exist? Where is awareness located? Is it in our mind or in our consciousness? How about mental phenomena such as happiness or sadness? Do they exist if we cannot observe them? If they exist in our consciousness, how do we study them? Can we use the same approaches and methods to study physical and mental phenomena, or should we use different ones? If so, is the knowledge produced by different methods 'scientific' knowledge? Or does it matter? These are some of the main questions that the phenomenological movement, which became prominent in the nineteenth century, have sought to answer.

The term 'phenomenology' comes from the Greek word 'phainomenon', which means 'appearance', and from 'ology', meaning 'the study of'. Therefore phenomenology is the study of things, events, actions, ideas, images and so on as they appear to us, and not whether or not they exist in reality.

Phenomenology has been practised for centuries, in particular by Hindu and Buddhist philosophers, when they reflected on states of consciousness, although they did not actually use the term 'phenomenology' itself (Stanford Encyclopaedia of Philosophy, 2013). The term 'phenomenologia' was introduced by Christoph Oetinger in 1736 and was later used by Johann Lambert, Immanuel Kant and others (Stanford Encyclopaedia of Philosophy, 2013). It was introduced into the discipline of psychology (since psychology deals with concepts such as consciousness, perception, experience, cognition and so on) by Frantz Brentano (1874). However, it is Edmund Husserl, a German philosopher in the late nineteenth and early twentieth centuries, who is credited with being the father of the phenomenological movement.

Husserlian phenomenology

Building on the work of other philosophers, in particular Bolzano (1835) and Brentano (1874), Husserl proposed a new 'scientific' way to study consciousness. His books, in particular *Logical Investigations* (Husserl, 1970), laid the foundation that a number of twentieth-century philosophers have drawn upon, expanded or adapted. Briefly, Husserlian phenomenology has three main features: intentionality, phenomenological reduction and eidetic reduction.

Intentionality

In the natural sciences (for example, biology or physics), objects are normally studied by viewing them as external to individuals. For example, a piece of rock can be studied under a microscope, and it is the same piece of rock no matter who studies it. Hence, there is a separation between 'mind' (of the person who studies it) and matter (the rock). While this principle applies to physical objects, it is rejected by those who believe that objects or phenomena exist when individuals are conscious of them. When we direct our attention to an object or phenomenon, we become aware of it. The act of directing our attention to an object or phenomenon is called 'intentionality'.

The term 'intentionality' has little to do with 'intention'; it is the act of consciously experiencing a phenomenon. For example, if we are walking along the street and do not notice that someone has snatched a handbag from another person, we have not had the experience of 'witnessing such an act'. It is only when our attention has been directed (by ourselves) to the phenomenon that we become aware of it.

For Husserl, there are three parts to intentionality: the intentional act, the intentional object and the intentional content. The intentional act in the above example is the act of witnessing the robbery. This is what is called the 'lived experience' (not hearing or reading about it). The intentional object is simply the event that is experienced, in this case 'the robbery'. The intentional content is what is actually experienced by the individual who witnessed the robbery. For example, he or she may be shocked, frightened, outraged or unmoved. How different people experience this event depends on a number of factors: what they see, hear, and perceive, and also how they interpret the event. Hence different people may experience the same event differently. The goal of Husserlian phenomenology is to study how people experience phenomena in their consciousness (the intentional content).

Phenomenological reduction

In the natural sciences, researchers carry out their study in a detached and objective way. Husserl believed that phenomenology should also be a rigorous science. He used the terms 'phenomenological reduction' or 'époque' to describe the process of 'bracketing' or 'suspending' previous knowledge of the experience in order for us to reveal what the phenomenon really means for us, not how we are expected to experience it.

In everyday life, we perceive phenomena through cultural and social lenses. We look for examples of what happened before (precedents) in order to interpret new experiences. Our perceptions may be influenced by our (and others') expectations, and by what we hear and read. Bergum (2003), in her study of birthing pain, gives examples of assumptions, theories and explanations that people may hold regarding childbirth pain. These include the idea that pain should be denied or relieved, that pain is only negative or that pain can be explained. What Husserl proposed was to go 'back to the things themselves', to find out what constitutes the experience, without the layers of interpretations. Husserl's view was that by suspending all these influences and beliefs, we might be able to reveal the experience itself in its 'naive' and 'pure' state. To reveal the experience as it really is for us (what it really means) in its pre-reflective, pre-assumption and pre-theoretical form, we must, according to Husserl, adopt a phenomenological attitude and not a natural attitude (i.e. the normal way in which we use previous experience or knowledge to interpret things).

Eidetic reduction

The product or outcome of phenomenological studies using a Husserlian approach is the 'essence' of phenomena. For Husserl, any phenomenon has a universal essence that represents it and is recognised by all those who experience it. Two processes are crucial to reveal the essence of a phenomenon. The first is bracketing. The second is 'imaginative variation', which is a process of examining what people say about the phenomenon (they experience) and selecting only what represents it. It is a mental process of eliminating the characteristics and properties that are not absolutely necessary to form the essence of the phenomenon. Eidetic reduction means reducing these experiences to what is absolutely necessary to describe the phenomenon.

Aristotle distinguished between the 'essential' and 'accidental properties' of a person or a thing (Stanford Encyclopedia of Philosophy, 2013). The colour of a chair, whether it is red or blue, or the material it is made of (for example, wood or plastic) does not tell us what a chair 'essentially' is. In this case, 'colour' and 'material' are accidental properties. What then is the essence of a chair? Consider this example about the 'essence of a chair' (from a chair's perspective) by Megy (2004):

> Some of us have four legs, some only three, some rock back and forth while others stay still. While many may think that a chair is just something for a person to sit on, our real meaning goes much deeper. Chairs serve as a human body rescue.

From this description, we can identify a number of properties such as the number of legs, those that rock or stay still and what their functions are (to offer body rescue). 'Imaginative variation' consists of identifying as many properties of a chair as possible (from different people who have the experience of a chair). This is followed by a process of *reducing* the list to what is absolutely *essential* to represent a chair (hence the term eidetic reduction). For example, a chair does not have to be made of wood only; it can be made of any material. The particular type of material is accidental but not essential to represent the essence of a chair.

To some individuals, a chair may represent comfort or relief. For others, it may represent 'oppression' if they were tied to a chair and tortured (for example, in a war situation). Are 'comfort', 'relief' or 'oppression' essential or accidental to what a chair represents to 'all' those who have a concept of a chair? Without a back, a chair would be a 'stool'. If more than one person can sit on it, it could be a 'bench'. Through this process of elimination, only the properties or structures (the term used by Husserl) are kept to describe the essence of a chair. In Husserlian phenomenology, the essence of a phenomenon is constructed from the particular (responses or individuals) to the universal (properties or structures).

In summary, Husserlian phenomenology rejects the division between 'matter' and 'mind' and endorses the idea of the existence of phenomena in the consciousness of individuals. Husserl believed in objectivity (achieved through bracketing) and generalisability (through essences that have universal application). It seems that, with his aim of using phenomenology as a philosophy to develop a rigorous human science, he kept some elements of positivism.

Together, these three features constitute what Husserl called 'transcendental phenomenology', which means going beyond the experience to get to the core or essence of the phenomenon. Husserlian phenomenology has been used by others to develop what is commonly known as the 'descriptive phenomenological research method'.

Post-Husserlian phenomenology

A number of philosophers took phenomenology further and in different directions. Among the most influential is Martin Heidegger, whose book *Being and Time* (Heidegger, 1927) provides a different understanding of how to study human consciousness of phenomena. His writing is complex, making it difficult to understand and convey to others. What follows is an attempt to identify some of his key ideas that researchers have used to develop their own research approaches.

According to Heidegger, the key to understanding how we experience phenomena is to understand our own existence in the world. He used the term '*Dasein*', which means 'existence in the world or being in the world'. By the time we experience things, we already exist in the world, and how we experience is also influenced by living and being in it. What we are conscious (or not conscious) of affects our perception or experience of phenomena. For example, an early childhood experience of 'being punished' may affect a person's behaviour in later life without him or her being aware or conscious of it.

Heidegger's view is that our experience of phenomena is neither 'pure' nor 'objective' but coloured by previous experience and knowledge. Husserl also recognised this but suggested that we go beyond these influences by bracketing them. Heidegger, who was a research assistant to Husserl, rejected the notion of bracketing, and recommended instead that we explore how people interpret their experience. He was aware that when we study the experience of others, we also interpret what they say or do. By 'being with' each other, participants and researchers bring their own subjective interpretations to the encounter, and together they co-create knowledge.

Heidegger also combined phenomenology with hermeneutics (the science of interpretation of texts). In an interview situation, the dialogue between participants and researchers, when transcribed, becomes contemporary texts that can be interpreted in the same way that scholars use hermeneutics to interpret biblical and other classic texts.

Other philosophers, frequently mentioned by nursing and other health researchers, include Merleau-Ponty and Gadamer. Merleau-Ponty (1962) focused on the role of the body in experiencing phenomena, hence the term 'embodied' experience. According to Husserl, consciousness is the place where objects or phenomena are experienced. Merleau-Ponty believed that the body is the primary site or instrument through which the experience enters our consciousness. Fuchs (2007) explains that 'subjective experiences are not be found "in the psyche" nor "in the brain", but extend over body, space and the world of a person'.

Hans-Georg Gadamer comes from a hermeneutical background and was inspired by the work of Heidegger. According to Gadamer (1995), each of us has our particular 'horizon' (or understanding of the world) shaped by our personal history and culture. To understand others, we need to examine ourselves, in particular our assumptions and prejudices. When two people discuss a particular issue, they bring together their 'horizons'. Gadamer (1995) describes this encounter (as in an interview) as the 'fusion of horizons'. Translated into a research situation, the interviewer and the participant engage in a conversation in which both contribute towards producing a new understanding of the phenomenon they are exploring. Heidegger and Gadamer, among others, have influenced the development of what has been called the 'interpretive phenomenological research method'.

Phenomenological research methods

These phenomenologists were philosophers not researchers, and they did not provide instructions or procedures for doing phenomenological studies. In fact, Gadamer (1995) was critical of modern approaches to humanities that modelled themselves on the natural sciences. He rejected the notion that there is one correct interpretation of phenomena. Giorgi (2000) points out that these philosophers (see above) were involved in the phenomenological movement as philosophers and not researchers.

Thus, researchers, looking at Husserl's work for how to do 'bracketing', or at the writings of Heidegger on how to interpret, would be disappointed. Their philosophical ideas and principles, however, provide the basis that researchers can use to develop their own research methods.

Two distinctive phenomenological research methods seem to have evolved in and used nursing and health research: the descriptive (based on Husserl's work) and the interpretive (based on the work of Heidegger and Gadamer). Merleau-Ponty's work has also been used to underpin both the descriptive and the interpretive methods.

The phenomenological descriptive method

Three researchers from Duquesne University in the USA (van Kaam, 1966; Colaizzi, 1978; Giorgi, 2000, 2009) are credited with developing a descriptive method based on Husserlian philosophy. Of these, Amadeo Giorgi is the most prolific writer as well as the foremost proponent of the descriptive approach. Giorgi (2000) distinguishes between philosophical phenomenology and scientific phenomenology. To stress this distinction, he calls his contribution 'a modified Husserlian approach' (Giorgi, 2009). He recognises that, in Husserl's phenomenology, it is the person with the lived experience who should do phenomenology, by communicating to others what he or she really experiences (without layers of interpretation). Used in this way, phenomenology is more appropriate for psychological analyses of human beings (Giorgi, 2009), as in a therapeutic session between a therapist and a client. On the other hand, phenomenology as a research method is the closest researchers can get to the lived experience of participants since researchers cannot possibly experience every phenomenon that they study (Giorgi, 2009).

In his book *The Descriptive Phenomenological Method in Psychology*, Giorgi (2009), who has a psychology background, provides a step-by-step guide on how to do phenomenological descriptive studies. In developing his descriptive method, Giorgi's aim is to produce 'scientific' knowledge that is 'general, systematic, critical and methodical' (Giorgi, 2009), in the form of essences or structures of consciousness. The key feature of his approach is phenomenological reduction or bracketing.

Bracketing is both an attitude as well as a strategy on the researcher's part to describe only what participants reveal about their experiences without any form of interpretation or pre-judgement. It is the process of withholding or suspending any pre-knowledge in order to understand participants' experiences with fresh eyes. Giorgi (2009) explains the meaning of bracketing:

> It is not a matter of forgetting the past; bracketing means that we should not let our past knowledge be *engaged* while we are determining the mode and content of the present experience. Indeed, quite often one is very aware of the past as one tries not to let it influence an on-going experience.

He acknowledges that bracketing 'can be difficult at times but not impossible' (Giorgi, 2009). He gives the example of jurors in a criminal trial being asked by the judge to disregard or ignore a piece of evidence in their deliberations. Bracketing is a contested issue in phenomenological research. This is further discussed later on in this chapter. For a discussion of the implications and challenges of bracketing in a study, see Hamill and Sinclair (2010).

Steps of phenomenological descriptive studies

Giorgi's descriptive method consists mainly of the following, interlocking steps (Giorgi, 2008, 2009, 2012):

1   Collecting phenomenological data
2   Reading whole descriptions
3   Breaking descriptions into meaning units
4   Transforming meaning units
5   Identifying the essential features of phenomena
6   Integrating features into structures (essences) of phenomena.

Bracketing underpins the whole research process of descriptive phenomenological studies. What follows is an outline of each of these steps. For a more in-depth understanding of the process of this approach, readers are strongly advised to read Giorgi (2009).

Step 1: Collecting phenomenological data

Phenomenological studies are about lived experience only, and not about views, opinions, attitudes or beliefs. The aim of this step is to obtain participants' descriptions of their experience (for example, what is the experience of waiting for examination results?). Not every description from a participant will constitute phenomenological data. Using the above example, it is likely that opinions on how long one should wait to get results, or what is the best way to communicate results, would be offered by participants. These are incidental not phenomenological data. Examples of the latter would be their account of the creeping anxiety as the time for releasing the results approaches or the building anticipation (butterflies in the stomach, and so on). The focus should be on what waiting for results means to the participants.

Methods of data collection in phenomenological descriptive studies are mainly interviews and written descriptions. Interviews should be long enough to obtain concrete descriptions and should be recorded (with permission from the participants) to allow a detailed analysis of the transcripts. According to Giorgi (2008), one participant is not enough to provide data; he recommends at least three. To obtain rich and varied descriptions, it is likely that more participants would be required. The ultimate sample size is decided when data saturation is achieved (see Chapter 15).

Step 2: Reading whole descriptions

The idea here is to obtain an overall 'feel' of the whole experience of each participant, in much the same way as one reads a whole letter or assignment to make sense of the totality of what it contains. As Giorgi (2009) explains:

> The phenomenological approach is holistic since it realizes that meanings within a description can have forward and backward references and so analysis of the first part of a description without awareness of the last part are too incomplete.

Reading whole transcripts is also part of data analysis in other qualitative approaches. The idea of reading the 'whole' is to avoid fragmentation of the data.

Step 3: Breaking descriptions into meaningful units

Experiences have different aspects or facets. For example, participants may talk about different ways they experience phenomena, different ways they react or how their experience evolves. In academic writing, sentences and paragraphs are used to help readers to follow descriptions or arguments. The idea is to break down lengthy papers into meaningful segments. One sentence can sometimes contain more than one meaning. Take this sentence, for example: 'It was during my daily morning walk in the park that I noticed something strange.' Although this is one sentence, it contains two meaning units: I walk every morning/I noticed something strange. Meaning units are chunks of descriptions, each conveying a different idea. In a well-written academic paper, sentences and paragraphs provide a structure for readers to follow the description or discussion. Conversations with participants (especially in phenomenological interviews) are unfortunately not as structured, and researchers have to work hard to break down what is said into different meaning units.

Step 4: Transforming meaning units

After the meaning units have been identified, researchers 'start interrogating each meaning unit to discover how to express in a more satisfactory way the psychological implications of the lifeworld description' (Giorgi, 2009). According to Giorgi, one has to adopt the attitude of the particular discipline one belongs to in order to transform the meaning units. As he explains:

> A psychological attitude is required to develop these potentialities for psychology just as a physicist's attitude is necessary to develop the perspective of physics or a mathematical attitude to develop mathematics. (Giorgi, 2009)

This process of transforming raw data into psychological or sociological expressions is intensively 'laborious' and 'difficult to implement' (Giorgi, 2009). One can add that there is a risk of seeing the data through the lenses of existing psychological or sociological concepts or theories.

Step 5: Identifying the essential features of phenomena

The transformed meaning units are grouped into essential features or themes. This is the stage when the method of imaginative variation is used to identify the features that are essential to represent the phenomenon. It is called imaginative variation because this is a mental exercise to decide which features, when combined together, form the essence. Therefore the researcher has to try a number of permutations (the act of changing the order of a given set of elements) before deciding what features are or are not essential.

Step 6: Integrating and presenting the essence of phenomena

The final step is to bring together the essential features to convey the essence of the phenomenon. This is the process of putting the 'parts' back to constitute the 'whole'. The outcome of a descriptive phenomenological study is the 'essence' of the phenomenon. Giorgi (2009) uses the term 'structure' in place of 'essence' as he believes that essence, as described by Husserl, has universal applicability, while structure is 'general' and context-specific.

The use of literature or self-knowledge is not permitted in the analysis of data in the descriptive method (Giorgi, 2009). The analyses and findings should therefore be presented separately from the discussion in reports or journal articles. In this way, readers will be able to distinguish between findings and interpretation or reflection. After the findings have been presented, they can be discussed in the context of existing literature.

Rigour in descriptive phenomenological study

Rigour in this process is ensured by an internal validity check (Giorgi, 2008), whereby the researcher 'goes back to the transformed units and checks that all essential intuitions are at least implicitly included in the structure'. The credibility of the findings is enhanced when the analysis is explained in sufficient detail for someone knowledgeable in the field and in phenomenology to either confirm or challenge the findings (Giorgi, 2009). Through bracketing and an analysis of the description of concrete experiences, Giorgi (2009) is confident that descriptive phenomenological studies 'can achieve at least the same degree of objectivity that quantitative analyses reach'. For an example of a descriptive phenomenological study, see Research Example 29.

Interpretive phenomenological methods

Two approaches that are popular within nursing, psychology, education and the health and social sciences in general are the 'hermeneutic phenomenological approach' (van Manen, 1990) and 'interpretive phenomenological analysis' (IPA) (Smith, 1996; Smith et al., 2009). Although the two approaches put emphasis on interpretation, they are also different in terms of what they focus on.

Research example 29

A descriptive phenomenological study, using Giorgi's approach

Lived experiences of self-care among older physically active urban-living individuals
Sundsli et al. (2013)

This study aimed to describe the lived experiences of self-care and features that influenced health and self-care among older urban home-dwelling individuals who were physically active.

Ten participants aged 65 years and over took part in an interview in their own homes. At the start of the interview, they were asked to talk about a situation when they had experienced that physical activity was important to them in their daily lives.

Comments

1 Giorgi's steps were followed in order to identify meaning units and formulate a general structure (essence) of the phenomenon as follows:

> The participants lived active every-day lives and were frequently physically active. They were part of a supportive, inclusive and promoting fellowship and had the opportunity to travel. They utilized their competence and experienced making themselves useful. It was a privilege to be part of a family life as a husband, wife, parent and/ or grandparent. They acknowledged physical and mental limitations, yet they felt they were in good health.

2 No literature or self-knowledge was used to analyse and present the findings (as per Giorgi's method).

3 In the discussion section, the authors used existing literature to put the findings into the context of what was known, how they contributed to new knowledge and how they could be used by health professional and politicians to enhance older people's self-care and health.

Hermeneutic phenomenological approach

In his book *Researching Lived Experience*, van Manen (1990) explains clearly the purpose of his approach, its philosophical underpinnings, the process of data collection and analysis and how to write up the findings. The main difference between his approach and Giorgi's is that van Manen makes use of self-knowledge, the literature and other relevant sources to reflect upon and interpret participants' phenomenological experience, while in Giorgi's descriptive approach there is a conscious attempt not to interpret these experiences.

Van Manen draws from a number of philosophers including Husserl, Heidegger, Merleau-Ponty and Gadamer. His approach combines hermeneutics with phenomenology, and he sees phenomenology as the study of 'essences'. However, for him, 'essence' is not 'some ultimate core or residue of meaning' (van Manen, 1990). As he explains:

> A good description that constitutes the essence of something is construed so that the structure of a lived experience is revealed to us in such a fashion that we are now able to grasp the nature and significance of this experience in a hitherto unseen way.

Selecting a research question

To van Manen, a question for a phenomenological study is more than a question: it reflects the researchers' life-long interest in a particular phenomenon, and this interest often arises out of their personal or professional lives. Van Manen's own background is in teaching and learning and, in his book (van Manen, 1990), he gives numerous areas of education that are suited to phenomenological investigation. Similarly, phenomenological questions can also arise from the daily practices of nurses, social workers and other health professionals. These questions are about 'lived experience', not about the participants' views, opinions, beliefs or attitudes.

Process of data collection and analysis

Van Manen sees the hermeneutic phenomenological method as a 'scholarship', drawing from 'a body of knowledge and insights, a history of lives of thinkers and authors'. Methods of collecting data consist of interviews, written descriptions of experiences (often in a diary format) and close observation (mainly for the purpose of collecting anecdotes). To provide a rich understanding of the lived experience of participants, interpretive phenomenologists 'often use literary sources (poetry, novels, stories, plays etc.)'.

Data analysis in the hermeneutical phenomenological method involves the process of reflecting (on the part of the researcher) and starts with reading the initial transcripts and identifying key themes. Themes are the main messages or ideas that a text conveys. They are not always explicit but may emerge out of our understanding and interpretation of what is happening in the story or narratives. Identifying themes is an activity that we engage in, for example when we watch a film or read a book. Apart from what goes on in the story (the descriptive part), we identify key messages from it (the interpretation part). For example, for those who have seen the stage or film version of *Les Miserables* (a novel by the eighteenth-century French writer, Victor Hugo), there are a number of key themes such as oppression of the poor, social injustice and poverty, redemption and forgiveness, the power of love, liberty and freedom, courage and self-sacrifice. Different individuals may identify different (for example, guilt and opportunism) as well as similar themes, according to their interpretation of the film.

In hermeneutical phenomenological research, the 'text' is not a classic one (such as Shakespeare's *Romeo and Juliet*) but is created by the interaction (for example, in an interview situation) between participant and researcher. Therefore the main difference between hermeneutics and hermeneutical phenomenological research is that, in the latter, the researcher and the participant create the text for the purpose of research, whereas in the former the text already exists (for example, theological manuscripts). Although classic texts were not written for research purposes, they offer insights that researchers may find useful to understand human phenomena.

According to van Manen, once the initial themes have been identified, the researcher returns to the participants to carry out further 'hermeneutical conversations', in which both researcher and participant 'collaborate' to find out whether the researcher's interpretation fits the experience of the participants. This, in some sense, ensures the 'fittingness' of the findings, although van Manen (1990) also recommends discussing these emerging findings in research seminar groups and/or with friends.

When the main themes are put together, they inform us of the nature of the phenomenon we are investigating. Research Example 30 shows how a hermeneutical phenomenological study was carried out.

A hermeneutical phenomenological study

Disclosure experience in a convenience sample of Quebec-born women living with HIV *Rouleau et al. (2012)*

The aim of this qualitative study was to describe the disclosure experience of French-speaking, Quebec-born women living with HIV. As the authors explain, 'the study was geared to identifying the essence of disclosure (gain an understanding of the whole) from a phenomenological viewpoint'.

Although an interview guide was used, the researchers let the participants express themselves freely in their own words to allow a deeper exploration and a richer description and understanding of their experiences. The hermeneutical phenomenological approach of van Manen was used. This consisted of 'reflection and writing'. 'Reflection consisted of discovering themes within the experiences' and 'writing reflected the interpretation and thoughts of the researcher' and her 'openness to all forms of language'.

The analysis of data, collected from seven participants, revealed 29 sub-themes and seven major themes. These themes were used to form the essence of the phenomenon of disclosure by women living with HIV, which was summed up by the authors as follows:

> For these women, disclosure of their HIV-positive status meant living the ambivalence of a paradoxical process of revealing/concealing, in a state of profound suffering, exacerbated by stigma, while also being enriched by the benefits attained.

Comments

1. In this study, the authors show clearly how the essence of the phenomenon of disclosure was developed from the seven major themes.

2. The authors explained that they did not carry out second interviews, as recommended by van Manen, because of 'the delicate and demanding nature of disclosure' and 'the difficulties encountered in setting up the first meeting'. This shows that researchers have to adapt their selected approach to their own particular circumstances.

Research example 30

Interpretive phenomenological analysis

Another research method that combines phenomenology with hermeneutics (interpretation) is IPA (Smith and Osborn, 2003; Smith et al., 2009; Smith, 2010). Although its roots are in psychology, it is fast becoming popular in the health professions, including nursing. The aim of IPA is 'to explore in detail how participants make sense of their personal and social world' (Smith and Osborn, 2003).

The focus of IPA is on participants' experience, and the outcome is a detailed, in-depth and thick description of the experience, rather than on producing an 'objective statement of the object or event itself' (Smith and Osborn, 2003).

Both Giorgi and van Manen explore individuals' experiences in order to understand phenomena. For example, if we take 'learning' as a phenomenon, Giorgi's aim would be to describe objectively what the essence of learning is, while van Manen would draw upon participants' experiences and other sources to construct a descriptive account of what constitutes 'learning'. Phenomenology is the study of phenomena as experienced by individuals. Giorgi's and van Manen's aim is to enhance our understanding of phenomena. Participants' experiences are important in so far as they help to give us insight into phenomena. Smith, on other hand, seems to be less concerned about phenomena and more focused on the experience itself. He does not seek to find the 'essence' of the phenomena; rather, he is interested in the many different ways in which people experience them. He treats each experience as a particular case. As Smith et al. (2009) explain:

> IPA is committed to the detail examination of the particular case. It wants to know in detail what the experience for *this* person is like; what sense *this* particular person is making of what is happening to them. This is what we mean when we say IPA is idiographic. IPA studies usually have a small number of participants and the aim is to reveal something of the experience of each of those individuals. As part of this, the study may explore in detail the similarities and differences between each case. It is possible to move to more general claims with IPA but this should only be after the potential of the case has been realized.

Smith uses phenomenology in a broad sense to justify his focus on people's experience as it 'appears' to them. He also uses hermeneutics in a general sense, to interpret participants' experience.

The process of IPA

Smith and Osborn (2003) offer clear and detailed guidance on how to carry out IPA, but they emphasise the point that the approach is flexible and open to adaptation. The research question in IPA is usually 'framed broadly and open' (Smith and Osborn, 2003). The sample is normally small to allow for an in-depth exploration of individual cases. The main method of data collection is the semi-structured interview, which Smith and Osborn (2003) describe as an interaction that allows the researcher and the participant to engage in a dialogue whereby initial questions are modified in the light of participants' responses, and the investigator is able to probe interesting and important areas that arise. According to Brock and Wearden (2006), a number of other data collection methods, such as written narrative accounts, diaries, email discussions and focus groups, have been used in IPA studies.

Data analysis consists mainly of identifying themes and master themes. Interpretation is at the heart of the analysis process and takes into account that 'meanings are constructed by individuals within both a social and personal world' (Smith and Osborn, 2003). In IPA studies, participants' experience should also be examined in the context of their 'mental and emotional state' (Smith and Osborn, 2003).

With its 'loose' interpretation of phenomenology and hermeneutics, its focus on individuals' experience and its use (or partial use) of a case study approach, IPA appeals to the person-centred approach of nursing and the health professions. In their discussion and critique of IPA, Pringle et al. (2011) conclude that:

> Interpretative phenomenological analysis offers an adaptable and accessible approach to phenomenological research intended to give a complete and in-depth account that privileges the individual. It enables nurses to reach, hear and understand the experiences of participants. Findings from IPA studies can influence and contribute to theory.

For examples of IPA studies and how they can be evaluated, see Smith (2011). Research Example 31 shows how IPA was used in one nursing study.

A study using IPA

Termination of pregnancy services: experiences of gynaecological nurses *Nicholson et al. (2010)*

To explore the experiences of gynaecological nurses involved with termination of pregnancy, Nicholson et al. (2010) interviewed seven nurses working in a termination of pregnancy service. They used IPA to analyse their data and identified eight 'superordinate themes' which, together, represented the experience of these nurses.

IPA was selected because 'this approach is concerned with making sense of individuals' personal perceptions or accounts of their experience. It acknowledges that the process is complicated by the researcher's own conceptions and therefore involves the researcher reflecting on their interpretations of participant accounts'.

Comments

1 They justified their small sample size on the basis that Smith and Osborn (2003) suggest five or six as a reasonable number of participants for a study using IPA methodology.

2 Although Nicholson et al. did not use the term 'case study', they introduced elements of a case study approach in that all these nurses worked in the same service, and they also used a questionnaire to collect data. Case studies can make use of more than one method of data collection. In IPA, researchers can use elements of a case study approach, as the aim is to explore individual cases in depth.

Research example 31

Value and limitations of phenomenological research

Van Manen (2007), reminding us of Heidegger's statement that phenomenology 'never makes things easier, but only more difficult', explains how phenomenology can be useful in practice:

In doing phenomenological research, through reflective methods of writing, the aim is not create technical intellectual tools or prescriptive models for telling us what to do or how to do something. Rather, a phenomenology of practice aims to open up the possibilities for creating formative relations between being and acting, between who we are and how we act.

Phenomenology has the potential to offer real insight into people's perceptions and feelings. Phenomenology, as a philosophy, has provided a rationale to justify why we need to focus on people's experience. The actual and direct contribution of phenomenology to nursing practice and patient care, however, remains to be explored. So far, nurses have used phenomenology mostly for research purposes. Carel (2011) explains that while phenomenology can illuminate the illness experience, it has been 'under-utilized in the philosophy of medicine as well as in medical training and practice'. In nursing, Parse (1999) developed the 'human becoming theory' to guide nursing practice. Much of Benner's work (based on post-Husserlian phenomenology) on nursing expertise is also informed by interpretive phenomenology (see, for example, Benner, 1985). However, there is little evidence in the literature that phenomenology, as a philosophy, is widely used to enhance the clinical encounter between nurses and patients.

The large number of phenomenological studies that have been carried out has no doubt added to the body of knowledge that constitutes nursing. How the findings of these studies influence nursing practice is not known. 'Essences' of phenomena may be of interest to researchers and philosophers, but they have limited direct applicability in the world of clinicians. While lengthy descriptive accounts of experience may provide useful insights, they may not suit the busy world of nurses and other health professions, where evidence summaries are thought to be the best way to access research information. More work needs to be done to realise the valuable potential of phenomenology in enhancing patient experience. Such contributions, however, may be intangible and subtle rather than measurable.

Examples of phenomenological studies in nursing include 'African American adolescent males living with obesity' (Ashcraft, 2013), 'Valuing knowledge from patient experience' (Gidman, 2013) and 'Undergraduate nursing students caring for cancer patients' (Charalambous and Kaite, 2013).

Summary

Anyone contemplating the use of phenomenology for a research project is faced with the challenge of making sense of what phenomenology as a philosophy is and how to translate it in research practice. In this chapter, three popular phenomenological research methods have been outlined. Giorgi's approach follows Husserlian philosophy using bracketing in order to describe objectively and systematically the essence of phenomena. Van Manen combines post-Husserlian phenomenology and hermeneutics to provide a description of the essences of phenomena. The main difference between the two approaches is that Giorgi avoids interpreting the experience of participants, while van Manen deliberately draws from self-knowledge and other sources (including literature) to interpret participants' experience. Smith's IPA uses phenomenology and hermeneutics in their broadest sense and combines them with elements of a case study approach to make sense of people's experience of events in their lives. Smith focuses more on 'experience' than on the 'phenomenon'. All three authors provide guidelines and/or examples of their approaches.

This chapter has introduced readers to the key principles and concepts of the main schools of phenomenology and outlined how researchers have attempted to translate philosophy into research practice. Choosing between the different phenomenological research methods requires a grasp of what each can offer and how they fit the aim of the study.

References

Ashcraft P F (2013) African American adolescent males living with obesity. *Public Health Nursing*, **30**, 1:29–36.

Benner P (1985) Quality of life: a phenomenological perspective on explanation, prediction and understanding in nursing science. *Advances in Nursing Science*, **8**, 1:1–14.

Bergum V (2003) Birthing pain. Retrieved from www.phenomenolgyonline.com/sources/textorium/bergum-vangie-birthing-pain (accessed 5 July 2013).

Bolzano B (1835) *Theory of Science* (ed. Jan Berg). (Dordrecht: D. Reidel, 1973).

Brentano F (1874) See the English translation in Rancurello A C, Terrell D B and McAlister L L, *Psychology from an Empirical Standpoint* (London: Routledge, 1995).

Brock J M and Wearden A J (2006) A critical evaluation of the use of interpretative phenomenological analysis (IPA) in health psychology. *Psychology and Health*, **21**, 1:87–108.

Carel H (2011) Phenomenology and its application in medicine. *Theoretical Medicine and Bioethics*, **32**, 1:33–46.

Charalambous A and Kaite C (2013) Undergraduate nursing students caring for cancer patients: hermeneutic phenomenological insights of their experiences. *BMC Health Services Research*, **13**:63.

Colaizzi P (1978) Psychological research as the phenomenologist views it. In: R Valle and M King (eds) *Existential-phenomenological Alternatives for Psychology* (New York: Oxford University Press).

Fuchs T (2007) Psychotherapy of the lived space: a phenomenological and ecological concept. *American Journal of Psychotherapy*, **61**, 4:423–39.

Gadamer H-G (1995) *Truth and Method*, 2nd edn revised (New York: Continuum).

Gidman J (2013) Listening to stories: valuing knowledge from patient experience. *Nurse Education in Practice*, **13**, 3:192–6.

Giorgi A (2000) The status of Husserlian phenomenology in caring research. *Scandinavian Journal of Caring Sciences*, **14**:3–10.

Giorgi A (2008) Concerning a serious misunderstanding of the essence of the phenomenological method in psychology. *Journal of Phenomenological Psychology*, **39**, 1:33–58.

Giorgi A (2009) *The Descriptive Phenomenological Method in Psychology: A Modified Husserlian Approach.* (Pittsburg, PA: Duquesne University Press).

Giorgi A (2012) The descriptive phenomenological psychological method. *Journal of Phenomenological Psychology*, **43**, 1:3–12.

Hamill C and Sinclair H (2010) Bracketing – practical considerations in Husserlian phenomenological research. *Nurse Researcher*, **17**, 2:16–24.

Heidegger M (1927) *Sein und Zeit (Being and Time)*, trans. J Macquarrie and E Robinson, 1966. (New York: State University of New York Press).

Husserl E (1970) *Logical Investigations*, Vols I and II, trans. J N Findlay. (New York: Humanities Press) (German original, 1900).

Megy J (2004) The essence of a chair. Retrieved from www.writework.com.essay/essence-chair (accessed 11 April 2013).

Merlean-Ponty M (1962) *Phenomenology of Perception* (New York: Humanities Press) (French original, 1945).

Nicholson J, Slade P and Fletcher J (2010) Termination of pregnancy services: experiences of gynaecological nurses. *Journal of Advanced Nursing*, **66**, 10:2245–56.

Norlyk A and Harder I (2010) What makes a phenomenological study phenomenological? Analysis of peer-reviewed empirical nursing studies. *Advancing Qualitative Methods*, **20**, 3:420–31.

Paley J (1997) Husserl, phenomenology and nursing. *Journal of Advanced Nursing*, **26**:187–93.

Paley J (1998) Misinterpretive phenomenology: Heidegger, ontology and nursing research. *Journal of Advanced Nursing*, **27**:817–24.

Paley J (2005) Phenomenology as rhetoric. *Journal of Advanced Nursing*, **12**, 2:106–16.

Parse R R (1999) *Illuminations: The Human Becoming Theory in Practice and Research* (Sudbury MA: Jones & Bartlett).

Pringle J, Drummond J, McLafferty E and Hendry C (2011) Interpretative phenomenological analysis: a discussion and critique. *Nurse Researcher*, **18**, 3:20–4.

Rouleau G, Côté J and Cara C (2012) Disclosure experience in a convenience sample of Quebec-born women living with HIV: a phenomenological study. *BMC Women's Health*, **12**:37.

Smith J A (1996) Beyond the divide between cognition and discourse: using interpretative phenomenological analysis in health psychology. *Psychology and Health*, **11**:261–71.

Smith J A (2010) Interpretive phenomenological analysis. *Existential Analysis*, **21**, 2:186–92.

Smith J A (2011) Evaluating the contribution of interpretive phenomenological analysis. *Health Psychology Review*, **5**, 1:9–27.

Smith J A and Osborn M (2003) Interpretative phenomenological analysis. In: J A Smith (ed.) *Qualitative Psychology: A Practical Guide to Methods* (London: Sage).

Smith J A, Flowers P and Larkin M (2009) *Interpretive Phenomenological Analysis: Theory, Method and Research* (London: Sage).

Stanford Encyclopaedia of Philosophy, 2013. *Phenomenology*. Retrieved from http://plato.standford.edu/entries/phenomenology/ (accessed 26 February 2013).

Sundsli K, Espres G A and Soderhamn O (2013) Lived experiences of self-care among older physically active urban-living individuals. *Clinical Interventions in Aging*, **8**:123–30.

van Kaam A (1966) *Existential Foundations of Psychology* (Pittsburg, PA: Duquesne University Press).

van Manen M (1990) *Researching Lived Experience* (Ontario: State University of New York Press, Albany).

van Manen M (2007) Phenomenology of practice. *Phenomenology and Practice*, **1**, 1:11–30.

Grounded Theory 13

> Induction for deduction, with a view to construction.
> Auguste Comte

Introduction

Grounded theory, in its different versions, is a frequently used qualitative approach in nursing and health research. This chapter provides an introduction to grounded theory, traces its origin, outlines its main features and highlights the differences between Glaser's and Strauss's approaches. Methods of data collection and data analysis in grounded theory are explained. Finally, some of the criticisms and challenges of the grounded theory approach are presented.

The meaning of grounded theory and its value to nursing

The term 'grounded theory', which was coined by Glaser and Strauss (1967) in their seminal work *The Discovery of Grounded Theory*, describes a research methodology whereby hypotheses and theories emerge out of, or are developed from, data. It is therefore an inductive approach to research, in contrast to the deductive approach whereby data are collected and analysed in order to test theories (see Chapter 2). Strauss and Corbin (1990) provide a clear answer to the question of 'What is grounded theory?:

> A grounded theory is one that is inductively derived from the study of the phenomenon it represents. That is, it is discovered, developed, and provisionally verified through systematic data collection and analysis of data pertaining to that phenomenon. Therefore, data collection, analysis, and theory stand in reciprocal relationship with each other. One does not begin with a theory, and then prove it. Rather, one begins with an area of study and what is relevant to that area is allowed to emerge.

Grounded theory itself is not a specific theory but a term to describe theories that are 'grounded in data'. A distinction can be made between 'grounded theory' and 'grounded theory method'. The former is a generic term to mean theories that are developed from data. The term 'grounded theory method' applies to the principles, procedures and techniques of 'how to do' grounded theory research.

Developing theories from data (collected from participants) pre-dates Glaser and Strauss's work. Anthropologists and ethnographers have, for centuries, developed theories by living among, and observing, people in their natural environments (Parahoo, 2009). For example, Goffman's theory of 'total institution' (Goffman, 1961) was developed based on participant observation in a psychiatric institution. However, he did not explain in detail the principles he used to develop this theory, although he gave some accounts of what he did. Glaser and Strauss (1967) were the first researchers to provide a detailed framework and technique that can be used to help others to develop theories from data. For a definition of theory, see Chapter 8.

At the core of nursing is the interaction between nurses, clients and families. Grounded theory, with its roots in symbolic interactionism, is well suited to exploring these and other interactions. For example, Annells (2007) conducted a grounded theory study about 'seeking relief from flatus as relevant client-nurse action and interaction', and Sun et al. (2009) carried out a grounded theory study of 'action/interaction strategies used when Taiwanese families provide care for formerly suicidal patients'. Grounded theory can make an important contribution towards our understanding of core concepts in nursing such as recovery, rehabilitation, health promotion, care-giving, autonomy and competence among others. As a practice-based discipline, nursing requires knowledge for its day-to-day practice, as well as theoretical knowledge to continue to build its pool of knowledge. Grounded theory has the potential to do both.

Versions of grounded theory

There is a lot of discussion about what grounded theory is, what methods and techniques there are to choose from and what, indeed, can be called grounded theory. No other approach in qualitative research has spawned such a large volume of literature in the last decade or so. According to Dey (1999), there are probably as many versions of grounded theory as there are grounded theorists!

With hindsight, it was inevitable that others would build on the original work or offer their own interpretation of grounded theory after the original publication of Glaser and Strauss (1967). What was surprising, however, was the 'breakaway' move by Strauss with the publication of the *Basics of Qualitative Research* (Strauss and Corbin, 1990). Glaser reacted by stating that Strauss and Corbin had developed another method, which he called 'full conceptual description', not grounded theory (Glaser, 1992). Glaser commented that the analysis framework or model proposed by Strauss and Corbin (1990) 'forces' the theory rather than allows it to 'emerge' (Glaser, 1992).

The 'disagreement' between the originators of grounded theory was followed by what Morse et al. (2009) termed 'the second generation of grounded theorists' (that is, students of Glaser and Strauss). These included Clarke's (2005) situational analysis and Charmaz's (2006) constructivist grounded theory methods.

Glaser's version of grounded theory (which is often referred to as 'classic grounded theory') has been described as having positivistic undertones in its emphasis on 'discovering' theories as if they exist independent of our interpretation. Charmaz (2006), on the other hand, takes the view that reality is constructed (hence constructivist grounded theory). In Charmaz's version, grounded theories are the product of interactions between researchers and participants (in their socio-cultural context). For his part, Glaser (2012) calls constructivist grounded theory 'a misnomer'. For fuller discussions of the different versions of grounded theory, see Melia (1996), Glaser (2012) and Seidel and Urquhart (2013).

Researchers sometimes provide an account of the 'trials and tribulations' of selecting an appropriate version of grounded theory for their studies. To gain an insight into researchers' rationale for making a choice, see Cooney (2010), who explains how she selected between a Glaserian and a Straussian approach and gives the reasons for her choice. Similarly, Hunter et al. (2011) describe their journey in deciding which of three approaches they selected for a study of the psychosocial training needs of nurses and healthcare assistants working with people with dementia in residential care.

Key features of grounded theory

The key features of grounded theory (its essence) can be explored by distinguishing between grounded theory as outcome and grounded theory as process. In this section, reference is made to the original work of Glaser and Strauss (1967). Where appropriate, the differences between Glaser and Strauss are also highlighted.

Grounded theory as outcome

While all qualitative approaches can lead to theory development, grounded theory is the only methodology that places explicit emphasis on discovering theory. The outcome of grounded theory research is a substantive theory that Glaser and Strauss (1967) describe as 'a theory developed for a substantive or empirical area'. Examples of a substantive area or topic include 'Information-seeking behaviour of senior nursing students' (Duncan and Holtslander, 2012), 'Nurses' collaboration with patients with chronic obstructive pulmonary disease on non-invasive ventilation' (Sørensen et al., 2013) and 'Recovery from the effects of severe persistent mental illness' (Henderson, 2010). The unit of analysis in grounded theory is not individuals but incidents or events involving human interactions (Glaser and Strauss, 1967). Substantive theories reveal the processes of these interactions and the meanings that the 'actors' give to them.

Glaser and Strauss (1967) distinguish between a substantive and a formal theory. The latter is a theory at a higher level on generalisation. Glaser (2007) explains how a substantive theory of 'becoming a nurse' can pave the way to a formal theory of 'becoming a professional':

> a well-known theory of becoming a nurse (Davis and Olesen, 1970) is easily formalized by comparing it constantly to other data and theory about becoming a doctor, becoming a lawyer, becoming a pilot, becoming an accountant, etc. to arrive at a theory of becoming a professional.

For a fuller and more in-depth discussion of substantive and formal theories, see Glaser (2007).

An example of a substantive theory comes from a study of the information-seeking behaviour of patients newly diagnosed with cancer in the immediate post-diagnosis period (McCaughan and McKenna, 2007). They explain:

> A substantive theory describing the transitions from 'being traumatized' by the diagnosis, through a phase of trying to 'take it on', through to 'taking control' is tentatively offered. It provides a theoretical framework to understand newly diagnosed cancer patients' changing, varied and continuing needs and their efforts to regain some control over their lives. Their information-seeking behaviour seemed a journey of 'never-ending making sense' with on-going discovery and new information needs as they struggled with the effects of the disease and treatments.

This theory may provide nurses with a framework to assess the readiness of patients to receive information and to assist them in their efforts to regain some control over their disease and their lives.

Grounded theory as process

A number of principles and techniques have been developed by Glaser and Strauss (1967) to explain how theories can be generated from data. The process of doing grounded theory, also known as the grounded theory method, consists of a number of key features:

- a reliance on emergence;
- the simultaneous collection and analysis of data;
- constant comparison;
- theoretical sensitivity and theoretical sampling.

Reliance on emergence

'Trust in emergence' is perhaps the most well-known of Barney Glaser's mantras. This is because he believes that, for a theory to be truly grounded in data, researchers should ensure that it reflects what is in the data, and not the researchers' views or preconceptions. Reliance on emergence is the fundamental principle that underpins the grounded theory method. The grounded theory method is primarily inductive (that is, it develops theory from data). However, as patterns and trends in the data begin to emerge, researchers can test or verify them using a deductive process. While the grounded theory method allows a certain measure of deduction (that is, it tests the ideas and hypotheses as they emerge), the emphasis is always on induction. Only what emerges from the data can be tested, and not the researcher's preconceptions. As Glaser (1978) explains:

> Grounded theory is, of course, inductive; a theory is induced or emerged after data collection starts. *Deductive work in grounded theory is used to derive from induced codes conceptual guides* as to where to go next for which comparative group or subgroup, in order to sample for more data to generate the theory.

Glaser (1978) also warns against 'forcing' or 'premature closure'. By forcing he means using the data to fit the preconceptions or prior knowledge of researchers. Premature closure, on the other hand, can occur when the initial ideas or patterns that emerge out of the data are not sufficiently explored to enable the theory to fully describe the phenomenon under investigation.

Glaser and Strauss (1967) recommend that researchers do not review the literature prior to undertaking a grounded theory study. This is because they do not want prior knowledge or existing theories or conceptualisations to influence the emerging theory. Knowledge or awareness of existing frameworks is often used subconsciously to analyse data. For example, in a study exploring the perceptions of causes of depression, the themes that 'emerged' closely reflected the factors that are known in the literature to be associated with depression. One can ask whether the researcher's prior knowledge of causes of depression influenced what she 'saw' in the data. Human beings use prior knowledge or experience as a frame of reference to understand new situations or events. While it is impossible put aside or forget everything we know about a topic we want to study, one should constantly make efforts to view phenomena from the perspectives of participants and reflect on how these perceptions are similar to or different from how we would see or interpret them. For more discussion of the use of literature in grounded theory studies, see Walls et al. (2010) and Dunne (2011).

Simultaneous collection and analysis of data

In an informal conversation, we listen to and process ('analyse') what the other person is saying so that we can respond appropriately. Afterwards, we may look back on the conversation, especially if we are unsure of our understanding of what was said. Similarly, in grounded theory, data collection and analysis take place simultaneously. This enables the researcher to think of questions on the spot, as the need arises. The recorded data are analysed throughout the process of data collection. Glaser (2004) recommends that data be analysed 'the first night after field notes are collected'. Of course, at the end of data collection, the recorded data and other notes taken are systematically analysed as well. In grounded theory, one does not collect all the data before they are analysed. When this happens, researchers are overwhelmed by large amounts of data and it becomes difficult to make sense of them. In fact, the main themes, patterns, trends, stages and transitions should already have emerged by the time the final analysis takes place.

Constant comparison

Comparing and contrasting is what we do all the time. As Silver (2010) explains:

> Comparative thinking is one of our first and most natural forms of thought. When we are infants, one of the first differences we must identify is that between mother and other. Without the ability to make comparisons – to set one object or idea against another and take note of similarities and differences – much of what we call learning would quite literally be impossible.

Constant comparison is at the heart of the grounded theory method. It is a process that eventually leads to the development of substantive or formal theories. Constant comparison consists of a number of strategies such as identifying the core category and the basic social processes that are linked to it.

There is no doubt that, in other types of qualitative research, we compare and contrast responses from the same participant and between participants. What is different is that constant comparison in grounded theory happens throughout the study and that the comparison is deliberate and systematic. It takes place as soon as data collection starts and ends after the substantive theory has been formulated. Even then, it is compared with other similar theories. However, constant comparison is most obvious during the coding stages.

According to Glaser (1978), there are three levels of coding: open, selective and theoretical. In the open coding stage, the researcher carries out line-by-line and sentence-by-sentence analysis, and as many codes, their properties and dimensions are constructed. For example, a code could be 'support' and the properties could be types of support (friends, family and colleagues) and their dimensions, and the degree of support (less, token or more substantial). This type of coding requires conceptual thinking and the ability to find similarities and differences. In a study of 'how nurses facilitate patients' transitions from intensive care', Häggström et al. (2012) identified 300 concepts in the open coding phase.

At the end of open coding, a 'core category' is identified. The core category captures the essence of what is happening in the way participants attempt to resolve what they are undertaking. Madill (2008) explains what a core category is:

> A core category is the main theme, story-line, or process which subsumes and integrates all lower-level categories in a grounded theory, encapsulates the data efficiently at the most abstract level, and is the category with the strongest explanatory power.

For example, in the study by Häggström et al. (2012), the core category was 'being perceptive and adjustable'. This is what, according to the authors, represented and encapsulated nurses' responses in their efforts to facilitate patients' transitions. Similarly, in a study of the process of breast cancer survivorship, Sherman et al. (2012) identified 'reclaiming life on one's own terms' as the core variable.

According to Glaser (2005), deciding a core category tests the analyst's skills and abilities. He goes to explain the process of identifying the core category:

> As s/he constantly compares incidents and concepts s/he will generate many codes, while being alert to the one or two that are core. S/he is constantly looking for the 'main theme', for what – in his or her view – is the main concern or problem for the people in the setting; for that which sums up, in a pattern of behaviour, the substance of what is going on in the data, for what is the essence of relevance in the data.

Once the core variable (sometimes called 'core category') has been selected, the analysis moves into the second stage: selective coding. Here the researcher looks for basic social processes. Grounded theory is suitable for studying phenomena involving social interactions. Human beings use a number of interactive processes such as making decisions, seeking information, taking control of situations and recovering from illness. These processes are dynamic and take place in a social context. In the selective coding stage, the researcher tries to identify the social processes that are linked to the core variable.

There are often processes within processes. For example, in Wuest and Merritt-Gray's (2001) study of the 'experience of women who have left abusive male partners and not gone back', the basic process of reclaiming self comprised four sub-processes: counteracting abuse, breaking free, not going back and moving on. 'Moving on' was itself made up of four other processes: figuring it out, putting it in its rightful place, launching new relationships and taking on a new image.

Finally, in the theoretical coding stage, the substantive theory is developed by integrating the basic social processes with the core variable. This is when relationships between the processes are explained, as well as the sequences in which they happen and the conditions for moving from one stage to another. Not all the movements are linear and unidirectional; they are often interactive (moving back and forth between stages). The reasons (conjectures) for why and when movement (transition to another stage) occurs are also explained. For example, in McCaughan's and McKenna's (2007) study of information-seeking among newly diagnosed cancer patients, a substantive theory described how their journey of 'never-ending making sense' (the core category) developed through the stages of 'being traumatised', 'taking it in' and 'taking control' (the basic social processes).

To broaden the scope of the emerging theory so that it can include as many variations as possible, grounded theory researchers should look outwards (to the literature and other sources) for ideas with which to make comparisons. Referring to their study of *Awareness of Dying*, Glaser and Strauss (1967) explain how an observation by one of the research team relating to the role of families in the care of people who were dying in another country contributed to a theory that reflected what actually happened in the US setting:

One of us noted that in Malayan hospitals, families work in caring for dying patients. This observation was interesting because up to this point we had considered the family member, in the United States, as either being treated as another patient (sedated, given rest) or just ignored as a nuisance. Reviewing our American data, though, we discovered that the family is used in several ways for the care of dying patients ... We then proceeded to study it at our home base, where we had more time for the inquiry.

In contrast with Glaser (1992), Strauss and Corbin (1990, 1998) proposed data analysis and interpretation strategies in the form of the paradigm model in order to develop theories from data. The model operates at three coding levels: open, axial and selective. These also constitute the three stages of coding, and each builds on the previous one, although there are opportunities to go back and forth once the preliminary coding of the three phases has been completed.

'Open coding' is the first stage when the data (transcripts, notes and so on) are broken down into small units, each with a new meaning. Strauss and Corbin (1990) recommend 'line-by-line' coding. In this first stage, the researcher does not consciously look for relationships between the codes but searches for properties, types and dimensions. The aim is to classify and categorise the codes and group them into themes.

Axial coding, with which Glaser (1992) takes the most issue, is the second phase and level. The researcher searches for relationships between codes and themes to start to make sense of what is happening in the data. Kelle (2005) explains this succinctly:

During axial coding the analyst tries to find out *which types* of phenomena, contexts, causal and intervening conditions and consequences are relevant for the domain under study. If, for instance, social aspects of chronic pain are investigated the researcher may try to identify typical action contexts which are relevant for patients with chronic pain as well as characteristic patterns of pain management strategies. Thereafter it can be examined which pain management strategies are used by persons with chronic pain under certain conditions and in varying action contexts. This may lead to the construction of models of action which capture the variance of the observed actions in the domain under study and which can provide the basis for a theory about action strategies generally pursued in certain situations.

The final stage is selective coding, when a core category (a term that has the same meaning as Glaser's) is identified. All the other variables are integrated at this stage to form the substantive theory. Data analysis is a laborious process during which the researcher interacts with, and reflects on, the data. There are various papers in the literature dealing with the issues arising from data analysis, using Strauss and Corbin's (1990) approach. For a detailed discussion of the differences between Glaser's and Strauss and Corbin's coding strategies, and examples of the challenges faced by researchers in doing axial coding, see Kendall (1999), Kelle (2005), Larossa (2005) and Madill (2008).

Theoretical sensitivity and theoretical sampling

Theoretical sensitivity is crucial if the emerging theory is to be as 'fully formed' as possible and to offer new insight into the phenomenon being studied. One of the ways in which researchers can further explore and test some of the tentative hypotheses emerging out of the data and further extend the scope of the theory is through theoretical sampling.

In grounded theory, the researcher's ability to think conceptually is crucial to the development of the subsequent theory. Glaser and Strauss (1967) point out that 'the root source of all significant theorising is the sensitive insights of the observer itself'. Thinking conceptually means thinking 'outside the box', creatively and abstractly. It is the ability to see meaning beyond the obvious (for example, to see the symbolic meaning in what participants say or do). Theoretical sensitivity leads to new questions about relationships and differences between concepts or gaps in the emerging theory.

An example of theoretical sensitivity comes from a study of the implementation of preventive protocols in dental practices in New South Wales, Australia (Sbaraini et al., 2011). After a few interviews, the researchers found that dentists talked about the concept of 'reliable' and 'unreliable' patients. They decided to 'theoretically sample' for both types of patient because they wanted to explore these concepts further and to compare the dentists' perspectives with the perspectives of the patients themselves.

Theoretical sampling is a grounded theory technique to explore new avenues and test emerging hypotheses. In the study of information-seeking among newly diagnosed cancer patients, McCaughan and McKenna (2007) reported that participants in the initial interviews talked about traditional healers – priests and hairdressers – as sources of information that they accessed. McCaughan and McKenna decided to interview some of these to get their perspectives on information-giving and to test some of the ideas emerging out of the data. The challenge for researchers when they theoretically sample groups of participants other than the original sample is not to be distracted. This can be achieved by keeping the focus on the core variable. For example, McCaughan and McKenna decided to interview lay healers in order to understand their role in the cancer patients' never-ending journey of making sense of their disease and treatment (the core variable).

In grounded theory, the number of participants cannot be pre-planned and fixed at the start of the study; the final number will be known only at the end of the study (Glaser and Strauss, 1967). However, there comes a time when sampling has to stop, and the criterion for judging this is theoretical saturation. According to Glaser and Strauss, 'saturation means that no additional data are being found' and that the researcher 'sees similar instances over and over again'. However, they stress that saturation can never be attained by studying one incident in one group.

Theoretical sensitivity is facilitated by the use of 'theoretical memoranda'. These are notes taken to record the conceptual thinking of the researcher (with particular reference to emerging ideas and concepts and questions that arise during the course of the study) and the actions and decisions taken to explore them. Memoranda serve also as a reflective diary and an audit trail. Sbaraini et al. (2011) wrote extensive conceptual memoranda that they used to record their impressions about the participants' experiences and to systematically question some of their pre-existing ideas in relation to what was said in the interview. Below is an excerpt of a memorandum written after interviewing a practice manager (Sbaraini et al., 2011):

Conceptual memo

Believing + Embracing + Developing = Adapting?

In these dental practices the adaptation to preventive protocols was all about believing in this new approach to manage dental caries and in themselves as professionals. New concepts were embraced and slowly incorporated into practice. Embracing new concepts/paradigms/systems and abandoning old ones was quite evident during this process (old concepts = dentistry restorative model; new concepts = non-surgical approach). This evolving process involved feelings such as anxiety, doubt, determination, confidence, and reassurance. The modification of practices was possible when dentists-in-charge felt that perhaps there was something else that would be worth doing; something that might be a little different from what was done so far. The responsibility to offer the best available treatment might have triggered this reasoning. However, there are other factors that play an important role during this process such as dentist's personal features, preconceived notions, dental practice environment, and how dentists combine patients' needs and expectations while making treatment decisions. Finding the balance between preventive non-surgical treatment (curing of disease) and restorative treatment (making up for lost tissues) is an every moment challenge in a profitable dental practice. Regaining profit, reassessing team work and surgery logistics, and mastering the scheduling art to maximize financial and clinical outcomes were important practical issues tackled in some of these practices during this process. These participants talked about learning and adapting new concepts to their practices and finally never going back the way it was before. This process brought positive changes to participants' daily activities. Empowerment of practice staff made them start to enjoy more their daily work (they were recognized by patients as someone who was truly interested in delivering the best treatment for them). Team members realized that there were many benefits to patients and to staff members in implementing this program, such as, professional development, offering the best care for each patient and job satisfaction.

Finally, to claim that a study used the grounded theory method, there should be evidence of all these four key features discussed above.

Data collection methods

In grounded theory studies, the main methods of data collection are interviews and observations. Documents and other artefacts such as songs, paintings, poems, stories and sculptures can also be useful. Glaser (2001) explains (what is now his famous dictum), that in grounded theory, 'all is data':

It means exactly what is going on in the research scene is the data, whatever the source, whether interview, observations, documents, in whatever combination. It is not only what is being told, how it is being told and the conditions of its being told, but also all the data surrounding what is being told. It means what is going on must be figured out exactly what it is to be used for, that is conceptualization, not for accurate description. Data is always as good as far as it goes, and there is always more data to keep correcting the categories with more relevant properties.

Rigour in grounded theory studies

Glaser and Strauss (1967) stressed that, for grounded theory studies, 'normal evaluation criteria of reliability and validity may not be appropriate and judgements should be based on the detailed elements of the strategies for collecting, coding and presenting the data'. This means that if the procedures are well followed (in particular, if researchers 'trust in emergence'), the rigour will have been maintained. Cooney (2011), for example, states that, 'researchers should trust in the grounded theory methodology and know that their studies will be rigorous if they apply the methodology correctly'.

The process of grounded theory methods, whether based on the original version (Glaser and Strauss, 1967) or the revised versions (Strauss and Corbin, 1990; Charmaz, 2006) has been extensively described in the literature. Researchers are required to show how they apply the key principles and techniques (for example, constant comparison, theoretical sampling and so on) of their particular grounded theory version. By showing how the core category, the basic social processes and the substantive theory have emerged out of the data, they create their own audit trail.

Glaser (2004) rejects the notion that concepts such as 'trustworthiness' and 'credibility' (Lincoln and Guba, 1985) are applicable to grounded theory studies. Instead, Glaser and Strauss (1967) listed the four criteria by which a substantive theory, developed by the grounded theory method, should be evaluated. These are fit, workability, relevance and modifiability. 'Fit' relates to how the theory actually represents the phenomenon being studied. Glaser (2004) does not recommend 'member checking' (whereby interpretations of what participants said are taken back to them for verification or confirmation). 'Relevance' means that the theory is recognisable by those who are directly involved with its use: practitioners and other academics. 'Workability' relates to how the theory can be used to explain similar situations and predict how people may react in similar circumstances. 'Modifiability' of the theory means that it can be further developed, adapted or changed. In this sense, the theory developed by grounded theory methods provides the foundation for contributing to knowledge in that particular substantive area.

For a fuller discussion of rigour in grounded theory studies, read Chiovitti and Piran (2003), Glaser (2004) and Cooney (2011).

Criticism of grounded theory

Although grounded theory is widely used as an approach in nursing, health and social research, it is not without its critics. Glaser's version of grounded theory gives the impression that there are theories out there waiting to be discovered. According to Charmaz (2006), the 'theory' that is developed is co-constructed by the participants and researchers. She believes that if different researchers studied the same phenomenon, it is quite likely that different theories would be produced.

Thomas and James (2006) went further and argued that 'what is contrived is not in fact theory in any meaningful sense, that "ground" is a misnomer when talking about interpretation and that what ultimately materializes following grounded theory procedures is less like discovery and more akin to invention'. One can say that Glaser (1992) puts too much trust or faith in 'emergence'. Preconceptions heavily influence the findings and theories that researchers produce. To recommend that a literature review is not carried out prior to a grounded theory study is like asking alcoholics not to be exposed to alcohol, rather than recognising that they have an alcohol problem. Another reason why 'trust in emergence' may not be enough is because researchers need to be able to think conceptually in order to produce anything resembling a theory. While thinking conceptually may be intuitive to some people, others require considerable training to do so.

Finally, the literature on grounded theory, which has grown considerably over the last two decades, has added to the confusion experienced by those contemplating the use of this method in their research. Much time is spent choosing from among a host of versions of grounded theory, and, worse still, considerable anxiety is generated when researchers wrestle with grounded theory jargons. Some find it hard to distinguish their core categories from their basic social processes, or their selective from axial coding. While Glaser does his best to explain and promote the methodology, he sometimes adds to the confusion, as when he states that he uses the words 'code, concept, property or category as synonymous' (Glaser, 2011). For a fuller criticism of grounded theory, see Allan (2003) and Thomas and James (2006).

Evaluating grounded theory studies

There is no doubt that, despite these criticisms of grounded theory, it is widely used as an approach to research in such fields as sociology, psychology, business, marketing, health and nursing, among others. However, every grounded theory study looks different in terms of how it is carried out. Researchers seem to mould the approach to their needs, with the result that most tend to use an adapted form of grounded theory, despite identifying the particular version that underpins their study. To evaluate grounded theory studies, one can look for evidence of these key features of grounded theory studies: a reliance on emergence, a simultaneous collection and analysis of data, constant comparison, theoretical sensitivity and theoretical sampling. A substantive theory should also be evident.

Ultimately, the quality of the findings is not reduced if some of the procedures of the stated approach are not used. Sandelowski and Barroso (2003) explain that 'the mere fact that a study presented as a grounded theory study contains no coherent conceptual rendering of data, but, rather a thematic survey of them does not by itself undermine the credibility of these findings'.

For anyone new to grounded theory, there are a number of useful papers in the literature that explain the process that the researchers followed (see, for example, Sbaraini et al., 2011). Research Example 32 describes a grounded theory study by McMillan et al. (2012) of older people after a fall-induced hip fracture repair.

A grounded theory study

A grounded theory of taking control after fall-induced hip fracture *McMillan et al. (2012)*

The aim of the study was 'to explore the post-discharge concerns of older people after fall-induced hip fracture repair'. The findings were expected to increase the understanding and awareness of issues that may impact on recovery and rehabilitation.

According to the authors, Glaser's approach to grounded theory was chosen as the aim was to generate a theory around a core category and to explain how people resolve their main concern related to the post-discharge concerns of older people after a hip fracture repair. The rationale for selecting this particular version of grounded theory was not provided.

Comments

1 Initially, potential participants were approached and those who volunteered were interviewed. This was followed by theoretical sampling that allowed the researchers to source those with particular experiences that would develop an 'emerging theory'.

2 Data were collected by semi-structured face-to-face interviews. The initial topic guide included broad questions relating to how participants managed at home. Later questions became more focused as categories started to emerge. The authors also gave examples of questions in earlier and later interviews.

3 The authors explained that constant comparison and theoretical sampling ensured the rigour of the study. Following Glaser's advice, member checking was not carried out, nor was an extensive literature consulted prior to the study.

4 'Taking control', which emerged as the core category, comprised processes moving through three stages: 'going under', 'keeping afloat' and 'gaining ground'. The authors explained that this adds 'a new dimension to our understanding of recovery from hip fracture'.

Research example 32

Grounded theory, as an approach to qualitative research, has much to offer towards a body of knowledge for nursing and health practice. It is a unique among qualitative approaches in its focus on developing theory from data. The key features and the process of grounded theory for developing substantive theories have been explained. The different versions of grounded theory, however, create dilemmas for researchers as they grapple with an ever-increasing number of grounded theory terminologies. Grounded theory is not without its critics, who point out that theories are researchers' interpretations of phenomena, and what is supposed to 'emerge' is in fact theories constructed by researchers.

Summary

References

Allan G (2003) A critique of using grounded theory as a research method. *Electronic Journal of Business Research Methods*, **2**:1–9.

Annells M (2007) A grounded theory: seeking relief from flatus as relevant client-nurse action and interaction. *Gastroenterology Nursing*, **30**, 4:269–76.

Charmaz K (2006) *Constructing Grounded Theory: A Practical Guide Through Qualitative Analysis* (Thousand Oaks, CA: Sage).

Chiovitti R F and Piran N (2003) Rigour and grounded theory research. *Journal of Advanced Nursing*, **44**, 4:427–35.

Clarke A E (2005) *Situational Analysis: Grounded Theory After the Postmodern Turn* (Thousand Oaks, CA: Sage).

Cooney A (2010) Choosing between Glaser and Strauss: an example. *Nurse Researcher*, **17**, 4:18–28.

Cooney A (2011) Rigour and grounded theory. *Nurse Researcher*, **18**, 4:17–22.

Davis F and Olesen V (1970) *Becoming a Nurse* (Glencoe, IL: Free Press).

Dey I (1999) *Grounding Grounded Theory: Guidelines for Qualitative Inquiry* (San Diego, CA: Academic Press).

Duncan V and Holtslander L (2012) Utilizing grounded theory to explore the information-seeking behaviour of senior nursing students. *Journal of the Medical Library Association*, **100**,1: 20–7.

Dunne C (2011) The place of the literature review in grounded theory research. *International Journal of Social Research Methodology*, **14**, 2:111–24.

Glaser B (2007) Doing formal theory. In: A Bryant and K Charmaz (eds) *The Sage Handbook of Grounded Theory* (London: Sage).

Glaser B (2011) Getting out of the data: grounded theory conceptualization. Retrieved from http://www.groundedtheory.com/gt-books.aspx (accessed 13 January 2014).

Glaser B (2012) Constructivist grounded theory. *Grounded Theory Review*, **11**, 1:1–14.

Glaser B G (1978) *Theoretical Sensitivity Advances in the Methodology of Grounded Theory* (Mill Valley, CA: Sociology Press).

Glaser B G (1992) *Basics of Grounded Theory: Emergence vs Forcing* (Mill Valley, CA: Sociology Press).

Glaser B G (2001) *The Grounded Theory Perspective: Conceptualization Contrasted with Description* (Mill Valley, CA: Sociology Press).

Glaser B G (2004) "Naturalistic inquiry" and grounded theory. *Forum: Qualitative Social Research*, **5**, 1:Art. 7.

Glaser B G (2005) Basic social processes. *Grounded Theory Review*, **4**, 3:1–27.

Glaser B and Strauss A (1967) *The Discovery of Grounded Theory* (Chicago: Aldine).

Goffman E (1961) *Asylums: Essays on the Social Situation of Mental Patients and Other Inmates* (New York: Anchor Books).

Häggström M, Asplund K and Kristiausen L (2012) How can nurses facilitate patients' transitions from intensive care? A grounded theory of nursing. *Intensive and Critical Care Nursing*, **28**:224–33.

Henderson AR (2010) A substantive theory of recovery from the effects of severe persistent mental illness. *International Journal of Social Psychiatry*, **57**, 6: 564–73.

Hunter A, Murphy K, Grealish A, Casey D and Keady J (2011) Navigating the grounded theory terrain. Part I. *Nurse Researcher*, **18**, 4:6–10.

Kelle U (2005) 'Emergence' vs. 'forcing' of empirical data? A crucial problem of 'grounded theory' reconsidered. *Forum: Qualitative Social Research*, **6**, 2:Art. 27.

Kendall J (1999) Axial coding and the grounded theory controversy. *Western Journal of Nursing Research*, **21**, 6:743–57.

Larossa R (2005) Grounded theory methods and qualitative family research. *Journal of Marriage and Family*, **67**:837–57.

Lincoln Y and Guba E (1985) *Naturalistic Inquiry* (London: Sage).

Madill A (2008) Core category. In: L M Given (ed.) *The SAGE Encyclopedia of Qualitative Research Methods* (London: Sage).

McCaughan E and McKenna H (2007) Never-ending making sense: towards a substantive theory of the information-seeking behaviour of newly diagnosed cancer patients. *Journal of Clinical Nursing*, **16**:2096–104.

McMillan L, Booth J, Currie K and Howe T (2012) A grounded theory of taking control after fall-induced hip fracture. *Disability and Rehabilitation*, **34**, 26:2234–41.

Melia K M (1996) Rediscovering Glaser. *Qualitative Health Research*, **6**, 3:368-78.

Morse J M, Stern P N, Corbin J, Bowers B, Clarke A E and Charmaz K (2009) *Developing Grounded Theory: The Second Generation* (Walnut Creek, CA: Left Coast Press).

Parahoo K (2009) Grounded theory: what's the point? *Nurse Researcher*, **17**, 1:4–7.

Sandelowski M and Barroso J (2003) Classifying the findings in qualitative studies. *Qualitative Health Research*, **13**, 7:905–23.

Sbaraini A, Carter S M, Evan R W and Blinkhorn A (2011) How to do a grounded theory study: a worked example of a study of dental practices. *BMC Medical Research Methodology*, **11**:128.

Seidel S and Urquhart C (2013) On emergence and forcing in information systems grounded theory studies: the case of Strauss and Corbin. *Journal of Information Technology*, **28**, 3:237–60.

Sherman D W, Rosedale M and Haber J (2012) Reclaiming life on one's own terms: a grounded theory of the process of breast cancer survivorship. *Nursing Forum*, **2**, 3:E258–68.

Silver H F (2010) *Compare and Contrast: Teaching Comparative Thinking to Strengthen Student Learning*. Strategic Teacher PLC Guides (Alexandria, VA: Association for Supervision and Curriculum Development).

Sørensen D, Frederiksen K, Groefte T and Lomborg K (2013) Nurse–patient collaboration: a grounded theory study of patients with chronic obstructive pulmonary disease on non-invasive ventilation. *International Journal of Nursing Studies*, **50**:26–33.

Strauss A and Corbin J (1990) *Basics of Qualitative Research: Grounded Theory, Procedures and Techniques* (Thousand Oaks, CA: Sage).

Strauss A and Corbin J (1998) *Basics of Qualitative Research: Techniques and Procedures for Developing Grounded Theory* (Thousand Oaks, CA: Sage).

Sun F K, Long A, Huang X Y and Chiang C Y (2009) A grounded theory study of action/interaction strategies used when Taiwanese families provide care for formerly suicidal patients. *Public Health Nursing*, **26**, 6:543–52.

Thomas G and James D (2006) Re-inventing grounded theory: some questions about theory, ground and discovery. *British Educational Research Journal*, **32**, 6:767–95.

Walls P, Parahoo K and Fleming P (2010) The role and place of knowledge and literature in grounded theory. *Nurse Researcher*, **17**, 4:8–17.

Wuest J and Merritt-Gray M (2001) Beyond survival: reclaiming self after leaving an abusive male partner. *Canadian Journal of Nursing Research*, **32**,4:79–94.

14 Ethnography

Opening thought

Culture is the process by which a person becomes all that they were created capable of being.

Thomas Carlyle

Introduction

A quick search of the relevant nursing databases up to December 2013 showed that ethnography, as a qualitative research approach, is less often used in nursing research than grounded theory or phenomenology. Yet nursing is essentially a cultural and social activity. When the word 'culture' is mentioned, one often thinks about people from other societies. However, culture is about ourselves as well as about others.

In this chapter, the meaning of ethnography, the beliefs underpinning its practice and the historical shifts in ethnographic practices will be explored. The key features of ethnographic studies, the process of the ethnographic method, and the ethical, political and practical issues and challenges involved in doing ethnography will also be briefly discussed.

Studying behaviour in context

Suppose a researcher decides to study how newly qualified nurses take on their first nursing post in a hospital. She can interview 10 or 12 nurses about their lived experience of this phenomenon. The participants may be recruited from a list of nurses who have recently been appointed as staff nurses. These nurses do not need to come from the same hospital, or to know one another. This will be a controlled situation in which participants will be interviewed in a designated place, at a pre-arranged time, for about 1 hour each. The interviews may be tape-recorded and the transcripts most likely analysed when all the interviews have been completed. The participants will have had time to reflect on their experience prior to the interview and they may be selective in what they share with the researcher. They will provide an account of their experience, which may be subject to distortion due to the time lapse between what happened and when it is reported (a retrospective view). The researcher has no way of knowing what actually took place in the clinical areas where these nurses work. The data from these interviews can be useful in providing an insight into the experiences of a number of individual nurses, with no connection between them. The researcher will be able to identify themes and describe what it means to start working as a qualified nurse from these nurses' perspectives. This type of study would probably suit a phenomenological approach.

On the other hand, the researcher may decide to observe how newly qualified nurses take on their new nursing roles and how they fit (or not) into existing teams. She will be able to observe the strategies they use when under pressure and how they relate to other members of staff and patients. She will have opportunities to talk with nurses at the time that the 'events' happen. She may observe differences between what nurses say and do. Others who are relevant to the study can also be observed and asked questions. However, there may be difficulties and challenges – for example, the researcher may get in the way of the nurses' work and/or could be excluded from observing certain activities. She will have less control over the research situation than in the previous example of interviewing nurses retrospectively. However, the collection of data at the site where the action takes place can provide a holistic understanding of what is being studied. The researcher would, in this case, be using what is commonly known as an 'ethnographic' approach.

Bjerknes and Bjork (2012) carried out such a study in Norway (an ethnographic study of nurses taking on the nursing role in a hospital setting). As they explain:

> An ethnographic design was used, drawing upon observations, interviews, and the analysis of documents. This was a qualitative design, monitoring the nurses in their encounters with colleagues, physicians and patients in clinical situations. The combination of different data sources is often highly productive and the resulting analysis and findings can be more complete when a number of different information sources are used to explore a question.

What is ethnography?

Ethnography is a qualitative approach that explores the behaviour of people in their natural environment using observation as well as a range of other methods of data collection. It is not about the study of individuals on their own, but about how they think and behave as members of groups or sub-groups. The term 'ethnography' is made up of 'ethno', meaning a group of people sharing the same characteristics, and 'graphy', meaning writing or description. Therefore ethnography means a description of groups and what goes on in groups. Underpinning ethnography is the belief that each group (large or small) has its own culture that binds the members together, sets the rules of how they should behave, defines their roles within the group and distinguishes them from others outside the group.

'Culture' is a term used to describe the values, goals, habits, customs and rituals shared by people who belong to the same groups. Each culture has its own rules and norms of how things should be done and why, what is acceptable or unacceptable behaviour, what is highly regarded or rewarded and how transgression is dealt with. Leininger (1995) explains that nursing culture 'is the learned and transmitted life-ways, values, symbols, patterns and normative practices of members of the nursing professions.' As a profession, nurses have their own world views and, in many aspects, are different from other health professionals, although they may work in multidisci-plinary teams. Within nursing itself, each clinical area may have its own culture.

To illustrate what is meant by culture in a nursing setting, we can look at the example of two wards in the same hospital. Ward A is characterised by the staff's belief in searching for new ways to improve practice, in collegiality, openness and respect for one another. The organisational structure allows for everyone to be included in decision-making, resulting in staff feeling valued and supported. Ward B is characterised by a belief in keeping the status quo. New ideas are not welcome. Staff feel unsupported and disempowered. The organisational structure is hierarchi-cal, and there is a lack of transparency in terms of how decisions are made. Staff on these two wards have a lot in common; they are from the same region, work in the same hospital, speak the same language and are trained in the same way. By compar-ing the characteristics of these two wards, one can say that they have different cultures, which in turn can impact on patient care.

The term 'emic' is used to describe the insiders' view. In the example above, we can observe the behaviour of staff (insiders) on each ward and try to understand, from their perspectives, why they behave the way they do. The term 'etic' is used to describe the view of the outsider (researchers) of what happens in the group being observed. In ethnography, researchers focus on the emic.

Ethnography can be used to explore sociocultural factors that affect the health-related behaviour of individuals. The rationale for focusing on sociocultural factors in a health context is because they have a significant effect of the health of individuals. According to the National Institutes of Health (2013):

> Social and cultural factors influence health by affecting exposure and vulnerability to disease, risk-taking behaviors, the effectiveness of health promotion efforts, and access to, availability of, and quality of health care. Social and cultural factors also play a role in shaping perceptions of and responses to health problems and the impact of poor health on individuals' lives and well-being.

Origins of ethnography

Ethnography has its roots in cultural anthropology. It was adopted by early European anthropologists such as Bronislaw Malinowski (1922), Margaret Mead (1928) and Edward Evans-Pritchard (1937), who went to distant places (for exam-ple, the South Pacific and Africa) to study the behaviour and customs of the 'natives'. They immersed themselves in the culture of their hosts and participated, to varying degrees, in the daily activities and rituals of these people. They were fascinated by the 'exotic', the 'unusual' and the folklore of these societies.

Anthropologists lived in these tribes for long periods and often visited them many times after their initial study. This type of ethnography is sometimes referred to as traditional ethnography. Malinowski is an icon of ethnographic studies, and his book *Argonauts of the Western Pacific* (Malonowski, 1922) is a compelling read for those embarking on an ethnographic study.

Later, American sociologists such as William Foote Whyte and Erving Goffman used the ethnographic method to study communities and groups in the sociologists' own societies. Whyte (1955) used participant observation (see Chapter 18) to study young men in an Italian community in Boston, USA. His book *Street Corner Society* is a classic work for budding and experienced ethnographers as well, not least because of his thoughtful reflections on the methodology he used.

Goffman's ethnographic study of psychiatric patients in a mental hospital is another seminal work that, despite its limitations, has been hugely influential in understanding 'total institutions' such as mental hospitals and the behaviour of 'inmates' and their carers. This is how Weinstein (1982) described Goffman's participant observational study:

> Goffman's work on asylums was one of the first sociological examinations of the social situation of mental patients, the hospital, world as subjectively experienced by the patient. He posed as a pseudo-employee of the hospital for a year, an assistant to the athletic director, and gathered ethnographic data on selected aspects of patient social life.
>
> Goffman claimed that it was necessary for him to present a 'partisan view' in order to describe the patient's situation faithfully. The main focus of the book is the world of the patient, not the world of staff.

Contemporary ethnography

It was inevitable that ethnography would evolve and change from its early roots in cultural anthropology and its focus on people in distant lands, since the world itself has changed beyond recognition in that time. Social scientists and others realised that the ethnographic method can be used to study people in their own countries and communities, closer to home. The concept of a group as a unit of study evolved from being distant tribes to any cluster of people who share some of the same characteristics by nature of their work, leisure, interests, activities, attitudes or beliefs. Schools, hospitals, prisons, birdwatchers, football clubs, music societies, support groups, cafés, airports and virtual online groups can all be legitimate units of ethnographic study. In a world of technologically driven changes, online ethnography (the study of virtual groups on the internet) is increasingly becoming an important method of learning about people (see, for example, Garcia et al.'s, 2009, study of the internet and computer-mediated communication).

There has been a shift from the 'exotic' and 'unusual' to the everyday concerns of people within the researchers' own communities. For example, Evans-Pritchard was interested in 'the magic and rituals of the Asande people in Central Africa' and Malinowski studied 'the sexual life of savages in North-Western Melanesia'.

However, ethnography is also useful for studying issues closer to home. Cruz and Higginbottom (2013) explain that 'focused ethnography' has emerged as a relevant methodology that can be used by researchers to understand specific societal issues that affect different facets of practice. For example, Ward-Griffin et al. (2012) carried out an ethnographic study to explore the 'relational experiences of family caregivers providing home-based end-of-life care'. Higginbottom et al. (2013) provide some useful guidance on how to conduct focused ethnography in health-care research.

Researchers doing contemporary ethnography can, more or less, select the particular issue or topic (for example, how new residents settle in nursing homes) prior to entering the field. Few projects will now be funded or get ethical approval if the research questions are not well formulated in advance. On the other hand, traditional ethnography tended to be guided by what attracted the attention of researchers after they had spent some time in the study setting.

While many anthropologists continue to pursue their interest in cultural issues abroad, others study the more 'mundane' topics such as café 'society' (Laurier et al., 2001). As the authors explain:

> Café society is something that many of us as customers and/or social scientists take for granted. Cafés are places where we are not simply served hot beverages but are also in some way partaking of a specific form of public life.

Market researchers have also realised the importance of studying the consumer behaviour of people in their own homes. Colyer (2013) relates how a director at a well-known international company justified observing people at home:

> We had a business requirement to understand a segment of the market we had traditionally spent less time exploring. We wanted to get closer to the reality of these consumers and their lives and specifically what and where they drink at home. For this particular project, it felt less appropriate to rely solely upon consumer recall in focus group environments and more important to get into consumers' homes to observe more closely the reality of the occasions and the motivations.

One could say that ethnography has literally 'come home'!

Doing ethnography closer to home means that researchers do not necessarily have to live in the communities where they conduct their studies. They can spend periods of time with the participants and still live at home. In this respect, more researchers can do ethnography than was possible previously, when ethnographers had to be absent from their own homes for months or even years.

Politically and ethically, contemporary ethnographers are required to reflect more on the effects of their work on participants. There are now more safeguards to protect the rights of individuals than there were at the time of the early cultural anthropologists who sometimes adopted Eurocentric and colonialist attitudes towards those they studied. They often presented these people as 'inferior', 'bizarre' and 'primitive' (Smith, 2001; Cruz and Higginbottom, 2013). The title of one of

Mead's books – *Coming of Age in Samoa: A Psychological Study of Primitive Youth for Western Civilisation* – is a perfect example of portraying participants as 'primitive' compared with 'civilised' Westerners, thus suggesting the superiority of one people over the other. Today, such a title is likely to be controversial, if not offensive.

In contemporary ethnography, researchers working closer to home are more able or inclined to sympathise or even empathise with participants, not least because they share common characteristics. Goffman (1961), for example, used the word 'partisan' to indicate that he was on the side of the patients in his study of mental institutions. After all, patients in psychiatric hospitals are the same as everyone else in society in all respects except for the fact that the former have some form of mental illness.

'Critical ethnography' emerged as a form of research in which researchers take a political stance in favour of the oppressed. They use the research process to work collaboratively with participants as co-researchers to challenge and address power inequality. Participants are therefore in some ways empowered by the research process. The aim of critical ethnography and the beliefs that underpin its practice are explained by Madison (2012):

> Critical ethnography begins with an ethical responsibility to address processes of unfairness or injustice within a particular *lived* domain. By 'ethical' responsibility, I mean a compelling sense of duty and commitment based on moral principles of human freedom and well-being, and hence a compassion for the suffering of living beings.

For an example of a study using a critical ethnographic approach, see Liu et al. (2012).

Contemporary ethnography allows for the use of a range of theoretical and philosophical perspectives by researchers to interpret and present their findings (Harris and Holmes, 2013). These include symbolic interactionism (see, for example, Carlson, 2013), hermeneutic phenomenology (see, for instance, Keim-Malpass and Steeves, 2012) and feminism (see, for example, Saewyc, 2003). Even the introduction of positivist elements in ethnography, such as questionnaires as one of the data collection methods, is advocated by some researchers (Whitehead, 2004). Although questionnaires can be used alongside observations and interviews to collect data, ethnography remains, overall, a qualitative approach because it seeks to see the world from the perspectives of the participants using primarily unstructured, interactive and flexible methods.

Key features of ethnographic studies

With all these changes, one can ask what remains of traditional ethnography for a study to be described as ethnographic. Three essential features seem to emerge from the literature (see, for example, Genzuk, 2003; Lambert et al., 2011):

1   The focus of the study is on how people think and behave in the groups they belong to, in their natural environment.

2   The primary method of collecting data is unstructured, holistic observation (participant and/or non-participant) in the natural environment where the study is being carried out. Holistic observation means that everything (what is seen, heard, read or felt) is data.

While observation as a data collection method is essential in ethnography, researchers can use other methods as well, in particular interviews. However, interviews on their own are not sufficient for a study to be ethnographic as they rely solely on reported and not observed accounts. Similarly, administering questionnaires to participants in their own homes does not make a study ethnographic, unless what is observed in these homes is used as data and analysed.

3   Adequate time is spent in the natural environment, with the participants. This is for the purpose of familiarising oneself with the groups, gaining trust, building relationships and immersing oneself sufficiently to gain an in-depth understanding of what is going on. It is difficult to specify what constitutes 'sufficient' time as gaining trust and grasping what is happening vary from setting to setting. Some groups accept outsiders less readily than others. Only after one enters the setting and starts to get to know some participants can one judge how long it will take to get 'accepted'.

For a study to be described as ethnographic, all three features have to be present.

The ethnographic process

Questions or aims in ethnographic studies

As previously explained, the ethnographic approach is suitable for questions relating to the thoughts and behaviour of participants in their particular setting. For example, St-Amant et al. (2012), in their ethnographic study, explored by means of interviews and participant observations how decisions in home-based dementia care were made. Intensive care units (Slatore et al., 2012), emergency departments (Fry, 2012) and online blogs (Keim-Malpass and Steeves, 2012) are examples of other settings where ethnographic studies have been undertaken. Below are examples of the questions and aims explored in ethnographic studies in nursing and other health professions:

- To explore the relational experiences of older adults with advanced cancer and their family caregivers and home care providers within the sociocultural context of home-based end-of-life care (Ward-Griffin et al., 2012).
- To examine the role of ward-based advanced nurse practitioners and their impact on patient care and nursing practice (Williamson et al., 2012).
- To examine forms of communication and power relations surrounding communication on medication among nurses, and between nurses and patients during handover (Liu et al., 2012).

Methods of data collection

In ethnographic studies, researchers can use a range of methods (formal or informal) including observations (participant or non-participant), interviews (face-to-face and focus groups) and data sources (such as documents, photographs, videos, paintings, sculptures, drawings, writings, poems and songs). However, the prime method of data collection in ethnography is observation.

Participant and non-participant observation

Layder (1993) describes the benefits sociologists derive from such an approach:

> The method of 'participant observation' allows the closest approximation to a state of affairs wherein the sociologist enters into the everyday world of those being studied so that he or she may describe and analyse this world as accurately as possible. Participant observation represents the ideal form of research strategy because this method requires that the sociologist for all intents and purposes 'becomes' a member of the group being studied.

Madden (2010) goes further in explaining that 'good ethnographers use their whole body as an organic recording device'.

Non-participant observation is useful when it is not possible or feasible to participate in the activities of those being studied. Even those who choose to do participant observation may not be able or allowed to get involved in everything the participants do, or it may not be appropriate to observe certain events (such as when someone is very distressed). Although with non-participant observation the researcher may not come close to experiencing what the group members do, this can provide useful data as well. In participant observation, getting involved in the action may restrain the researchers in terms of taking notes. Participating in one activity may hinder the researcher's ability to have an overview of what is happening in the setting. In practice, however, researchers can use both types of observation in the same study. Williamson et al. (2012) used non-participant observation to study the role of ward-based advanced nurse practitioners, and Brooks (2008) explored nursing and public participation in health by means of non-participant observation. See Chapter 18 for more discussion on the different types of observation used in research.

Talking with participants

In ethnographic studies, researchers talk with participants as they observe them. Although multiple sources of data are used, they are not used in isolation but are in fact part of the ethnographic process of collecting data in context. For example, if a researcher observes a participant looking at photographs, she may have a conversation with him during which she notices that the man feels uncomfortable when looking at particular photographs. In this case, one can say that the researcher simultaneously engages in a number of ways (observation, interview and artefacts) to gain access to understanding this individual's behaviour.

While formal interviews can be set up with participants, this may not be the best way to collect data in ethnographic studies. The ethnographer normally spends time and effort to get accepted in the group and to be as informal as possible. Moving between formal (as in an interview situation) and informal (as in having a 'chat' with participants) roles can confuse participants. In Whyte's (1955) study of an inner city Italian community, he was advised 'to go easy' with the 'who, what, when, where questions'. He was told that 'if people accept you, you can just hang around and you'll learn the answers in long run without even asking the questions'. Whyte explains that he found this advice to be 'true':

> As I sat and listened, I learned the answers to questions that I would not even had the sense to ask if I had been getting my information solely on an interview basis. I did not abandon questioning altogether, of course. I simply learnt to judge the sensitiveness of the question and my relationship to the people that I only asked a question in a sensitive area when I was sure that my relationship to the people involved was very solid.

While formal interviews serve the researcher's purpose of getting answers to specific questions, they should not be the main method in ethnography, since interviews are reports of what happened. Ethnography provides a unique opportunity to 'see' what happens. As Whyte (1955) explains:

> A man's attitudes cannot be observed but instead must be inferred from his behaviour. Since actions are directly subject to observation and may be recorded like other scientific data, it seems wise to try to understand man through studying his actions.

A number of studies have used face-to-face interviews (Kennedy and Lyndon, 2008; Ward-Griffin et al., 2012; Williamson et al., 2012) and focus groups (Liu et al., 2012; Brooks, 2008) in ethnographic studies to complement data from observations. See Chapter 17 for more discussion on interviewing. For a study using multiple methods including document analysis, non-participant observation, face-to-face interviews, focus group, video and audio recordings, see Brooks (2008).

Participants in ethnographic studies

Unlike in other research designs (for example, grounded theory, phenomenology or surveys), researchers in ethnographic studies do not normally select, in advance, all the participants for their study. They depend on who agrees to be observed or interviewed as the study progresses. The term 'key informant' is used in ethnographic studies to describe the main person or persons who can provide insights into the group's behaviour and can help the researcher to gain access to others, events or activities. An ethnographic site can have more than one key informant. In a study of the oral health of Latino pre-school children in rural California, Barker and

Horton (2008), recruited 30 key informants from a range of health professionals and policy-makers. They were chosen because they 'had relevant knowledge or insight into the issues of interest, and provide a perspective important for properly contextualising observational data and the comments of study participants'.

In traditional ethnography, it was not possible to report precisely the number of people who took part in a study. Living in and researching a community brings the researcher into contact with a large number of people, some who are directly involved, and some who are involved on the periphery. In focused ethnography, researchers decide, in advance, the number of participants to be interviewed or observed (see, for example, Higginbottom et al., 2013). Data saturation determines whether this number is increased or decreased. For a further discussion of samples and sampling issues in qualitative studies, see Chapter 15.

Data analysis

As with other qualitative approaches, data collection and analysis should take place as the study proceeds. Field notes are important in recording data, the researcher's thoughts and new lines of enquiry. Notes should be written in between observations, as note-taking may make participants uncomfortable or curious as to what is being written. Notes should also comprise a thick description of the context in which the events are taking place, as it is difficult to remember the relevant details of a situation later on.

Different researchers observing the same phenomena in the same group setting are likely to 'find' different things. With ethnography, the temptation to pass judgement on others is great. Researchers should ensure that they support their findings with descriptions of the context of what happened or what was said by the participants. In practice, ethnography is a product of the 'fusion' of the 'emic' and the 'etic' perspectives. The researcher gains access to the participants' world view and uses her own (outsider's) world view to make sense of it. It is not simply that she sees their world through her 'lens'. Rather, through the process of spending time with participants, she has the opportunity to see it from their position. She reflects upon and questions her own preconceptions and/or what is in the literature. The result is a new product that reflects the researcher's new interpretation of what goes on in the group and the meanings that participants give to their actions.

Rigour in ethnographic studies

The use of multiple methods to collect data should, in principle, contribute to the validity of the findings since it is possible to compare what participants say and what they do (and to seek clarification for inconsistencies). However, this is not sufficient to ensure validity. Other strategies used to ensure rigour are reflexivity and member checking. Reflexivity is the act of examining one's own assumptions, prejudices and decisions to find out how these may have affected data collection, analysis and interpretation. Madden (2010) makes a case for the importance of methodological reflexivity:

There is a need to account for the inevitability of the ethnographer's influence on the research process and to manage the tension between objectivity and subjectivity in order to produce better portraits of the human condition. Dealing rigorously with reflexivity is an important aspect of contemporary ethnography.

Member checking involves finding out what participants think of the researcher's interpretations. Williamson et al. (2012) explained that, in their study, 'when analysis was completed, the preliminary findings were shown to the advanced nurse practitioners and ward nurse participants to ensure that views and events were reported accurately'. For rigour in qualitative studies, see Chapter 20.

Reporting findings

Ethnographic findings should be written in such a way that readers can feel, when particular events or incidents are described, as if they had been there. According to Harris and Holmes (2013), 'a 'quality' ethnography is one which speaks to the reader; one which conveys the reality of participants' lives and one which stimulates the reader to question their own value position'. One may add that if a detailed and rich account is given, readers can also question the interpretation of the researcher.

Below is an example of thick description from a study of diabetes in the United Arab Emirates by Baglar (2013), in which the author relates a scene from her observations to describe the customary practice of commensality (social group eating together):

> Large platters of meat and rice are brought by maids; lentils, vegetables, and salads are also available. Bottles of Pepsi are passed around as guests are constantly enjoined to eat more; refusals are met with apparent amazement: 'But you've hardly eaten, what's wrong?' With this a further spoonful is added to one's plate. A large fruit platter, chocolate cake, cream, trifle, and ice cream complete the dessert course. The host's sister begins to serve dessert, again, encouraging everyone to 'just try some.' Almost everyone does, including, after persuasion, a young teenager who is morbidly obese. There is no doubting the popularity of the calorie laden 'Western' type foods; dates and fruit remain virtually untouched.

Through observing a number of instances of social eating and talking with people in her study, Baglar (2013) concluded:

> As relationships are cultivated and honor exchanged, contradictory demands are placed on people with diabetes who strive to fulfil their social obligations while attempting to comply with health advice. The cultural requirement to participate in commensality, and the obligations inherent in gift giving, make it difficult for those with diabetes to reduce their food intake generally, refined carbohydrates and sugars in particular. The commensality is so crucial, I argue, is what makes it extremely challenging for individuals to follow advice. It is, of course, not merely the absolute neces-

sity for commensality that creates difficulties for the people I met, but rather the frequency with which episodes of hospitality take place and the quality and quantity of food consumed at these events that is effectively impossible to avoid. The link between food (particularly sugar) and honor is clear from the examples given and offers some insight into the motives for the quantity and quality of food consumed. The inexorable consumption of high fat, highly refined globalized foodstuffs, coupled with low levels of physical activity and high levels of stress are, I believe, evidence of chronicities of modernity in the UAE, producing an environment highly conducive to the development of type 2 diabetes.

Such insights show how rituals, practices, norms of behaviour, pressures and relationships are influential in explaining what, how, when and why some people in that community consume, in large quantity, the types of food that can contribute to obesity and diabetes.

For more discussion of issues of quality in ethnographic research, see Harris and Holmes (2013).

Ethics of ethnography

All research has ethical implications. Ethnography, however, has particular implications because researchers often have little control over the type and number of participants and the events they want to observe. A good ethnographic study is one in which the researcher uses her instincts, skills, experience and common sense in deciding what to observe and who to talk to as the study proceeds. While researchers may have an idea of who and what to observe (one of the requirements of ethical approval committees), in practice ethnographic research plans do not run according to intentions. As Madden (2010) points out:

> At every phase of ethnographic research, there is an ethical backdrop. In designing research, ethnographers need to make ethical decisions about its structure, in conducting research ethnographers will make ethical decisions as they negotiate the field situation, and as they analyse and write up their data, ethnographers will make ethical decisions about what material to include or exclude, and about the evolving issues of privacy and confidentiality that arise in the writing process. Even after ethnographers have departed the field, they will have ethical issues to consider about the nature of their departure and on-going association with their participant group.

The challenge of obtaining informed consent from participants selected in advance of the study and all those who visit the site when researchers carry out their observation can be significant. Liu et al. (2012) explained that they had to ask for written consent from 76 nurses and 27 patients, and verbal consent from all other individuals who interacted with the targeted participants at the time of observation. The ethical issues involved in interviewing and observing participants are further discussed in Chapters 17 and 18, respectively.

Criticisms and challenges of ethnographic research

Despite being a method of choice for exploring people's behaviour in their natural environment, ethnography is not without its challenges, problems and limitations. Obtaining ethical approval is not easy since it is not possible to state in advance precisely what will happen during an ethnographic study. It is not feasible to ask for everyone's informed consent, especially in a busy setting (for example, an emergency unit).

Immersing oneself in any setting and gaining the trust of the participants is time-consuming and perhaps not conducive to part-time researching. Getting accepted by key informants and gaining access to events and activities can be as much a matter of how the researcher is perceived, and of luck. It requires considerable skill to get accepted, especially in settings where outsiders are viewed with suspicion. Researchers usually have to obtain access to a particular setting from managers or employers; this can itself raise suspicions about what the real 'agenda' of the researcher and the managers is. There is also a real risk that the researcher could be drawn into existing conflicts or be 'manipulated' by one faction against another. The final report is likely to please some and not others, as group members may not all share the same views about themselves and about what they do.

'Thick description' does not suit the article format of journal articles, which impose word limits. Publications in the form of monographs and books are viable options, but they may not suit the busy practitioner. The challenge for researchers to summarise the findings in an easily digestible format is real. The final product of an ethnographic exploration is still one person's view of the culture of others. There is a real risk of misrepresenting the group and thereby causing harm to the very people who may have generously welcomed and helped the researcher.

Summary

Ethnography has evolved from its roots in cultural anthropology. It has been adapted for use in contemporary ethnographic studies of issues closer to home. New branches, such as focused ethnography, critical ethnography and online ethnography, have emerged as a response to contemporary needs and interests. The main features of ethnographic studies are its focus on the thoughts and behaviour of individuals in a group context and its reliance on observation as the main collection method, in conjunction with the use of other sources of data such as interviews, documents and artefacts. A degree of immersion in the setting is also crucial to help researchers to get as close as possible to where the action is and the meaning that participants give to their behaviour. Despite the ethical, political and practical challenges, the ethnographic approach is a potent way to get access to what people experience and to gain a first-hand glimpse of the world from their viewpoint.

References

Baglar R (2013) 'Oh God, save us from sugar': an ethnographic exploration of diabetes mellitus in the United Arab Emirates. *Medical Anthropology*, **32**, 2:109–25.

Barker J C and Horton S B (2008) An ethnographic study of Latino pre-school children's oral health in rural California: intersections among family, community, provider and regulatory sectors. *BioMedCentral Oral Health*, **8**:8.

Bjerknes M S and Bjork I T (2012) Entry into nursing: an ethnographic study of newly qualified nurses taking on the nursing role in a hospital setting. *Nursing Research and Practice*, 2012:art. id 690348.

Brooks F (2008) Nursing and public participation in health: an ethnographic study of a patient council. *International Journal of Nursing Studies*, **45**:3–13.

Carlson E (2013) Precepting and symbolic interactionism – a theoretical look at preceptorship during clinical practice. *Journal of Advanced Nursing*, **69**,2:457–64.

Colyer E (2013) Take a closer look at your customers. Retrieved from http://www.brandchannel.com/features_effect.asp?1ofid=167 (accessed 27 June 2013).

Cruz E V and Higginbottom G (2013) The use of focussed ethnography in nursing research. *Nurse Researcher*, **20**,4:36–43.

Evans-Pritchard E (1937) *Witchcraft, Oracles and Magic Among the Azande* (Oxford: Oxford University Press).

Fry M (2012) An ethnography: understanding emergency nursing practice belief systems. *International Emergency Nursing*, **20**, 2:120–5.

Garcia A C, Standlee A I, Bechkoff J and Cui Y (2009) Ethnographic approaches to the internet and computer-mediated communication. *Journal of Contemporary Ethnography*, **38**:52–84.

Genzuk M (2003) *A Synthesis of Ethnographic Research*. Occasional Papers Series (Los Angeles: Center for Multilingual, Multicultural Research, Rossier School of Education, University of Southern California).

Goffman E (1961) *Asylums: Essays on the Social Situation of Mental Patients and Other Inmates* (New York: Doubleday Anchor).

Harris J and Holmes C A (2013) Issues of quality in ethnographic research. Retrieved from www.edu.txtshr.com/docs/index-35677.html (accessed 13 January 2014).

Higginbottom G M A, Pillay J J and Boadu N Y (2013) Guidance on performing focused ethnographics with an emphasis on healthcare research. *Qualitative Report*, **8**, 17:1–16.

Keim-Malpass J and Steeves R H (2012) Talking with death at a diner: young women's online narratives of cancer. *Oncology Nursing Forum*, **39**, 4:373–8.

Kennedy H P and Lyndon A (2008) Tensions and teamwork: the relationship of midwives and nurses in a tertiary setting. *Journal of Obstetric, Gynecologic and Neonatal Nursing*, **37**:426–35.

Lambert V, Glacken M and McCarron M (2011) Employing an ethnographic approach: key characteristics. *Nurse Researcher*, **19**, 1:17–24.

Laurier E, Whyte A and Buckner K (2001) An ethnography of a neighbourhood café: informality, table arrangements and background noise. *Journal of Mundane Behaviour*, **2**, 2L:195–232.

Layder D (1993) *New Strategies in Social Research* (Cambridge: Polity Press).

Leininger M (1995) *Transcultural Nursing: Concepts, Theories, Research and Practice* (Columbus, OH: McGraw Hill).

Liu W, Manias E and Gerdtz M (2012) Medication communication between nurses and patients during nursing handovers on medical wards: a critical ethnographic study. *International Journal of Nursing Studies*, **49**:941–52.

Madden R (2010) *Being Ethnographic. A Guide to the Theory and Practice of Ethnography* (Thousand Oaks, CA: Sage).

Madison D S (2012) *Critical Ethnography: Method, Ethics and Performance*, 2nd edn (California: Sage).

Malinowski B (1922) *Argonauts of the Western Pacific* (London: Routledge & Kegan Paul).

Mead M (1928) *Coming of Age in Samoa: A Psychological Study of Primitive Youth for Western Civilisation* (New York: William Morrow).

National Institutes of Health (2013) *Social and Cultural Factors in Health* (Bethesda, MD: NIH Office of Behavioral and Social Sciences Research).

Saewyc E M (2003) Influential life contexts and environments for out-of-home pregnant adolescents. *Journal of Holistic Nursing*, **21**, 4:343–67.

Slatore C G, Hansen L, Ganzini L et al. (2012) Communication by nurses in intensive care units: qualitative analysis of domains of patient-centred care. *American Journal of Critical Care*, **21**, 6:410–8.

Smith L T (2001) *Decolonizing Methodologies: Research and Indigenous People* (Dunedin, New Zealand: University of Otago Press).

St-Amant O, Ward-Griffin C, De Forge R T et al. (2012) Making decisions in home-based dementia care: why context matters. *Canadian Journal on Aging*, **21**, 4:423–34.

Ward-Griffin C, McWilliam C L and Oudshoorn A (2012) Relational experiences of family caregivers providing home-based end-of-life care. *Journal of Family Nursing*, **8**, 4:491–516.

Weinstein M W (1982) Goffman's asylums and the social situation of mental patients. *Journal of Orthomolecular Medicine*, **11**, 4:267–76.

Whitehead T L (2004) What is ethnography? Methodological, ontological and epistemological attributes. Ethnographically Informed Community and Cultural Assessment Research Systems (EICCARS) Working Paper Series. Retrieved from http://www.cusag.umd.edu/documents/WorkingPapers/EpiOntAttrib.pdf (accessed 8 January 2013).

Whyte W F (1955) *Street Corner Society: The Social Structure of an Italian Slum* (Chicago: Chicago University Press).

Williamson S, Twelvetree T, Thompson J and Beaver K (2012) An ethnographic study exploring the role of ward-based advanced practitioners in an acute medical setting. *Journal of Advanced Nursing*, **68**, 7:1579–88.

Samples and Sampling

Introduction

One of the important decisions in designing a study is what data to collect and from whom. When the study population is too large, as is often the case, researchers have to resort to strategies to obtain the same information from a smaller group of people. In this chapter, we will explore the meaning of samples, identify a number of sampling techniques and discuss their strengths and limitations. In particular, we will explore the use of samples in quantitative and qualitative research.

Samples and populations

One of the crucial tasks in designing a research project is to decide on the number and characteristics of the respondents who will be invited to take part in the study. It is not always possible to include the entire population in a study, not least because of the costs involved. Having more respondents means that researchers spend more time in collecting and analysing data, so the life span of the project itself is increased. It is also easier to collect more, and in-depth, data from a smaller than a larger number of people. For these reasons, researchers sometimes select a proportion of the total number of potential respondents from whom to collect data. A proportion or subset of the population is known as the sample. The selection method or technique is called sampling. A carefully selected sample can provide data representative of the population from which the sample is drawn.

A population can be defined as the total number of units from which data can potentially be collected. These units may be individuals, organisations, events or artefacts. In a study on the use of evidence by staff nurses in medical wards in the UK, all staff nurses (individuals) working in this type of ward in the UK constitute the population under study. If a study is to find out which types of dressing are used in surgical wards in a particular health district, the population is all surgical wards (organisations) in that district. All the dressings would constitute a population of artefacts. In a study of psychiatric patients' eating behaviour at meal times over a period of 3 months in one hospital, all the meal times (events) during the 3-month period make up the population. And in a historical study of how nurses were portrayed in newspapers in the nineteenth century, all the newspapers (artefacts) during this period make up the population. In layman's language, 'population' is mainly used to describe people, but in research terms it has a wider meaning. For the purpose of this chapter, the individuals, organisations, events and artefacts that make up a population will be referred to as 'units'. It is sometimes important to use the entire units of a population in a study. For example, the decennial Census of Population, undertaken by the Office of National Statistics, comprises data from all households in the UK.

In theory, all the units of a population (also called the theoretical population), could potentially take part in a study, but in practice this may not be possible for various reasons. A researcher asking questions of patients with Alzheimer's disease in a ward will quickly realise that not all patients are able to take part. She may decide to include only those who are at an early stage of the disease. Additionally, she may exclude those who are restless and aggressive. In stipulating the inclusion criteria (an early stage of disease) and exclusion criteria (restlessness and aggressive behaviour), the researcher has defined the target population, that is, the population to be studied or, as it is commonly referred to, the study population (see Research Example 33 below). The target population is, therefore, the group that a researcher aims to draw a sample from. This population or group is defined by taking into account how they can be accessed and who can realistically take part.

The units of a population are never totally homogeneous (that is, sharing the same characteristics). Although all staff nurses in medical wards work in the same type of clinical setting, they are not a homogeneous group because they differ in such variables as age, gender, years of experience and qualifications. Depending on the research question and the resources, the researcher may want to include only full-time day staff nurses with 3 years' experience and may exclude those who are educated at graduate level. In practice, researchers must have good reasons for including and/or excluding units of population and must also clearly define these criteria. For example, 'patients in the early stages of Alzheimer's disease' needs to be operationally defined.

The target population, once defined, becomes the population of interest from whom the data can potentially be collected. In fact, the target population is a subset of the theoretical population. Sometimes all the units in the target population are included in the study, but more often a sample or subset of the target population is selected. When this happens, it is to the target population rather than the theoretical population that generalisations may be made.

In a study of 'postoperative pain', MacLellan (2004) used the following inclusion criteria to define her population: gynaecological, orthopaedic, urological and general surgical patients on the planned theatre lists of two selected hospitals. The exclusion criteria were: patients 'admitted to the intensive care unit or high dependency unit, confused, unable to use a 10-cm Visual Analogue Scale (VAS) or did not consent' (MacLellan, 2004). Therefore her findings are generalisable to those who match the characteristics of the participants included in this study. To maximise the generalisability of research findings, researchers should, as much as possible, be as inclusive as possible.

Sample frame

A list of all the units of the target population provides the frame from which a sample (if required) is selected. Therefore the sample frame contains the same number of units as the target population. There are some ready-made sample frames. For example, if a researcher decides to explore the learning styles of current nursing undergraduates at one university, the sample frame would be a list of the names of all nursing undergraduates who are currently studying there. The researcher would simply cross out the names of those who did not meet the inclusion criteria. Examples of ready-made lists that may potentially be used as sample frames are the Nursing and Midwifery Council register, a general practitioner's list of patients and a postcode address file. There are some drawbacks in using existing registers or lists as they may be incomplete, biased or not up to date. For a study using a sample frame, see Research Example 33.

It is not always possible or desirable to construct sample frames. For studies on sensitive issues such as sexually transmitted diseases, drug addiction or crime, ready-made lists are, understandably, not available. Participants are often recruited by means of newspaper adverts and newsletters, from support groups or by word of mouth. Sample frames are necessary when the researcher seeks to draw representative samples and thereafter to generalise from the data. It is important to note, however, that in qualitative research the concept of generalisation has a different meaning from what it does in quantitative research, and that sample frames are rarely used by qualitative researchers. This will be discussed later in this chapter.

Selected and achieved samples

The units in the sample selected by the researcher are the ones invited to take part in the study. However, not everyone invited is available, willing or able to take part. People change addresses and cannot be traced; others are too busy or are uninterested. Whatever the reasons, the selected sample loses some units and becomes the achieved sample. Although the achieved sample is normally smaller than the selected sample, some researchers may exceptionally decide to replace units in the original sample that did not take part by other units from the target population. Research Example 33 gives an example of how a selected sample was reduced to an achieved sample.

Sample frame, target population and achieved sample

Comparison of nurse practitioners' perceptions of required competencies and self-evaluated competencies in Taiwan *Chang et al. (2012)*

The sample frame in this study was the list or register of all nurses who 'qualified for the first annual nurse practitioner national licence exam'. Their names and addresses were obtained from the Department of Health database.

In this study, the researchers decided to 'target' all these nurses rather than select a sample. Therefore all nurses on this database constituted the 'target population'.

Of the 582 questionnaires distributed (the total number of nurses on the database), 374 completed questionnaires were returned, giving a response rate of 64.2 per cent. The achieved sample in this case is 374 nurse practitioners.

Types of sample

There are two basic types of sample:

- probability
- non-probability.

In a probability sample, every unit in the target population has a greater than zero chance of being selected. For example, if a sample of 10 students is to be selected from a target population of 50, each student will have a 1 in 5 (or 20 per cent chance) of being selected. In probability samples, the chance of selection for each unit is known in advance.

The main characteristic of a probability sample is that it is randomly selected from the target population. The term 'random', in the layman's sense, usually means haphazard, as when an interviewer picks out people as they come out of a doctor's surgery. Those who look approachable to the interviewer or those who do not seem to be in a hurry may be chosen. Apart from being subjective, this method of sampling has no sample frame. Therefore the chance of being selected for all those attending the surgery on that particular day is not known. In research terms, the random selection of units for a sample is carried out according to a specified objective method, such as giving each unit a number, putting all the numbers in a box and blindly picking out one number at a time until the required size of the sample has been drawn (although there are more 'scientific ways' to do this, as explained below). The aim, in quantitative research, is to select a sample representative of the target population.

Non-probability samples are made up of units whose chances of selection are not known in advance. In the example of people leaving a doctor's surgery, those who were available before the researcher arrived had a zero chance of selection, and the chances (of being selected) of those who were interviewed are also not known, as the potential number of all those who could have been interviewed is not known.

Qualitative researchers often use non-probability samples because, according to them, the purpose of qualitative research is to contribute to an understanding of phenomena. They therefore choose the sample that can best provide the required data, whatever the sampling method is. In fact, qualitative researchers sometimes substitute the term 'sampling' with 'recruitment'. The use and nature of samples in qualitative research is further discussed in a later section.

If the purpose of the study is to examine the relationships between variables and make generalisations, a probability sample should be selected. On the other hand, if the purpose is to explore phenomena in depth, researchers need to ensure that the participants in the sample have experience and/or views that can be useful in achieving this objective. The emphasis is less on representation and more on what they can contribute. Other factors that researchers take into consideration include the availability of, and access to, potential participants and the resources allocated to the study.

In quantitative research, decisions about samples and sampling are not taken after the research question and the methods of data collection are known: all three must be considered at the same time as they depend on one another. Sampling also has implications for the analysis of data. For example, inferential statistics (see Chapter 19) are based on the assumption that random samples of populations have been used to generate the data (Williamson, 2003). Watson (2004), for example, explained that inferential statistics 'can apply to a convenience sample but any claims should be attenuated by warnings about the extent to which the results may be generalised'.

In qualitative research, the aim is to explore and develop a conceptual and theoretical understanding of phenomena. Researchers should select participants who have experience of these phenomena by whatever ethical means are possible. While there is a degree of flexibility about whom and how many participants to recruit to a study, they must be carefully selected to reflect the range of possible experiences. Decisions about samples and the sampling method in qualitative research can be taken both prior to and during the data collection stage.

Types of probability sample

There are four types of probability sample:

- simple random sample;
- stratified random sample;
- systematic random sample;
- cluster random sample.

Each of these sampling procedures requires a sample frame before a random selection can be drawn.

Simple random sample

The most common form of random sampling is one in which each unit in the sample frame is given a number; these are then put into the proverbial hat, and numbers are drawn one at a time until the size of sample, specified in advance, is reached. Each unit has an equal chance of being selected. Simple random sampling is so called because once a number is given to each unit, only one step is then needed: picking numbers. Once a number has been taken out of the hat, the chances of those remaining are altered from what they were at the start of the process. For example, if a researcher decides to draw a sample of 10 from a population of 50, the chance of selection of each unit at the start of the operation is 1 in 5. After five units have been selected, the chance of each of the 45 units remaining in the hat being selected is altered to 1 in 9.

Simple random sampling is mostly suitable for a population that is more or less homogeneous and from which any sample drawn is unlikely to be seriously biased. A homogeneous sample is one in which most participants (normally over 90 per cent) are similar in key characteristics such as ethnicity, gender, age or socioeconomic status. However, when the population has varied characteristics (that is, it is heterogeneous), it may be unwise to rely on simple random sampling to obtain a representative sample possessing the main variables being studied.

Stratified random sample

When the sample frame contains units that vary greatly in variables such as age, gender, education, experience or illness condition, it is possible that simple random sampling may not be the most appropriate form of sampling in order to achieve representation. If one or more of these variables are important for the study, it is wise not to trust the selection process to chance. There are reasons why variables should sometimes be assured of representation. For example, some illness conditions are more prevalent in one gender than another. Myocardial infarction is more common in men, and breast cancer in women. Any sample of patients with either condition must be stratified if gender representation is important for the study. Stratified random sampling consists of separating the units in the sample frame into strata (layers) according to the variables the researcher believes are important for inclusion in the sample, and drawing a sample from each stratum using the simple random sampling method.

For example, in a study of student nurses' satisfaction with support from lecturers, if the sample frame of 150 students comprises 75 students from year 1, 45 students from year 2 and 30 students from year 3, the researcher must seek the views of students of each of these three groups if the findings are to be generalised to the target population. A simple random sample may by chance under- or over-represent one or more of these groups, or may not even include any representative of one of the smaller groups. To ensure representation, the sample frame of 150 students is divided into its year-group composition before a proportionate sample from each group is drawn. The sampling method involves three steps as follows:

Step 1   Stratify the sample frame into its constituent groups

       e.g.   Year 1 students: 75 (50%)
              Year 2 students: 45 (30%)
              Year 3 students: 30 (20%)

Step 2   Decide on a sample size and the proportion for each stratum

       e.g.   Total sample size required = 50
              Sample size of year 1 = 50% of 50 = 25
              Sample size of year 2 = 30% of 50 = 15
              Sample size of year 3 = 20% of 50 = 10

Step 3   Draw a simple random sample of the required size from each stratum

       e.g.   Year 1 students = 25 out of 75
              Year 2 students = 15 out of 45
              Year 3 students = 10 out of 30

In this example, a proportionate stratified random sample of each stratum was drawn. This means that each unit from each of the strata had the same chance of selection (1 in 3). However, if the size of the year 3 sample is not large enough to represent the views of the students, the researcher may decide to increase the size of this sample in order to increase their representation. The sample then becomes a disproportionate stratified random sample.

If gender as a variable is also important for this study, the sample frame would have to be stratified into male students and female students before a proportionate or disproportionate random sample could be drawn from each stratum. The heterogeneity of the target population is not in itself the only reason for stratification. The decision to stratify depends on the research question and the variables of interest to the researcher. Research Example 34 describes a study where stratified random sampling was used.

Stratified sampling

Nurses' perceptions and attitudes towards computerisation in a private hospital
Chow et al. (2012)

The researchers in this study wanted to target different 'types' of nurse: 'full-time senior nurses, including ward-in-charge and senior registered nurse, registered nurses (RNs) and enrolled nurses (ENs) working in different units [general wards, intensive care unit (ICU) and specialist out-patient centres] of the hospital'. Stratified random sampling was used to ensure the representativeness of each of these sub-groups of nurses.

Computer software was used to randomly select an equal proportion of these nurses for the final sample.

Comment

Although the authors did not explain exactly how the sample was drawn, it is likely that a list of each of these sub-groups was compiled, from which the participants were selected.

Research example 34

Systematic random sample

Systematic samples are drawn by choosing units on a list at intervals prescribed by the researcher in advance. The most basic system is choosing every 'nth' number on a list until the required sample size is reached. A researcher may decide to interview the occupants of every third house on a street to find out about their health beliefs, or a teacher may pick out every fifth student on the register to ask about their views on the organisation and delivery of the course.

For a systematic random sample to be drawn, there must be a sample frame, and every unit on the frame must have a chance of being selected. If a systematic random sample of 10 is to be drawn from a sample frame of 50, every fifth number (50 divided by 10) on the list is chosen. To avoid starting with number 1 each time, the researcher can pick a number at random between 1 and 5 and proceed to choose every fifth number from it. Say number 4 is picked at random as the starting number, every fifth number (9, 14, 19, 24, 29, 34, 39, 44, 49) will be selected until a sample size of 10 (including the starting number, 4) is obtained. One of the limitations of this type of sampling is that lists may have biases of their own. It is possible that every fifth name on a list is male and that they could by chance be selected, therefore creating a gender bias in the sample.

The sample frame could also have patterns or trends. For example, at weekends (especially on Friday and Saturday nights) people may attend accident and emergency (A&E) units for different accidents or injuries than they do on weekdays. A chronological list of patients may, in this case, contain what is known as a 'periodic' or 'cyclical' trend. A researcher using the A&E's list of patients as a frame to draw a systematic random sample may, by chance, pick a disproportionate number of weekenders.

One way to offset this drawback is to rearrange the names on the list and therefore break any periodic cycles it may contain. A systematic random sample will not be random unless the sampling frame is first put into random order. Research Example 35 illustrates the use of systematic sampling.

Research example 35

Systematic sampling

Patient satisfaction with triage nursing care in Hong Kong *Chan and Chau (2005)*

The sample frame in this study was a list of all patients who attended the emergency department of an urban acute hospital in Hong Kong in 2001. After setting the inclusion and exclusion criteria and calculating the required sample size, a systematic sampling technique was used to select 92 participants.

The authors explain that every fifth person on the list was selected until the desired sample size was achieved. The first person was selected randomly using a table of random numbers. This gave every person on the list a chance to be selected, instead of selecting the first person all the time.

Cluster random sample

A cluster is defined in the *Oxford Dictionary* as 'a group of similar things'. The units of a study population are sometimes already in the form of clusters. For example, each district has a number of hospitals. Each hospital is a cluster of health professionals, and within hospitals each ward is also a cluster of nurses. When the population already exists in clusters, it is sometimes more practical and cost-efficient to sample the clusters first and then sample the units from the selected clusters.

Suppose that the aim of our study is to find out the knowledge of, and attitude to, primary nursing among nurses in hospitals in Wales. A simple random sampling will involve listing all staff nurses working in all the hospitals in the country. When the sample frame is ready and a simple random sample of staff nurses is drawn, it is possible that some hospitals will be overrepresented and others underrepresented. Researchers may have to travel to hospitals where two or three nurses have been selected. The whole exercise can be demanding, time-consuming and costly. A stratified random sample would ensure that each hospital is proportionately represented in the sample, but the cost of compiling a sample frame and travelling to all the hospitals can still be enormous. However, stratified random sampling is necessary if the purpose is to study differences between hospitals.

Cluster random sampling, on the other hand, involves randomly sampling the hospitals before drawing a random sample of nurses from each of the selected hospitals or using the whole population of the randomly selected hospitals. In the above example, if there are 20 general hospitals, a cluster random sample of eight hospitals could be drawn. Thereafter, a simple random sample can be drawn from a list of nurses in the selected hospitals. This type of sampling is known as multistage, as it involves more than one stage. In doing this, a more in-depth study can also be carried out with less cost. Cluster random sampling is appropriate when the clusters are more or less homogeneous and when the final number of clusters selected is not small. For example, choosing a random sample of two hospitals out of 10 may decrease the viability of generalising the findings to the 10 hospitals. Therefore cost alone should not be the deciding factor in choosing this type of sampling.

A combination of stratified and cluster sampling can also be used. In the above example, if both psychiatric and general hospitals were included in the study, these hospitals could be divided into strata representing each specialty before a cluster random sample of each stratum was drawn.

The use of cluster sampling is illustrated in Research Example 36. For a detailed and insightful example of multistage sampling involving cluster, stratified and simple random sampling, see Marsland and Murrells (2000).

Cluster sampling

Dying of cancer in Italy: impact on family and caregiver. The Italian Survey of Dying of Cancer *Rossi et al. (2007)*

To recruit a representative sample of the families and caregivers of persons who died of cancer, a two-stage probability sampling strategy was used. In the first stage, 30 of 197 local health districts (LHDs) were randomly selected. The second stage consisted of selecting families and caregivers from each of the selected LHDs. To ensure the required sample size (*n* = 2000) and adequate representation, a fixed proportion (8.4 per cent) was selected from each of the selected clusters (LHDs).

Comments

1 Each LHD is a cluster of potential participants. The number of clusters ($n = 197$) was too large for these researchers to recruit participants from. Therefore a decision was taken to randomly select 30 clusters. By using an objective method of selection (simple random sampling), every cluster had an equal chance of selection.

2 If all the families and caregivers of those who died of cancer in the 30 LHDs were included in the study, the sample size would still be too large. Therefore these researchers decided to allocate a 'quota' of 8.4 per cent to each cluster.

Types of non-probability sample

There are five types of non-probability sample, which can be divided into two broad and overlapping categories: purposive or judgemental, and convenience. The first involves judgement and choice on the part of the researcher, thereby giving her a degree of control over the composition of the sample. With convenience sampling, on the other hand, the researcher chooses according to who or what is available. In practice, this distinction is not rigid since both may approaches involve a degree of judgement and convenience.

The five types of non-probability sample are:

- accidental sample
- purposive sample
- volunteer sample
- snowball sample
- quota sample.

Accidental sampling

In accidental samples, only those available have a chance of being selected. Interviewing shoppers outside a supermarket on their health beliefs is one way to select an accidental sample. Only those visiting the supermarket at that time and on that day will have a chance of being selected. In this type of sampling, there is no sample frame.

There are occasions when accidental sampling is appropriate. For example, if a researcher wants to find out patients' views on the information they receive on admission to hospital, she may decide to interview the first 50 consecutive patients following admission. She does not have a sample frame as she does not know who will be admitted. No one outside the first 50 patients will have a chance of selection. By accident, the sample may comprise mostly those with minor problems or of a particular social class.

Accidental sampling can have implications for the data. For example, waiting at street corners to interview people about their satisfaction with the health services in the area could mean that only pedestrians will be chosen. Those who have cars, and who may perhaps be more affluent, may be excluded. With accidental sampling, there is degree of subjectivity involved in the selection, as the researcher does not always choose everyone who happens to be available. These who appear more approachable may be more likely to be interviewed.

Purposive or purposeful sampling

This method of sampling, used mainly in qualitative research, involves the researcher deliberately choosing who to include in the study on the basis that those selected can provide the necessary data. Thus, if she wants to investigate the leadership styles of hospital general managers, she can deliberately choose (hand-pick) managers with different styles in order to study the concept of leadership from different perspectives. For this, she may have to rely on her own judgement and/ or that of those she believes can help her to make the choice. In such a study, generalising the findings to the target population of managers is not the main concern of the researcher. Instead, she is seeking to contribute to the (conceptual or theoretical) understanding of leadership styles rather than finding out the percentage of managers who use different styles. The sample is deliberately chosen by the researcher on the basis that these are the best available people to provide data on the issues being researched.

In choosing a purposive sample, the researcher must be guided by her research question and not be tempted to choose samples out of convenience or leave it to others to make the selection. The use of purposive samples in qualitative research is discussed further in this chapter. Research Example 37 shows the use of purposive sampling.

Purposive sampling

Stories of young people living with a liver transplant *Taylor et al. (2010)*

The focus of this study was to explore adolescents' experience of living with a liver transplant. The authors wanted as many different perspectives as possible in order to fully reflect the phenomenon under investigation. Purposive sampling was used to select participants based on 'stage of adolescence', gender, presentation of liver disease (acute, chronic or metabolic) and time since transplantation.

Research example 37

Volunteer sampling

Perhaps the weakest form of sampling is one in which people volunteer to take part and are therefore self-selected. It is a sample of convenience over which the researcher has little control. There are two categories of volunteer. First, there are those who offer to take part in a study before coming into contact with the researcher or her associates. An example of this is when people respond to a notice board or newspaper advert asking for people to take part in a study (see Gagliardi, 2003, for an example of a recruitment advertisement for volunteers). The researcher exerts little or no influence on the prospective participant except perhaps when financial or other inducements are offered. The second type of volunteer is those who are part of a captive population, either as patients in a hospital or students on a course. It is more difficult to know whether these groups really volunteer and whether their actions are what van Wissen and Siebers (1993) term 'uncoerced voluntary participation'.

There are a number of reasons why a captive population may 'volunteer' to take part in a study:

- moral obligation – they may feel that the research will be of benefit to other patients;
- gratitude – in return for the care they receive;
- fear of reprisals – as if they refuse, they think they may be punished;
- fear of being labelled as uncooperative;
- the need to conform.

For these reasons, the validity of the data could be seriously questioned, especially if, in addition, the volunteer may not trust the confidentiality and anonymity of the data.

Volunteering is itself an act of cooperation and reflects the personality of those more likely to volunteer. They may be conformists and traditional in outlook and could thus bias the sample. Those who are self-selected may show more interest and motivation than those who do not. Therefore volunteer samples are limited because we know little or nothing of those who do not take part in the study. Research Example 38 shows how volunteers were recruited in one study.

Research example 38

Volunteer sampling

Racial discrimination experienced by Aboriginal university students in Canada
Currie et al. (2012)

Participants for this study were invited to respond to poster advertisements on campus and e-newsletters. They were given 50 Canadian dollars each for participating. The use of a volunteer sample was acknowledged by the authors as a limitation of this study.

The sample size was small ($n = 60$), and more women (70 per cent) responded to the invitation to participate. The authors explained that this may be because more female than male aboriginals study at universities in Canada.

Comments

It is not known to what extent the honorarium of CAD$50 influenced participation and what limitations this might have had on the findings. The ratio of male to female aboriginals in the university where this study was carried out was not given or known. Therefore there may be other reasons why there was a much higher proportion of women volunteers in this study.

With volunteer sampling, the researcher has little control over the composition of the sample.

Snowball sampling

In simple terms, this means that a respondent refers someone they know to the study, who in turn refers someone they know, until the researcher has an adequate sample. It is sometimes difficult for the researcher to identify people who could take part in a study because of the sensitivity of the topic or because the researcher may not have ready access to a sample. For a sample of drug-takers or petty criminals, the researcher may depend on initial contacts to direct them to others who may be willing to take part. However, snowball sampling is not used exclusively when sensitive topics are being researched or when potential participants are scarce. In qualitative research, the number of units in the sample is often not decided in advance. As the fieldwork progresses, the researcher may come across other potentially useful participants and enlist them as she goes along. One of the major drawbacks of snowball samples is that participants may refer people of similar backgrounds and outlook to themselves.

The use of snowball sampling is shown in Research Example 39.

Snowball sampling

'It's not me, it's them': how lesbian women make sense of negative experiences of maternity care: a hermeneutic study *Lee et al. (2012)*

In this study, the researchers used the snowball technique, which consisted of identifying key informants and then asking them to identify others to participate. According to Lee et al. (2012), this type of sampling 'ensured a data-rich sample in what was potentially a small and hard-to-identify population' (that is, lesbian women). The authors also acknowledged that this type of sampling might 'lead to recruitment of similar participants'.

Research example 39

Quota sampling

Quota sampling involves elements of purposive and stratified sampling without random selection. In this type of sampling, the researcher recognises the need for different groups in the sample to be adequately represented. In a survey of students' views on the resources and support they receive in a nursing department of a university, there are a number of groups that should be represented in the sample. These could include full-time and part-time students, students on all the courses offered, school leavers and mature students, and males and females. Thus, the researcher may allocate 20 to each group. Depending on the aim of the research, proportionate or non-proportionate samples can be used. In accidental sampling, it is left to chance who is included in the sample. In quota sampling, the researcher allocates places in advance.

Quota sampling involves two stages. In the first stage, the quota allocation is decided. For example, in a study of nurses' attitude to person-centred nursing, 25 places could be allocated to each of the following sub-group of nurses – male, female, newly qualified and those with over 5 years' experience post-training –

making a total of 100 nurses. Or the researcher could allocate the 100 places according to the proportion of each grade. The second stage involves selecting the sample. If there is a sample frame of nurses and a random sample of 20 in each grade is drawn, the quota sampling becomes a stratified random sampling, or after deciding on quotas the researcher can purposefully choose 20 nurses whom she believes will provide the data for the project. She can also wait at the exit of the nurses' cafeteria and interview those who are available until the quota for each of the sub-groups is met.

In quota sampling, the overriding concern of the researcher is to have various elements represented. However, the sampling procedure remains a non-probability one because there is no recourse to random selection. If there is random selection, it becomes a random stratified sample. In the above study, while the researcher is interested to find out the views of nurses in each sub-group, these nurses would not necessarily be representative of the rest of the nurses in the hospital, mainly because no random selection has been carried out. Research Example 40 illustrates the use of quota sampling in one study.

Research example 40

Quota sampling

Information-seeking behaviour of nurses: where is information sought and what processes are followed? *O'Leary and Ni Mhaolrúnaigh (2012)*

In this study, the authors wanted to interview different sub-groups of nurses. They use a quota sampling technique to ensure that the major sub-groups were represented. The composition of the sample was as follows: 10 general nurses working in acute hospitals, 5 general nurses working in community hospitals, 5 intellectual disability nurses, 5 mental health nurses and 3 public health nurses.

With quota sampling, researchers decide in advance the number of participants to be allocated in each group, rather than leaving it to chance.

Sampling in quantitative research

It is generally believed that, in quantitative research, samples are large and probability sampling is frequent, while qualitative researchers use small, non-probability samples. Although this is a fair description as far as sample size is concerned, it is not unusual to observe from research journals that many quantitative researchers use convenience samples, and some qualitative ones resort to random selection. Convenience samples are probably the most frequently used of all types of sample in both types of research.

Webb (2003) reviewed all papers published in 2001 and 2002 in the *Journal of Clinical Nursing*. She concluded that the vast majority of quantitative and qualitative studies used convenience samples. When Webb (2004) did a similar exercise for all 256 papers published in the *Journal of Advanced Nursing* throughout 2002, she found that 'virtually all the empirical studies were based on convenience samples'. Cowman and Conroy (2004) explain that, in real-life research, sample frames are rarely available, and as a result 'non-random samples are therefore the rule rather than the exception'.

In quantitative research, the data from randomly selected samples are generalised to the target population and sometimes beyond, to similar populations and settings. The purpose of research is not only to study the specific, but also to draw general principles and conclusions in order to apply them to similar situations outside the particular population and setting being studied.

Sampling in qualitative research

Qualitative researchers believe that the phenomena they study are culture-specific and time-bound, and that their findings are a result of the interaction between the researcher and the researched. This means that although the same phenomena may exist in other cultures, they are often manifested and experienced differently in different cultures or settings. Additionally, since the findings were obtained at a specific point in time (that is, they are time-bound), the study cannot be replicated and the findings are not necessarily generalisable to other settings. Therefore sampling for the purpose of generalising to other populations and settings is normally not the prime reason for researchers in the qualitative tradition,

There is a great deal of overlap and confusion in the way researchers describe their sampling strategies in qualitative research. Terms such as 'purposive', 'accidental', 'convenience' and 'theoretical' sampling are often used interchangeably. There is a need to understand the differences and similarities between them and the purpose for which they can be used. In a broad sense, all qualitative sampling methods can be described as 'selective' since they involve the subjective judgement of the researcher in the selection process. Beyond this, there are different types of selective samples including, among others, purposive sampling and theoretical sampling. A cursory examination of qualitative and mixed method studies in the literature shows different ways in which researchers sample their participants.

In some studies, the researcher selects among accessible and consenting participants those who can, in her judgement, contribute most towards understanding the phenomenon under investigation. The emphasis is on obtaining different perspectives from participants so that the phenomenon can be revealed in all its dimensions and facets. It is therefore helpful to select those who can offer insights into the phenomenon by virtue of having some experience or views about it. Particular attention is paid to those who hold different, conflicting or contradictory views, even if those individuals are not representative of the population or group to which they belong. Demographic characteristics such as gender, age, occupation, status or education are often taken into account, as people with different attributes may have different views.

This type of sample can be called purposive since participants are selected on purpose because they have enough experience and abilities to answer the research question. One can say that all samples are purposive because researchers always choose people who can answer the question (for example, they would ask mothers, not fathers, about the experience of giving birth). The difference between this and purposive sampling in qualitative research is that, in the latter, the researcher chooses on purpose those who have different characteristics and different contributions to make, while in the former this is left to chance.

Purposive samples are frequently used in phenomenological studies (see Chapter 12). The size of the sample and the individuals selected are decided upon at the start of the study. It is possible to increase the size of the sample if not enough data are forthcoming, or to stop sampling if the same data are being repeated. Larsson et al. (2003) describe how they selected their sample in their phenomenological study of 'Lived experiences of eating problems for patients with head and neck cancer during radiotherapy':

> The informants were undergoing radiotherapy for head and neck cancer at two oncology clinics in Sweden. The inclusion criterion was that informants were expected to experience eating problems because of side-effects of radiotherapy. In order to achieve a broad description as possible of the phenomenon under study, they were chosen to represent different categories of gender, age and civil status.

Another frequently used procedure in qualitative research is 'theoretical sampling'. The term comes from Glaser and Strauss (1967) and is mainly used in grounded theory studies (see Chapter 13). Strauss and Corbin (1998) define it as:

> data gathering by concepts derived from the evolving theory and based on the concept of 'making comparisons', whose purpose is to go to places, people or events that will maximise opportunities to discover variations among concepts.

The essential feature of theoretical sampling is that the researcher does not know, in advance, who to interview or observe. As the data are analysed, the emerging ideas (which need to be further explored) guide the researcher in her choice of other people (or documents or events) to collect data from. In McCaughan and McKenna's (2007) study of 'information needs and information seeking behaviour of newly diagnosed cancer patients', one of the emerging ideas from data collected at the beginning of the study was patients' frequent use of lay sources. It was important that the researchers followed up these sources (faith healer, hairdresser and so on) in order to understand the behaviour of these patients. Prior to the study, McCaughan and McKenna did not intend to include these lay sources in their sample, nor did they anticipate that they might have to.

As can be seen from the above example, data collected and analysed at the beginning of a grounded theory study guide the further selection of participants. Researchers using a grounded theory approach therefore need an initial sample to start with. They normally resort to a small purposive sample and thereafter use theoretical sampling. This tends to cause problems when they apply for funding, because they cannot state in advance all the sources of data that they will eventually use.

In ethnographic studies, the concept of samples and sampling have different meanings from these two types (purposive and theoretical) described above. This is mainly because ethnographic studies involve spending prolonged periods in particular settings. The number of people with whom the researcher comes into contact and the varying contributions that they make are not easily quantified or even described. The term 'key informants' refers to people whom the ethnographer relies upon for providing information and insights, and access to other people, events and artefacts (such as documents or other evidence). Everyone in the setting and any other source of information (within practical, legal and ethical limits) are potentially useful in providing data. Researchers have to convey this in their publications, as well as the reasons for selecting the setting where the study is being carried out.

Finally, in mixed methods studies, researchers may want to confirm the findings of a questionnaire by means of qualitative interviews. They may select a random sample of respondents in order to obtain representative views. However, if the purpose of selecting a representative (random) sample in this case is to generalise to the target population, one should remember that generalisability depends not only on random selection, but also on other factors such as predetermined, objective, structured and standardised methods of data collection and analysis.

To some extent, overlap and confusion in the use and description of qualitative sampling methods are inevitable because the different techniques share some of the same characteristics, such as subjective judgement in selecting participants, and flexibility to increase the sample size to learn more about a phenomenon or to stop the study when no new ideas are emerging. There is also scope to interview or observe the same participant on more than one occasion. However, one should also understand the differences between different types of sampling and the purpose, process and implications of using them. Coyne (1997) explains that 'distinctions between sampling strategies may be helpful for the neophyte researcher, but conforming to those arbitrary distinctions may not be helpful for the purpose of the qualitative study'. It is less important for researchers to correctly name the type of sampling used than to explain precisely how the sample was selected, the reasons for their decisions and the implications for the findings. For further discussions of sampling in qualitative research, see Crouch and McKenzie (2006) and Forman et al. (2008).

Critiquing samples and sampling

Although qualitative researchers may not claim that their data are generalisable to other settings, it is important for them to describe their samples and sampling method adequately for the reader to assess whether they are useful to other settings.

In quantitative research, the purpose of sampling is to collect valid and reliable data from a subset of the population that would be representative of the whole population. These findings are often expected to be generalisable to other similar populations and settings. The representativeness of the sample and the generalisability of the findings depend on at least four factors: the size and the characteristics of the sample, the method of sampling, the setting where the study was carried out and the response rate.

Sample size

Small samples in quantitative research are also unlikely to yield results of significance. In fact, academic journals may refuse to publish quantitative research projects in which small samples have been used, except if little research exists on the topic. A sample size of 10 out of a student population of 300 is clearly unlikely to be representative, even if the sample is one of probability. The degree of representativeness will increase with a sample of 50 and above.

A power calculation is carried out to determine the sample size required for statistical analysis to confirm or reject a correlation or causal relationships between variables. The size of the sample depends on the magnitude or extent of the anticipated changes. If the change is estimated to be large, a smaller sample is required than if the change is estimated to be small. For example, if, in a study assessing the effects of an educational programme on participants' knowledge scores, researchers expect an increase of 20 points (on a scale of 0 to 100), a small sample can detect these changes. On the other hand, if a drug is being tested for its effectiveness in reducing body temperature by 0.5 of a degree, a larger sample is required in order to ascertain that this change is statistically significant.

If a sample is too small, it may fail to detect that the experimental (new) intervention is more effective than the conventional one. In this case, it is the small sample size that may be responsible for showing no difference, when in fact there may be one. Why not use a large sample? Large samples are costly and time-consuming. It is also unethical to recruit more participants than necessary in a study.

Computer software has been developed for estimating the required sample size for a quantitative study. A simple online search will reveal many useful online sample size calculators (see, for example, http://www.surveysystem.com/sscalc.htm). For a paper on for how to calculate sample size, see McCrum-Gardner (2010).

In appraising a quantitative study, you should expect a justification of the sample size. Where correlational relationships are investigated, a statement of how the sample size was calculated should be provided. Equally important is the degree of 'fit' between the sample and the population from which it is drawn. This means that the sample must be similar in its characteristics to the overall population. For example, if in a study of stress among hospital nurses the composition of the target population is 50 per cent staff nurses, 30 per cent healthcare assistants and 20 per cent clinical managers, the sample should, more or less, reflect a similar proportion of these three groups. Certain variables, such as gender or age, may be more important in one study than in others; therefore the samples must reflect the target population in these key variables. The more homogeneous the target population, the more representative the sample is likely to be. Samples for heterogeneous populations need to be large and carefully selected. Stratified random sampling is often the answer.

In general, qualitative studies use small samples, but it is a misconception to think that 'numbers are unimportant in ensuring the adequacy of a sampling strategy'

(Sandelowski, 1995). However, size is not the starting point. It is the purpose for which the sample is required that should decide how many respondents are recruited. In in-depth studies, the sample is unlikely to be large. There have been cases where a sample of two or three respondents has been studied. It is possible, although unlikely, that such a sample size could yield a range of different perspectives if this is what the researcher is seeking. On the other hand, if researchers carry out qualitative interviews with 100 respondents, it is possible that saturation of data could be reached very quickly. The time and effort required to interview all the respondents could be better spent on more in-depth interviews with, for example, 50 of them, with the option of interviewing some of the same respondents more than once. The more varied the population from whom the data are required, the larger the sample size should be.

In quantitative studies, the focus is on how particular views or beliefs are distributed in a population. In qualitative studies, researchers are interested in the range of their experiences in order to obtain as complete an understanding of the phenomenon as possible. If these experiences are suspected to vary greatly in a population, or if the population that possess these experiences themselves vary in terms of demographic variables such as age, race, gender or social class, it makes sense that the sample should take this into account.

The flexible and enquiring nature of qualitative research makes hard and fast rules inappropriate. According to Sandelowski (1995), researchers have to make their own judgements. She explains that:

> Numbers have a place in ensuring that a sample is fully adequate to support particular qualitative enterprises. A good principle to follow is: An adequate sample size in qualitative research is one that permits – by virtue of not being too large – the deep, case-oriented analysis that is a hallmark of all qualitative inquiry, and that results in – by virtue of not being too small – a new and richly textured understanding of experience.

Sampling method

Although probability samples are likely to be more representative than non-probability samples, representativeness is not necessarily assured with random selection. The decision on which form of random sampling to use depends on, among other things, the availability of lists, the composition of the population and the research questions. Whatever the sampling methods, these must be described in enough detail for you to decide whether the sample has any bias. Just stating that a random or a convenience sample was drawn, without explaining how, is not helpful. It is important for researchers to say who selected the sample. This is often left to 'gatekeepers', managers and practitioners, resulting in researchers having little control over who is included in the study.

The setting

To generalise findings from research in one setting to another requires a careful consideration of how similar or different the settings are. The findings of a study of support for the informal carers of people with dementia in the USA may not be applicable to carers in the UK. Statutory, voluntary services as well as social networks are likely to be different in the two countries. Far from rejecting the results, this could serve as a basis for comparisons, thereby enhancing one's understanding of support for carers in general.

The setting in which the data are collected can also introduce bias into the findings. Researchers must provide you with adequate details of the context in which research has been carried out. The responses from a 'captive' population of patients (in hospital, receiving care) may not be the same as when they are interviewed in their own homes. The social and cultural factors in the environment in which the research is taking place must be taken into consideration.

Response rate

Another aspect of sampling that you need to monitor is the response rate. The lower the response rate, the less representative the achieved sample is likely to be of the target population.

Those who do not respond may have characteristics different from those who do. In a study of attitudes to homosexuality, it is possible that non-respondents are not interested in the topic or that they are homophobic and are so 'disgusted' that they do not take part. Some people may see non-responding as a form of protest.

It is difficult to define an acceptable response rate. Researchers usually compare their response rates with the 'norm' in similar studies. What is more important is for researchers to attempt to explain non-responses and their possible implications for the data.

Summary

In this chapter, we have looked at some of the common terms used in relation to samples and sampling. The uses, strengths and limitations of the main sampling methods in nursing research have been discussed. Samples are the sources of research data and as such must be carefully selected and soundly justified. Researchers must provide readers with adequate information on the composition of the target population and sample, as well as the sampling method, to enable them to evaluate the representativeness of the sample and the usefulness and possible generalisability of the findings.

References

Chan J N and Chau J (2005) Patient satisfaction with triage nursing care in Hong Kong. *Journal of Advanced Nursing*, **50**, 5:498–507.

Chang I W, Shyu Y I, Tsay P K and Tang W R (2012) Comparison of nurse practitioners' perceptions of required competencies and self-evaluated competencies in Taiwan. *Journal of Clinical Nursing*, **2**, 17–18:2679–89.

Chow S K, Chin W Y, Lee H Y, Leung H C and Tang F H (2012) Nurses' perceptions and attitudes towards computerisation in a private hospital. *Journal of Clinical Nursing*, **21**:1685–96.

Cowman S and Conroy R M (2004) A response to: Misrepresenting random sampling? A systematic review of research papers by G R Williamson (*Journal of Advanced Nursing*, 2003, 44:278–88). *Journal of Advanced Nursing*, **46**, 2:221–3.

Coyne I T (1997) Sampling in qualitative research. Purposeful and theoretical sampling; merging or clear boundaries? *Journal of Advanced Nursing*, **26**:623–30.

Crouch M and McKenzie H (2006) The logic of small samples in interview-based qualitative research. *Social Science Information*, **45**:483–99.

Currie C L, Wild T C, Schopflocher D P, Laing L and Veugelers P (2012) Racial discrimination experienced by Aboriginal university students in Canada. *Canadian Journal of Psychiatry*, **57**, 10:617–25.

Forman J, Creswell J W, Damschroder L, Kowalski C P and Krein S L (2008) Qualitative research methods: key features and insights gained from use in infection prevention research. *American Journal of Infection Control*, **36**:764–71.

Gagliardi B A (2003) The experience of sexuality for individuals living with multiple sclerosis. *Journal of Clinical Nursing*, **12**:571–8.

Glaser B and Strauss A (1967) *The Discovery of Grounded Theory: Strategies for Qualitative Research* (Chicago, IL: Aldine).

Larsson M, Hedelin B and Athlin E (2003) Lived experiences of eating problems for patients with head and neck cancer during radiotherapy. *Journal of Clinical Nursing*, **12**:562–70.

Lee E, Taylor J and Raitt F (2012) 'It's not me, it's them': how lesbian women make sense of negative experiences of maternity care: a hermeneutic study. *Journal of Advanced Nursing*, **67**, 5:982–90.

MacLellan K (2004) Postoperative pain: strategy for improving patient perspectives. *Journal of Advanced Nursing*, **46**, 2:179–85.

Marsland L and Murrells T (2000) Sampling for a longitudinal study of the careers of nurses qualifying from the English pre-registration Project 2000 diploma course. *Journal of Advanced Nursing*, **31**, 4:935–43.

McCaughan E and McKenna H (2007). Never-ending making sense: towards a substantive theory of the information-seeking behaviour of newly diagnosed cancer patients. *Journal of Clinical Nursing*, **16**:2096–104.

McCrum-Gardner E (2010) Sample size and power calculation made easy. *International Journal of Therapy and Rehabilitation*, **17**, 1:10–14.

O'Leary D F and Ni Mhaolrúnaigh S (2012) Information-seeking behaviour of nurses: where is information sought and what processes are followed? *Journal of Advanced Nursing*, **68**, 2:379–90.

Rossi G, Beccaro M, Miccinesi G et al. (2007) Dying of cancer in Italy: impact on family and caregiver. The Italian Survey of Dying of Cancer. *Journal of Epidemiology and Community Health*, **61**:547–54.

Sandelowski M (1995) Sample size in qualitative research. *Research in Nursing and Health*, **18**:179–83.

Strauss A and Corbin J (1998) *Basics of Qualitative Research: Techniques and Procedures for Developing Grounded Theory*, 2nd edn (London: Sage).

Taylor R M, Franck L S, Dhawan A and Gibson (2010) The stories of young people living with a liver transplant. *Qualitative Health Research*, **20**, 8:1076–90.

van Wissen K A and Siebers R W L (1993) Nurses' attitudes and concerns pertaining to HIV and AIDS. *Journal of Advanced Nursing*, **18**:912–17.

Watson R (2004) A response to: Misrepresenting random sampling? A systematic review of research papers by G R Williamson (Journal of Advanced Nursing, 2003, 44:278–88). *Journal of Advanced Nursing*, **46**, 2:220–1.

Webb C (2003) Research in brief. An analysis of recent publications in JCN: sources, methods and topics. *Journal of Clinical Nursing*, **12**:931–4.

Webb C (2004) Editor's note: Analysis of papers published in JAN in 2002. *Journal of Advanced Nursing*, **45**, 3:229–31.

Williamson G R (2003) Misrepresenting random sampling? A systematic review of research papers. *Journal of Advanced Nursing*, **44**:278–88.

Questionnaires

Introduction

In this chapter, we will take a close look at the questionnaire as a method of data collection in nursing research, in particular its value and limitations and the advantages and disadvantages of different modes of questionnaire administration. The strategies that researchers can use to ensure and enhance the validity and reliability of questionnaires are examined, and some of the ethical implications of this popular method of data collection are explored and discussed.

Use of questionnaires in nursing

The questionnaire is by far the most common method of data collection in social and health research. However, it is not useful just for research purposes. We have all, at some time or other, been asked questions or asked to fill in a form, for example when attending a general practitioner's surgery or an accident and emergency department. Nurses have a number of forms to complete as part of their work. The hospital admission form itself is a questionnaire seeking information such as the name, date of birth, next of kin, previous admissions, family medical history and any previous illness of the patient. Clinical specialties may have their own forms asking specific questions. For example, a 'preoperative screening chart' in one hospital asked questions about 'allergies, general health (hypertension, diabetes, cardiac disease), skin problems, dental problems and social habits'. Below is an extract from a 'clinical' questionnaire administered to patients at a fracture clinic.

Q5	Any past illnesses?	☐	Yes	☐	No
Q6	Do you have blackouts or faint easily?	☐	Yes	☐	No
Q7	Do you get breathless easily, i.e. asthma?	☐	Yes	☐	No
Q12	Do you have transport to and from hospital?	☐	Yes	☐	No

| Q13 | Do you live alone? | ☐ Yes | ☐ No |
| Q14 | Do you smoke? | ☐ Yes | ☐ No |

Most of these forms or questionnaires that nurses administer to clients serve two main purposes: diagnostic and record-keeping. The information gathered provides the basis for any subsequent diagnosis and treatment. It is useful for assessing clients' needs and helps in the formulation of care plans. Other general information is routinely kept by health centres and hospitals for administrative, accounting and planning purposes. It provides indicators of admissions, discharges, morbidity, mortality, resource allocation, uptake of services, deployment of personnel and so on.

These questionnaires were not designed primarily for the collection of research data, although patients' notes, care plans and other records are valuable sources of data for researchers conducting retrospective studies. Some of these questionnaires would not withstand a rigorous validity and reliability test, but they are usually useful for the purpose they serve: they provide the necessary information on which clinical and policy decisions can be made. There are, of course, methodological, ethical and legal issues involved in the use of information from patients' notes for research purposes.

What is a questionnaire?

A questionnaire can be described as a method that seeks written or verbal responses from people to a written set of questions or statements. It is a research method when it is designed and administered solely for the purpose of collecting data as part of a research study. It is a quantitative approach since it is predetermined (constructed in advance), standardised (the same questions in the same order are asked of all the respondents) and structured (respondents are mainly required to choose from the list of responses offered by the researcher).

Questionnaires can be used in descriptive studies, correlational studies and experimental studies (see Chapter 10). In descriptive studies, they may not only provide data that facilitate an understanding of the phenomena being investigated, but can also generate data from which concepts and hypotheses can be formulated. In correlational studies, questionnaires can provide data to support or reject hypotheses. In randomised controlled trials, questionnaires are used to measure, among other things, outcomes.

The questionnaire is, however, most frequently used in survey designs. In fact, the term 'questionnaire' is often used interchangeably with 'survey'. A distinction needs to be made between them. A survey is a research design that can comprise one or more methods of data collection, including questionnaires, interviews and/ or observations. For example, in a survey on the dental health of schoolchildren, data can be collected by asking questions (by means of either questionnaires or interviews) and by observing the presence or absence of dental caries in these schoolchildren. Some surveys can be carried out almost entirely by observations, as in the case of a 'survey on food intake', when the food intake is observed, weighed and analysed.

Questionnaires in nursing research

Questionnaires are efficient in providing data on the attributes of clients and staff, and are used in the evaluation of practice and policy and in the assessment of the needs of clients and staff. They have also been increasingly used in the measurement of concepts and constructs as varied as, for example, empathy, burnout, social support, pain, coping, hope, stress and quality of life. There are, of course, other methods that are equally, if not better, suited to the study of these phenomena. Researchers must always choose the most appropriate data collection method or methods in order to answer the research question(s).

Questionnaires have been used mainly to collect information on facts, attitudes, knowledge, beliefs, opinions, perceptions, expectations, experiences and the behaviour of clients and staff. The most common factual data collected by questionnaires are demographic ones, such as age, gender, occupation, social class and qualifications. These are very useful for constructing profiles of clients and staff and for exploring their correlation with other attributes, such as personality, attitudes or expectations. Other facts related to practice include physiological measures, such as temperature, pulse, respiration or blood pressure, and other occurrences, such as the amount of fluid intake, attendance at outpatient departments and frequency of bowel movements.

The attitudes, knowledge and beliefs of clients are studied because they can influence, among other factors, how people regard their health and illness, what services they use, how compliant they are with nursing and medical treatment and advice, and what actions they take to promote their health. The attitudes, knowledge and beliefs of health professionals can also influence their practice. For example, their knowledge of, and attitudes to, research may determine whether and how they utilise research. The opinions, perceptions, expectations and experiences of clients and practitioners are legitimate areas of enquiry because nursing is about meeting the needs of the client.

Although behaviour is best studied by observation, it is sometimes not feasible or practical to do this, as in the case of sexual practices and behaviours of dubious legal or moral status. Past behaviour, unless captured on film, cannot be studied by observation, nor can behavioural intentions. The questionnaire, on the other hand, can ask respondents to report on past, actual and potential behaviours, as perceived by them.

All the above phenomena that are commonly studied by means of questionnaires are important in helping professionals to better organise and deliver care and treatment. The data produced can also be useful in promoting health, preventing illness and disability and contributing to effective rehabilitation.

Question formats

Researchers have developed a range of question formats to collect valid and reliable data efficiently and to analyse them quickly. These are strategies designed to facilitate respondents in providing the necessary and relevant information in a short time and in a relatively painless way. The choice of question format depends mainly on the type of data that researchers want to collect. If they set out to find out from respondents which factors affect their job dissatisfaction, they could ask a type of question that is open enough to allow respondents to formulate their own responses. On the other hand, if researchers want to compare the degree to which staff are satisfied with their job, they may offer respondents a number of categories to choose from, such as 'very satisfied', 'satisfied', 'neither satisfied nor dissatisfied', 'dissatisfied' and 'very dissatisfied'. Common question formats in questionnaires include closed questions, open-ended questions, vignettes and rating scales.

Closed questions

Common formats of closed questions include:

- two-way questions
- checklists
- multiple-choice questions
- ranking questions.

Two-way questions, as the term suggests, offer a choice between two responses, as shown below:

Male ☐   Female ☐   (please tick one box)

A true/false or an agree/disagree as well as a yes/no option can also be offered, as in the following example:

	Please tick one box	
	True	*False*
The reliability of an instrument is the degree to which it measures what it is expected to measure	☐	☐
	Agree	*Disagree*
A knowledge of nursing theories is essential for the practice of nursing	☐	☐
	Yes	*No*
Do you think that every nurse should learn how to do research?	☐	☐

Checklists provide respondents with a list of responses from which to select. They can 'tick' as many items or statements as they think are applicable. The following example of a checklist question comes from McKenna et al.'s (2004) study of barriers to evidence-based practice in primary care:

Please tick the source(s) of information that you use to inform your practice on a day-to-day basis (tick as many as apply).

Media	☐	Evidence-based circulars	☐
Colleagues	☐	Clinical guidelines	☐
Conferences	☐	Protocols	☐
Central Services Agency	☐	Courses	☐
Journals	☐	Drug representatives	☐
Own judgement	☐	Other	☐

Sometimes the checklist is not exhaustive, and respondents are asked to add to it.

Multiple choice is another format used in questionnaires. This offers respondents a list of responses, normally in the form of statements, from which they can select the one most applicable to them:

Please tick one journal that you read most frequently.

Midwifery	☐
Journal of Advanced Nursing	☐
Scandinavian Journal of Caring Sciences	☐
Qualitative Health Research	☐
Journal of Clinical Nursing	☐
Journal of Community Nursing	☐
Nurse Education Today	☐
Nurse Researcher	☐

Researchers sometimes want to know how respondents prioritise their needs, whom they consult most or least for health advice or what interventions they find most or least useful. To obtain rapid answers, they ask respondents to rank from a list of responses. The following is an example of a ranking question on schoolchildren's knowledge of, and attitudes to, mental illness:

Where did you get information on mental illness from?
Please rank the items below by putting 1 to 6 in the boxes provided
(1 = most information, 6 = least information)

School teacher	☐
Television	☐
Books	☐
Internet	☐
Magazines	☐
Parents	☐
Friends	☐

Closed questions are asked when researchers consider that they know all the potential answers and only require respondents to select the one or ones that apply to them. Such questions are appropriate for demographic data and in cases where there are a more or less fixed number of alternatives. For example, a researcher can ask a closed question such as that shown below, when medication can only be given via these five routes:

By which route do you normally administer medication X? Please tick one box.

Oral   ☐
Sublingual   ☐
Rectal   ☐
Topical   ☐
Parenteral   ☐

Closed questions yield data that allow for a comparison between respondents as all the responses are in the same format. They can be pre-coded, thereby making analysis a relatively easy task. The main problem with closed questions is that the researcher may omit an important response and thereby obtain a result different from that had the response been included. If, for example, the researcher omitted 'magazines' from the list in the above ranking question, the schoolchildren in the survey would rank what is on offer and therefore provide different data from those obtained if 'magazines' had been included. Another example of forced choice is when a respondent is asked to rank in order from 1 to 6, when in reality he or she may want to rank two items at number 1. Researchers constructing closed questions must make sure that all possible choices are included, bearing in mind that respondents may be confused if they have to choose from too many categories.

The list of responses offered by the researcher may give the respondents an idea of what is normal. For example, by asking respondents to choose from a list of journals that nurses read, they may think that nurses normally read these journals, and that perhaps they should indicate that they do so as well. Therefore, checklists and multiple choices may unwittingly reveal to respondents what the norm is and thereby encourage them to give socially desirable answers.

These limitations can be to a large extent offset by careful and skilful construction of the questionnaire, by paying particular attention to the categories offered to respondents and by including questions in appropriate formats.

Open-ended questions

When researchers do not have all the answers and/or want to obtain respondents' views, they can formulate an open-ended question, as in the example below.

Please indicate below the main factors that contribute to your job satisfaction.

_____

_____

_____

_____

It is also possible to ask an open-ended ranking question in a different way:

Please list, in order of importance, four factors that contribute to your job satisfaction (1 = most important, 4 = least important).

1 _____

2 _____

3 _____

4 _____

Open-ended questions give respondents the opportunity to frame their answers in their own words. Questionnaires are designed to collect data quickly. However, too many open-ended questions will require more time and effort from participants, who may decide to skip these questions or provide superficial answers. There can be a large number of missing answers to open-ended questions, which can cast doubt on the generalisability of the findings. Nonetheless, researchers often find that the most interesting data come from these types of question.

Open-ended questions give respondents the opportunity to participate in, and interact with, the questionnaire in a way that closed questions do not. An open-ended question must be clear and unambiguous, or different respondents will interpret it differently. For example, in a questionnaire on job satisfaction, the researcher who wants to know the types of clinical area where respondents work (that is medical, surgical or care of the elderly) may ask 'Which type of ward do you work in?' The answers could be 'a 25-bedded ward', 'a mixed ward', 'a care of older people ward', 'an open ward' or 'a chaotic ward'. There is always the possibility with open-ended questions that the researcher understands the question differently from some of the respondents. The responses given above would not be useful to the researcher, as they do not answer the question in the way and form she wants.

Responses to open-ended questions can also vary in length. Some respondents continue their answers on the back of the questionnaire, whereas others give a response in a few words. The space provided for responses is sometimes an indication of how long the researcher expects them to be. However, some respondents have larger handwriting than others. A bigger problem may be in deciphering what is written and in making sense of what is said. Open-ended questions can generate large amounts of data. In a study by Wahlberg et al. (2003), respondents were asked one open-ended question: 'What problems have you experienced with telephone advice?' This generated 154 statements, which were later reduced to 24 'problem categories'. An analysis of responses from such questions can be time-consuming and difficult since responses are rarely made using the same terminologies, unlike the case with closed questions. The analysis of quantitative data is further discussed in Chapter 19.

Open-ended questions do not make a questionnaire a qualitative method, as some people believe. As I have explained elsewhere (Parahoo, 1993):

> questionnaire data are treated at face value; there is no opportunity to unravel the real meaning of each individual response. What people say and what they mean can be

different, and several interviews with the same person are sometimes necessary to collect meaningful data.

Open-ended questions are valuable in that they give respondents some freedom in expressing themselves rather than their being constrained by the 'straitjacket' style of closed questions.

Both closed and open-ended questions have their place in questionnaires. Researchers must use them judiciously and appropriately, and as much as possible use the strength of one to offset the limitation of the other.

Vignettes

Another imaginative strategy that can be used in questionnaires is asking people to respond to questions by providing them with short descriptions of a situation or event that closely resemble a real situation. Gould (1996) describes vignettes as:

> Simulations of real events which can be used in research studies to elicit subjects' knowledge, attitudes or opinions according to how they state they would behave in the hypothetical situation depicted.

This method is used in teaching and in examinations as well. For example, Chan et al. (2006) used videotaped vignettes to evaluate 'nursing practice models in the context of the severe acute respiratory syndrome epidemic in Hong Kong'. In examinations, students are given a brief description of an 'event' or 'case', and their knowledge is tested by focused questions. In research, vignettes have been used to study a number of phenomena such as 'attitudes towards older residents with long-term schizophrenia' (Hellzén et al., 2003), 'attitudes to adolescent self-harm behaviour' (Law et al., 2009) and nursing diagnosis (Hakverdioğlu Yönt et al., 2013).

One or more vignettes can be used in the same study, and questions to vignettes can be open-ended or structured. In a study by Hellzén et al. (2003), nurses were given 13 pairs of categorical statements to select 'the standpoint describing the way they should think and act towards the resident in the vignette by scoring their decisions on a two-degree scale'. For another study using vignettes to collect quantitative data, see Brown et al. (2011). On the other hand, vignettes were used in Long-Sutehall et al.'s (2011) grounded theory study of 'how nurses shape withdrawal of treatment in hospital critical care units' in relation to dying patients. The researchers explain that vignettes were chosen as they offered participants the 'opportunity to discuss sensitive issues from a non-personal, and potentially less threatening perspective'.

Some of the advantages of vignettes are that they require minimal resources and are easy to administer; participants do not need an in-depth knowledge of the topics but they can provide sufficient detail to reduce unwarranted assumptions, thus ensuring that all participants respond to the same stimulus (Paddam et al., 2010). The main disadvantage is that vignettes are hypothetical cases; in real situations, participants may react differently from when they are asked to provide an answer for which they do not expect any retribution. The lack of contextual information also makes the situation artificial, and vignettes are unable to convey emotion through sound or vision, such as tone of voice, facial expressions and body language (Paddam et al., 2010).

Rating scales

You may have come across a questionnaire in a popular magazine or newspaper in which readers are asked to 'tick' the appropriate boxes and add up their scores to find out how 'sexy', 'romantic' or 'intelligent' they are. If you have indulged in such an activity, you have in effect filled in a rating scale. If you have not, here is an extract from a newspaper from a scale 'Are you hot on gossip?'

1. After the party I like talking about how others there looked
    agree   A . . . ☐   disagree   B . . . ☐
6. I usually skip the gossip columns in newspapers
    agree   B . . . ☐   disagree   A . . . ☐
10. The saying 'There is no smoke without fire' is often wrong
    agree   B . . . ☐   disagree   A . . . ☐

There were 10 items in all, and readers were asked to add up their number of As and Bs. Those who scored eight or more As were described as:

> You are so interested in gossip that you often prefer rumour and speculation about others than the hard truth.

If their score was two As or fewer, they were described as:

> You probably prefer your own company to groups, and also realise that there are usually more mundane explanations for the events which grip and promote gossips.

While this may be light-hearted fun, the same principles apply to the construction of rating scales used in research and clinical practice.

Rating scales are sometimes referred to as questionnaires. There are, however, crucial differences between the two, especially with regard to their structure, design and purpose. Questionnaires, on the whole, contain a set of questions mostly in closed and open-ended formats. The responses to each of the questions are treated on their own and analysed separately, although researchers seek to correlate and cross-tabulate variables. Together, responses from all the questions provide an answer to the research question or hypotheses. Rating scales are made up of statements or items that respondents are required to rate. Each rated statement is given a score, and the total score, as shown in the 'gossip scale', is given an interpretation.

Researchers designing questionnaires carefully select questions that reflect the attributes of the concept or aspects of an issue or topic being studied. For example, for a questionnaire on job satisfaction, a researcher will make sure that the main components of job satisfaction, such as autonomy, pay, working environment, promotion prospects and good working relationships, are represented in the questionnaire. A rating scale is normally constructed by collecting a large number of statements on the phenomenon (for example, attitudes to authority), through an elaborate process, reducing them down to a smaller number that can be administered to respondents.

There are different types of rating scales and different techniques for developing them. Although the process may differ, they all have to undergo the following steps:

1 *Develop a large number (pool) of items or statements to indicate the strength of feeling of respondents towards the concept or issue being measured.* This is done by searching the literature and/or asking people (by means of individual interviews, focus groups or questionnaires). Examples of statements relating to research utilisation in clinical practice are 'Using research is a waste of practitioners' time', 'Using research does not always improve practice' and 'Research utilisation contributes a great deal towards enhancing practice.'

2 *Reduce the pool of items to a manageable number.* This is done with or without the help of a panel of experts or other respondents. Statements representing extreme views are usually eliminated.

3 *Carry out tests to ensure the validity and reliability of the provisional scale* by administering it to a sample of respondents.

4 *Modify the scale* as a result of these tests and repeat the tests as appropriate, until the researcher is satisfied that the scale can consistently measure what it is supposed to measure.

A number of tools such as Likert scales, semantic differential (SD) scales and visual analogue scales (VASs) are frequently used to measure phenomena of interest to nurses and other health professionals. These are discussed below.

Likert scale

A Likert scale is an instrument used to measure attitudes, beliefs, opinions, values and views (Sechrist and Pravikoff, 2001). The scale comprises a set of statements (some positive and some negative) about the concept being measured, and the respondents are asked to choose from an odd number of responses (usually five), including a neutral one. Typical responses are 'strongly agree', 'agree', 'neither agree nor disagree', 'disagree' and 'strongly disagree'. Scores for each item range from 1 to 5 (5 for positive and 1 for negative statements). The scale is structured such that negative items are mixed to prevent respondents getting in a 'rhythm' of 'ticking' boxes in the same column. The total scores represent the strength of particular attitudes or views.

This type of scale was named after Likert (1932), who developed it to measure attitudes. It is a useful tool to gauge attitudes among groups of people in a relatively short time and cheaply, although if the tool is developed from scratch it can be expensive. Its limitation is mainly related to the total scores, which can be the sum of a combination of the scores of individual items, therefore not particularly reflecting the strength of agreement with individual ones.

There is a difference between a Likert scale and a Likert-type scale. A Likert scale is developed systematically (similar to the process for a rating scale described above) and evaluated rigorously for validity and reliability. A Likert-type or pseudo-Likert scale involves the formulation of items or statements that the researcher believes represent the concept being measured, without going through the necessary steps to generate and validate items. The score of each item is usually reported individually. On the other hand, a Likert scale, rigorously developed, should provide a total score. In appraising a scale, readers should look for evidence of how it was constructed and its reliability scores. For example, Abou Samra et al. (2013) developed a Likert scale to measure students' intentions to pursue an educator role. As they explain, 'the initial scale items were generated using the social cognitive career theory constructs and were reviewed by an expert panel to ensure content validity'. Relevant statistical tests were carried out to ensure rigour in the construction of the scale.

Semantic differential scale

The SD scale, originally developed by Osgood et al. (1957), is another technique or method that has been developed to measure an attitude or feeling towards a concept or phenomenon. It can be described as a set of opposite adjectives that respondents select from to represent how they 'feel' about a particular item. The item is usually a statement, a word or a picture, and it is placed above the scale. Respondents are asked to 'tick' or put an 'X' on a line, or 'circle' a number, which can range from five to nine gradings.

Below is an example of the use of an SD scale in a study by Festini et al. (2009) of how the use of multicoloured, non-conventional attire designed by children themselves affects children's general perception of the nurses taking care of them. In this quasi-experimental study, the children were cared for by nurses wearing either a single-coloured or a multicoloured uniform. They were then presented with the scale below and asked to rate their perceptions of nurses, on a scale of 1 to 5:

How do you think your nurses are?:
1--------------------2--------------------3--------------------4--------------------5
Bad   Good
1--------------------2--------------------3--------------------4--------------------5
Disagreeable   Nice
1--------------------2--------------------3--------------------4--------------------5
Boring   Fun

The scale had more questions and pairs of adjectives than presented here. In this study, only five gradings were offered, and the middle one (3) represented a neutral attitude.

An SD scale has three components: a stem, steps and anchors. In the scale used in Festini et al.'s study, the stem is 'How do you think your nurses are?' (it can also be expressed as a statement). The steps are the five gradations to choose from. The anchors are the adjectives on each side of the lines (for example, boring/fun). Respondents are instructed to circle a number as quickly as possible. They are usually advised not to reflect or think rationally, but to give their immediate reactions, as it is their attitudes, feelings and emotions that are being measured. Such scales are used with the assumption that 'meanings often can be or are usually communicated by adjectives' (Waltz et al., 2010). The total score obtained by each respondent is an indication of the strength of their attitudes or feelings. These scores can then be subjected to statistical analysis.

In a study of the prevalence of stigmatising attitudes in the German public to obesity (Sikorski et al., 2012), participants were presented with a vignette and asked to put a X on a line of five gradings, with a pair of adjectives at each end. In this example, the stem was a vignette depicting an obese individual. The steps were the five gradings (one of which represents the strength of attitude of the participant). The anchors were the adjectives (for example, attractive/unattractive). This example shows that elements of vignettes and semantic differentials can be combined in a scale.

Visual analogue scale

Another measuring instrument, similar to the SD format, is the VAS. The VAS is described as a continuous scale comprising a horizontal (HVAS) or vertical (VVAS) line, usually 10 cm (100 mm) in length and anchored by two verbal descriptors, one at each end of the line (Hawker et al., 2011).

The main difference between the VAS and the SD technique is that, in the latter, the respondents are given a series of steps or gradations (between five and nine) to choose from. On the other hand, with the VAS, the response is recorded on a line representing a continuum between two points or anchors, thus allowing more freedom to respondents to put their 'X' in any position on the line.

An example of a horizontal and a vertical VAS is given in Figure 16.1. The line can be of different lengths, although the popular length is 100 mm. In a study of the 'relationships of dyspnoea, physical activity and fatigue in patients with chronic obstructive pulmonary disease', Woo (2000) used a vertical VAS to measure dyspnoea. He explains that the scale consisted of a 100 mm vertical line with anchors of 'no shortness of breath' at the bottom and 'shortness of breath as bad as can be' at the top. Although Woo does not give a reason for choosing a vertical rather than a horizontal VAS, he points out that 'evidence of the validity of the V [vertical] VAS has been indicated by its positive correlation with the horizontal VAS'.

The VAS has been particularly useful in measuring different types of pain, including acute pain (Rahman and DeSilva, 2012), menstrual pain (Rahnama et al., 2012) and chronic pain (Bennell et al., 2012). It is an easy tool for respondents to rate. The language is uncomplicated, and the scale takes little time to complete. It can also chart changes over time in the feelings or attitudes being measured. According to Pritchard (2010), the VAS has a number of advantages, 'the most important of which is that it is simple to use and therefore is unlikely to cause patients any further stress or anxiety'. Its disadvantage is that people with visual impairment or psychomotor disability may find it difficult to make their mark on

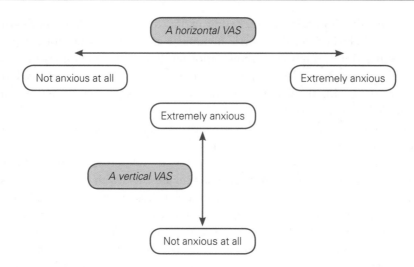

Figure 16.1   A horizontal and a vertical VAS

the line. The concept of a line measuring feelings may not be as easily understood by some respondents as it is by researchers.

The evidence for the reliability of the VAS is not conclusive. Bijur et al. (2001) found it to be 'sufficiently reliable' in a study measuring acute pain. In a study comparing the VAS with a numerical rating scale and a verbal rating scale for the measurement of pain in chronic pruritus, Phan et al. (2012) concluded that all these three scales showed high reliability. On the other hand, de Jong et al. (2005) found that both the VAS and an observation scale had poor inter-rater reliability when the two scales were used in the measurement of pain in children. Crichton (2001) explains that the VAS is a highly subjective form of assessment that is more useful when charting change within individuals than when comparing across a group of individuals at one time point.

Advantages and disadvantages of questionnaires

These depend partly on the mode of questionnaire administration. Questionnaires can be self- or researcher administered. A self-administered questionnaire is one in which respondents write their responses on the questionnaire without the researcher helping in any way. The latter is usually not present, but there are cases when the researcher is in the same room or in the vicinity. The questionnaire can be delivered personally or posted, hence the term 'postal questionnaire'. Alternatively, the researcher can read the questions and record the responses on the questionnaire. This can be either 'face to face' or over the telephone. This type of 'face-to-face' encounter is more like a structured interview (described in Chapter 17). Questionnaires can also be administered to a group of people, for example students in a classroom. Telephone surveys are popular in the social and health sciences, and questioning by telephone is extensively used in market research. Internet questionnaires are increasingly used for research purposes. One of the popular web survey is the SurveyMonkey software (https://www.surveymonkey.com/); this is how it is described on its website:

> SurveyMonkey is the world's most popular online survey tool. It's easier than ever to send free surveys, polls, questionnaires, customer feedback and market research. Plus get access to survey questions and professional templates.

Phenomena studied with the use of SurveyMonkey include: 'informatics competencies of students' (Choi and DeMartinis, 2013), 'stress and burnout in nurse anesthesia' (Chipas and McKenna, 2011) and the 'ethical concerns of nursing reviewers' (Broome et al., 2010).

The main advantage of questionnaires is that they can reach large numbers of people over wide geographical areas (especially in online surveys) and collect data at a lower cost than can other methods such as interviews and observations. Because they are structured and predetermined and cannot as a rule be varied, either in their wording or in the order in which they are answered, they have a fair degree of reliability. The data collected from all respondents are in the same form, and comparisons can be made between them without great difficulty. Closed questions and rating scales can be pre-coded and can thereafter be easily and quickly analysed, especially if computer packages, which are becoming increasingly more efficient, are used. Self-administered questionnaires have the advantage of keeping the respondents anonymous except in cases where the researcher deliberately uses a code to identify non-responders for follow-up purposes. They also allow respondents to answer in their own time and at their own convenience. They can have the time to check records, especially when they answer factual questions.

Finally, the questionnaire designer can improve the instrument by piloting it many times before administering it to respondents, thereby increasing its validity and reliability. It can also be useful for other researchers to borrow and adapt for use in their studies.

The main disadvantage with the self-administered questionnaire is that there is no opportunity to ask respondents to elaborate, expand, clarify or illustrate their answers. Respondents themselves have no opportunity to ask for clarification. They may understand questions differently from researchers, thereby not inspiring confidence in the validity of questionnaires. Developing and testing a questionnaire can be time-consuming and costly. It can also be a laborious process involving a number of stages and drafts.

Questionnaires tell us little about the context in which the respondents formulate their responses. In interviews, researchers can read the body language and take it as a cue to probe further, if appropriate. The data collected from questionnaires are sometimes superficial. They are devoid of the context that gives rise to them, and although researchers may attempt to measure important contextual variables, they typically separate the measured behaviour from its particular historical, social and cultural contexts (Mechanic, 1989).

Questionnaires do not suit everyone, in particular those who have difficulty in reading and comprehension and in articulating written responses. This may lead some respondents to confer with others or ask them to complete the questionnaires. The implications of this for knowledge and attitude questions are obvious.

Another serious problem with questionnaires is low response rates. There are a variety of reasons why people may not respond to questionnaires. 'Respondent burden' is the discomfort put on them by making use of their effort and time in completing questionnaires or taking part in research generally. Health professionals (as participants in research studies) can be prone to question fatigue. With increasing demands on their time and increasing emphasis on the need for research, it can be difficult for them to find time to reply to questionnaires. Various strategies can be used to increase response rates, including making respondents feel that their responses are valuable and ensuring that the questionnaire is easy to respond to, not too lengthy and well structured and presented. Other methods of data collection such as interviews and observations can also impose a burden on participants.

Some of the above disadvantages are inherent in the method, in that the questionnaire is by its very nature limited to collecting certain types of data, but many of the other disadvantages can be overcome through skilful construction. The questionnaire's popularity as a method of data collection suggests that, to many people, the advantages outweigh the disadvantages. Some of the limitations of questionnaires were also discussed in Chapter 3.

Validity and reliability of questionnaires

For questionnaires to be of use to practitioners and policy-makers, they have to produce valid and reliable data. The validity of a questionnaire is the extent to which it addresses the research question, objectives or hypotheses set by the researcher. For example, if a questionnaire is designed to assess patient satisfaction, it must 'assess' rather than 'explore' patient satisfaction with nursing care; all the questions, together, must also fully reflect the concepts of 'patient satisfaction' and 'nursing care'. It can happen that the questionnaire addresses only physical care and ignores other aspects, such as psychological, social and spiritual care. Therefore such a questionnaire can hardly be said to assess satisfaction with 'nursing care'. Two questions can be asked when assessing the validity of a questionnaire:

● Does the questionnaire answer the research question?
● Do the questions adequately represent the different attributes of the concepts or the different aspects of the issues being studied?

The reliability of a questionnaire refers to the consistency with which respondents understand, and respond to, all the questions. For example, if a question such as 'What type of accommodation do you live in?' is put to respondents, would all of them interpret the terms 'type', 'accommodation' and 'live' in the same way? Do all respondents use the terms 'house', 'flat' and 'studio' in the same sense? Some may reply that they live in 'comfortable' or 'cheap' or 'council' accommodation. Others may 'live' in more than one accommodation. It is clear, therefore, that the responses to this question will not be consistent if respondents interpret it differently. Two questions that can be asked when assessing the reliability of a questionnaire are:

● Are the questions or statements clear and unambiguous enough for a respondent to understand and to respond to them in the same way each time they are presented to him (except where respondents have different answers to give), and for the respondent to understand them in the same way as others do?
● Do all respondents interpret the instructions given by the researcher in the same way?

A questionnaire can be reliable without being valid, but it cannot be valid if it is not reliable. In the above example of a questionnaire assessing patients' satisfaction with nursing care, if the questions and instructions are interpreted in the same way by all the respondents, but the questionnaire content does not represent all the different aspects of nursing care, the questionnaire is reliable but not valid. If some respondents interpret the questions differently from others, their responses are not reliable and cannot also be taken as a valid assessment of 'patients' satisfaction with nursing care' as a result of the confusion over the meaning of some questions. Therefore reliability is a necessary but not a sufficient condition for validity.

Earlier in this chapter, we looked at the types of phenomena, such as facts, knowledge and attitudes, that nursing research questionnaires describe or measure. However, they present a number of difficulties to researchers. In theory, facts are believed to be the easiest type of data that questionnaires can collect; in practice, it may be quite different. Yet people can also be 'economical with the truth' for various reasons; facts can be 'coloured' to make the responses more socially desirable. For example, some people who cannot afford two meals a day may not want the world to know about it. Lydeard (1991) explains that:

prestige bias, social desirability, ego, or practical/ethical standards, all are different names for the same phenomenon, i.e. responders are modest/social drinkers that rarely smoke, brush their teeth with alarming frequency and never allow their children to watch dubious television programmes.

Memory distortion, memory gaps and selective memory can all be responsible for inaccuracies in self-reporting. Memory distortion can happen when, for example, a past event is seen to be worse or better than it was because the 'passing of time' has put a different perception on it. Memory gaps simply refer to the forgetfulness of events of little significance to the respondents, especially if they happened a long time ago. With selective memory, respondents choose to remember certain events, for example joyful ones, and repress others that are painful.

Events and activities that require respondents or researchers to make an assessment, as in the case of the 'amount of fluid intake' or the 'frequency of bowel movements', can be under- or overreported as these involve a subjective judgement.

These difficulties in, and limitations of, collecting reliable factual information must be borne in mind when evaluating data. However, they do not in themselves undermine the usefulness of questionnaires in the collection of such data. The reliability of questionnaires and scales can be greatly enhanced by systematic development and rigorous testing.

Measuring respondents' knowledge by questionnaire is a less challenging task than is measuring attitudes. However, there are particular problems that can threaten the reliability and validity of the responses. For example, self-administered questionnaires, as explained earlier, give opportunities for respondents to confer with others or consult other sources.

For interviewer-administered questionnaires, researchers often make an appointment with respondents and disclose in advance the remit of the questionnaire, thereby possibly giving them the opportunity to 'brush up' on the topic. Assessing the knowledge of health professionals, no matter what method is used, can be threatening to them even when the promise of confidentiality is offered. The response rate may understandably be low, and the number of partially completed questionnaires is often high. It is difficult to ascertain whether a non-response to a question means that the respondent did not know the answer, did not understand the question or simply chose to ignore it.

People often give an opinion when asked even if they have little or no knowledge of the topic or have not thought seriously about it. Multiple-choice and checklist questions offer the opportunity for guesswork. Many of the questions asked in a questionnaire can only be answered conditionally.

Studying behaviour and behavioural intention with the use of questionnaires can also be particularly difficult. Earlier, we mentioned some of the problems with self-reporting, including memory distortion, memory gaps and selective memory. Behavioural intention is the 'nut' that policy-makers, planners and opinion pollsters would dearly like to 'crack'.

The reliability of questionnaires depends largely on the question wording and questionnaire structure. McCorry et al. (2013) reported that almost 60 per cent of respondents in their study found that the term 'altered immunity' in the 'Illness Perception Scale' adapted for people with type 2 diabetes was confusing. They also indicated that items such as 'my treatment will be effective in curing my diabetes' and 'my symptoms come and go in cycles' were not applicable, as participants with type 2 diabetes 'did not endorse the concept of a cure for diabetes and they did not perceive themselves to have overt symptoms'.

Some of the threats to reliability come from questions that are ambiguous, double-barrelled, leading, double-negative and hypothetical. The question order and length of the questionnaire can also affect the responses. Terms such as 'often', 'sometimes' or 'happy' can mean different things to different people. Schaeffer (1991) gives this interesting illustration:

In the movie *Annie Hall*, there is a scene with a split screen. On one side Alvie Singer talks to his psychiatrist; on the other side Annie Hall talks to hers. Alvie's therapist asks him, 'How often do you sleep together?' and Alvie replies, 'Hardly ever, maybe three times a week'. Annie's therapist asks her, 'Do you have sex often?' Annie replies, 'Constantly, I'd say three times a week.'

As the author says, the fact that frequency can be reported in different ways is a source of concern for researchers. Below are examples of the types of question that can affect the reliability and validity of questionnaire data.

Double-barrelled:

Reading research reports can lead to cost-effective and evidence-based care:

Agree ☐   Disagree ☐

Leading:

In the UK, 30,000 people each year die from smoking-related diseases. Indicate your reaction to this statement by marking an X on the line below.

Very concerned ⬅━━━━━━━━━━━━━━━➡ Apathetic

Double-negative:

Are you not taking the sleeping tablets as prescribed?

Yes ☐   No ☐

Hypothetical:

Would you like free dental care?

Yes ☐   No ☐

Lengthy and uninteresting questionnaires not only affect response rates, but can also lead respondents to take them lightly. Self-administered questionnaires that are time-consuming to complete may cause fatigue and lack of concentration, especially in people who are not accustomed to reading and writing. The order of the questions, the way in which they are grouped and their sensitivity (or lack of it) can all affect the responses.

The reliability and validity of questionnaires can be greatly enhanced by careful preparation and skilful construction, paying particular attention to the needs and circumstances of potential respondents and anticipating how they would react. One thing to remember is that, despite all the efforts made to construct and administer a reliable and valid questionnaire, there will always be some respondents who will interpret terms or questions differently. Large samples can, to some extent, accommodate minor individual inconsistencies. There are a number of strategies that researchers can use in order to reduce bias and ambiguities and ensure the validity and reliability of questionnaires.

Assessing validity

There are a variety of validity tests that can be applied, the main ones described here being content validity, criterion-related validity and construct validity.

Content validity

This type of validity refers to the degree to which the questions or items in the questionnaire adequately represent the phenomenon being studied. If the questionnaire sets out to measure staff nurses' nutritional knowledge in relation to the care of diabetic patients, a content validity test would ensure that there are enough relevant questions covering all the major aspects of the nutritional knowledge that nurses are required to have for nursing this particular group of patients. Content validity also ensures that irrelevant questions are not asked.

Content validity can be illustrated by the example of a teacher setting questions on an examination paper for a particular module. All the questions together must address the whole content of the module. Padden (2013) explains how a panel of three 'judges' assessed the content validity of a scale to assess the level of 'reflection-on-action' in students' reflective journal entries:

> The expert panel was asked to rate the criteria described at each level for the degree of accuracy, using a Likert scale. Ratings ranged from 1 = not at all accurate to 4 = very accurate. Two of the three experts rated each of the six items at a score of 3 or 4, indicating that the descriptions were either quite accurate (rated as a 3) or very accurate (rated as 4). The third rater did not assign ratings but indicated in the overall assessment that the instrument was a 'reasonable framework' and cautioned against grading student journal entries. Additional feedback from each content expert regarding specific wording and suggestions for additional questions for feedback to students was included in the final draft of the instrument.

Another common method of validating the content of questionnaires is by calculating the content validity index. This is achieved by asking a group of experts to rate the relevance of items in the questionnaire (for example, by choosing between responses such as 'not relevant', 'somewhat relevant', 'quite relevant' and 'very relevant') and by calculating the degree of agreement or disagreement between them on individual items (Wynd et al., 2003). Mastaglia et al. (2003) explain how content validity could be ensured when developing an instrument. They provide a checklist for experts to rate questionnaire items in terms of clarity, content validity and internal consistency.

There is no statistical test for content validity, although an index of content validity can be calculated based on the degree of agreement of the panel members. The terms 'face validity' and 'content validity' are sometimes used interchangeably. Redsell et al. (2004) offer the following distinction between the two terms:

> Face validity: the extent to which the assessment instrument subjectively appears to be measuring what it is supposed to measure.

Content validity: the extent to which the instrument includes a representative sample of the content of a construct.

In effect, face validity involves giving the questionnaire to anyone, not necessarily an expert on the subject, who can 'on the face of it' assess whether the questions reflect the phenomenon being studied. Greater or lesser weight may be given to face validity depending on how it is accessed. Methods range from giving the questionnaire to colleagues to have a cursory review of items, to asking a number of participants in a survey to comment on the tool. Angel et al. (2012) assessed the face validity of the 'Nurses Self-Concept Instrument' with two stakeholders (academics in the areas of educational psychology with specialised expertise in self-concept and cross-cultural instrument development and validation). Face and content validity are the ones most frequently reported in the literature.

Criterion-related validity

Another way to find out about the validity of a questionnaire is to compare its findings with data collected on the same phenomenon by other methods, such as another questionnaire or clinical observations. The data from these other sources become the criteria against which data from the present questionnaire can be compared. If the data are similar, the questionnaire can be said to have criterion-related validity. There are two types of criterion-related validity: concurrent and predictive.

Concurrent validity refers to other current criteria (hence 'concurrent') with which comparisons can be made. For example, for a questionnaire measuring pain to have concurrent validity, the data from the questionnaire must correspond to other data, such as nurses' observations relating to requests for painkillers and other behaviours. If the questionnaire is able to distinguish those who have pain from those who do not, data from other sources, including nurses' observations, must tell a similar story about the same patients. If this happens, the questionnaire can be said to have concurrent validity.

Predictive validity refers to data available in the future that will confirm whether or not data from the present questionnaire are valid. For example, a questionnaire that can distinguish between those who have positive and those who have negative attitudes towards people with a learning disability will have predictive validity if their future behaviours are consistent with the findings of the questionnaire. For studies measuring the criterion validity of scales and instruments, see Allgaier et al. (2012) and Franzen et al. (2013).

Construct validity

This is the most difficult type of validity for a questionnaire to achieve. It refers to how well a questionnaire or scale measures a particular construct. Examples of constructs are self-esteem, burnout, social support and empathy. Each of these constructs is difficult to define, let alone measure. Researchers have to resort to the theoretical and research literature before they can break down each construct into attributes, which can thereafter form the items or questions on a scale. The construct validity of an instrument is its ability to measure the intended construct. It should be able to discriminate or differentiate between similar constructs.

It is difficult for a newly constructed questionnaire to achieve construct validity as it has to be tested in a multitude of settings and with different populations over a number of years. For examples of studies testing the construct validity of scales, see Franzen et al. (2012) and de Melo Ghisi et al. (2013).

Assessing reliability

A number of reliability tests have been devised to find out the consistency with which questionnaires collect data. Among the well-known ones are test–retest, alternate-form and split-half.

Test–retest

Test–retest simply involves administering the questionnaire on two occasions and comparing the responses. For example, an 'attitude towards mental illness' questionnaire can be administered to a group of chemistry students. The same questionnaire can then be readministered to the same group 3 weeks later. The second set of responses from each individual should not differ unless something has happened to change their attitudes. If a group of student nurses were given the same questionnaire on two occasions and had visited a psychiatric hospital in the interval between the two administrations, a difference in results could be explained. If nothing has happened in the period between the two administrations that might change respondents' attitudes, the scores must be the same; the questionnaire thus passes the test–retest and can be said to be reliable.

Bernhardsson and Larsson (2013) carried out a test–retest of their questionnaire by distributing a draft version to a sample of 64 participants on two occasions separated by 1–2-week interval.

Population test

The population reliability test (also known as equivalence) is carried out by asking the questions in different forms. Sometimes the order of the categories can be altered. For example, if we take the following three items from the questionnaire measuring evidence-based practice among physical therapists (Bernhardsson and Larsson, 2013), we could administer them in three different versions. Version A is the original, and Versions B and C are alternative ways in which the question could be asked. The third version (C) would remove what is known as a set response bias (the tendency of respondents to rate the item in a set pattern, for example to tick the first category that is offered).

Version A

I have fast and easy access to relevant evidence-based guidelines at my place of work.

☐ *Strongly disagree* ☐ *Disagree* ☐ *Neutral* ☐ *Agree* ☐ *Strongly agree*

I can integrate the patients' preferences with evidence-based guidelines.

☐ *Strongly disagree* ☐ *Disagree* ☐ *Neutral* ☐ *Agree* ☐ *Strongly agree*

Evidence-based guidelines are important to facilitate my work.

☐ *Strongly disagree* ☐ *Disagree* ☐ *Neutral* ☐ *Agree* ☐ *Strongly agree*

Version B

I have fast and easy access to relevant evidence-based guidelines at my place of work.

☐ *Strongly agree* ☐ *Agree* ☐ *Neutral* ☐ *Disagree* ☐ *Strongly disagree*

I can integrate the patients' preferences with evidence-based guidelines.

☐ *Strongly agree* ☐ *Agree* ☐ *Neutral* ☐ *Disagree* ☐ *Strongly disagree*

Evidence-based guidelines are important to facilitate my work.

☐ *Strongly agree* ☐ *Agree* ☐ *Neutral* ☐ *Disagree* ☐ *Strongly disagree*

Version C

I have fast and easy access to relevant evidence-based guidelines at my place of work.

☐ *Strongly disagree* ☐ *Disagree* ☐ *Neutral* ☐ *Agree* ☐ *Strongly agree*

I can integrate the patients' preferences with evidence-based guidelines.

☐ *Strongly agree* ☐ *Agree* ☐ *Neutral* ☐ *Disagree* ☐ *Strongly disagree*

Evidence-based guidelines are important to facilitate my work.

☐ *Strongly disagree* ☐ *Disagree* ☐ *Neutral* ☐ *Agree* ☐ *Strongly agree*

Another way of testing alternate forms of reliability is to substitute the wording of the question by equivalent terms without altering the meaning of the question.

Split-half test

This test involves dividing or splitting the instrument into two equal halves and finding out whether or not their scores are similar. For example, for an attitude rating scale with 10 statements, the researcher will take the total score of the first five and compare it with the score of the last five. If the scores are similar, the statements or test items are said to be homogeneous. No item has a greater value than any other in assessing an attitude. This means that all the items are designed to make the respondent react consistently in the same way if they possess a particular attitude. If this happens, the test shows high internal consistency.

The split-half test can only be carried out with questionnaires that measure a concept or phenomenon, and applies only to instruments for which there is a total score. Most questionnaires that set out to describe or explore particular phenomena do not fall into this category.

There are other tests for validity and reliability, but only those most frequently reported in the literature are described here.

To sum up, the validity of an instrument is established mainly by comparing its responses or scores with the scores of other sources (other research instruments, clinical observations or other records). On the other hand, the reliability of an instrument is tested mainly by comparing its own responses or scores (on different occasions, with different wordings or structure, and between items). For a study using the split-half test, see Kutlu et al. (2012).

Pilot-testing the questionnaire

Even before validity and reliability tests are carried out, researchers can refine their questionnaires by administering them to a small group of people similar in characteristics to the intended respondents. Those who have done so have been amazed at the types of error, not just typographical, that can be detected. The first and most efficient way to find out the quality of a questionnaire is to test or 'pilot' it. The responses will give the researcher a fair idea of whether all the respondents understand the questions in the same way, whether the format of the questions is the most suitable for this population, whether they understand the instructions and how relevant the questions are. She can also find out whether the length of the questionnaire and its structure are likely to affect the responses.

Researchers who take the opportunity to consider respondents' views on the above aspects of the questionnaire, listen to the problems encountered by them and seek to resolve some of the doubts the researchers have about their questionnaires, are likely to learn a lot about the strengths and weaknesses of their tools. Researchers are professionals whose 'language' and culture can be different from those of the potential participants in their study. It is important for them to realise that their questionnaires reflect their value positions and may create a different impression on respondents from the one they anticipate.

Critiquing questionnaires

Many authors of reports or articles do not give a detailed description of the questionnaires for readers to assess their validity and reliability. Only on rare occasions are questionnaires included as an appendix; often only a brief description of the number of items is given. Other information that is frequently missing includes pilot-testing, validity and reliability tests, reminders or follow-ups to increase response rates and information about non-responders.

When assessing the use of a questionnaire in a research study, you must look at how the questionnaire was developed, if this is the case. Did the researcher formulate the items only from her own experience and/or the literature? Content validity is likely to be enhanced if efforts were made to consult the literature or other instruments for relevant items to be included. If a questionnaire is borrowed and adapted, does the author comment on how the validity and reliability of the original instrument has been affected? You should also determine whether the questionnaire was piloted, with whom, how and with what results. More than one round of piloting is an indication that serious attempts have been made to refine it.

You must also find out other measures taken to enhance validity and reliability. How were face or content validity ensured? Was the questionnaire given to one or more 'experts' to comment and make suggestions? Construct validity, especially in studies that use existing, well-established tools, is sometimes reported. For most self-designed questionnaires, it is not fair to expect the author(s) to comment on concurrent, predictive or construct validity, as the data to establish these are not always readily available.

It is sometimes possible to evaluate the wording or formats of questions only when these appear in the article or report. When the questionnaire is available, you can assess its content validity, how appropriate or effective the question formats are and the possibility of biases in the wording. The structure of the questionnaire must facilitate rather than hinder respondents in providing answers. The questionnaire as a whole must make sense, and the questions should not jump from one topic to another and back again. You can find out whether the instructions are clear and whether the length and presentation are likely to encourage respondents to complete it.

One of the main sources of bias in studies using questionnaires is in a low response rate. This happens when the characteristics and attributes of non-responders are different from those of responders. Volunteer and accidental samples, in particular, can be different from those who did not volunteer. Such bias can be taken into account and corrected, to some extent, by statistical means. However, the nature and extent of non-respondent bias 'can only be made by collecting data directly from non-respondents' (Lynn, 2003). In a survey of 'general practitioners and their views of the NHS changes', Armstrong and Ashworth (2000) compared responders and non-responders. They found that the latter 'differed significantly from responders in many of their views'. When appraising the validity of findings in surveys, you should look for information on the characteristics of those who did not respond. However, finding out about non-responders can be costly and difficult since they can continue to refuse to respond.

Your task in assessing a questionnaire is to find out how valid and reliable it is in answering the research questions. However, it is important to remember that it is easier to critique a questionnaire than to construct one. Perhaps for this reason alone, researchers rarely attach their questionnaires to their articles.

Ethical aspects of questionnaires

The self-administered questionnaire is one of the few methods of data collection that can potentially keep respondents anonymous. This can be an advantage because it gives them the opportunity of making their views known without being identified, unless of course each questionnaire is numbered or coded for the purpose of sending reminders to those who have not replied. One way to maintain anonymity and increase response rates is to send a reminder to all participants regardless of who replied (which can be costly), but bias may be introduced if a respondent replies twice and this is overlooked by the researcher.

Confidentiality and privacy, as with other methods of data collection, must also be respected. However, both confidentiality and respect for privacy are easier to promise than to fulfil. Despite the best efforts and intentions of researchers, there are ways in which respondents can be identified by others or identify themselves. Privacy must mean what it says; that is, the questionnaire must be administered to the respondent alone and in a private place.

Researchers are expected to obtain informed consent from respondents. However, because the questionnaire seems to be less intrusive than the interview or observation and less interventionist than the experiment, there is a tendency to think that it can cause no harm. Obtaining approval from an ethical committee is often not thought to be necessary. Questionnaires, however, can be intrusive by asking people embarrassing and sensitive questions, and can invade privacy. They can open 'old wounds' with no one at hand to offer support. The following three consecutive questions taken from a real questionnaire on cervical screening exemplify the potential of questionnaires to do harm:

		Yes	No
Q9	Do you have any history of sexually transmitted disease?	☐	☐
Q10	Have you been sexually abused in the past?	☐	☐
Q11	Does your family have a history of cervical cancer?	☐	☐

Apart from being highly personal, these questions can trigger memories of traumatic experiences. These types of questions can potentially be very harmful. A respondent who has been sexually abused in the past can rightly ask why the researcher wants to know this and why she should tell anyone about it. This questionnaire may not be typical of questionnaires in general, but it shows that researchers can ignore, or be unaware of, the sensitive nature of their questions. The questionnaire, by psychologically assaulting respondents, can itself be an instrument of abuse.

Sheikh et al. (2001) explained the moral issues raised when research conducted at a distance uncovers information about participants which indicates that they may be at increased risk of harm. Their study on psychological morbidity among general practice managers raised a number of ethical and research dilemmas. They were concerned that 17 per cent of managers had 'scores indicative of depression, with 5 per cent of responders reporting that they entertained suicidal ideas' (Sheikh et al., 2001).

Evans et al. (2002) expressed concern that the 'likely impact of questionnaires upon patients is not often considered and therefore, the balance of benefit and harm not fully explored'. In their study of breast cancer among women, some respondents asked questions, for example, about risks of getting cancer and risks related to treatment. Evans et al. pointed out that debriefing opportunities are not readily available when questionnaires are used to collect data. Sheikh et al. (2001)

suggest that a warning might be added 'at the top of the questionnaire pointing out that the questions asked might bring to the surface distress which the participants might wish to discuss in the context of a confidential helpline'.

Questionnaires can make people feel guilty about their lifestyles, for example by asking them questions about healthy living. They can identify their lack of knowledge on particular topics. Knowledge questions can be threatening to health professionals as the data may fall into the hands of their employers. One can ask also whether it is ethically right for people to participate in studies and not be told what the findings are, as would be the case for most research studies. The latter are published in journals of which lay people are unaware, and which professionals themselves may not read.

Finally, online questionnaires (and online research in general) have the same ethical implications as face-to-face, telephone or postal surveys, but these may be manifested in different ways. For example, the lack of direct contact in online surveys means that researchers are unable to know who is really responding or whether or not they are upset. This is the same as in postal surveys. It is important that researchers apply the same ethical principles (outlined in Chapter 6) to online research as well. For advice on how to conduct ethically sound online research, see British Psychological Society (2007) and Barchard and Williams (2008).

Summary

The questionnaire is the most popular method of data collection in health and social research. Like other methods, it has a number of advantages and disadvantages. It is suitable mainly for collecting data on facts, knowledge, attitudes, beliefs and opinions when it is carefully prepared, constructed and administered. It is clear also that questionnaire data must not be taken at face value. Readers must assess the validity and reliability of the instrument where possible, and researchers must provide evidence of validity and reliability checks they have carried out. If used wisely, sensitively and ethically, the questionnaire has the potential to provide valuable data on which policy and practice decisions can be made.

References

Abou Samra H, McGrath J M and Estes T (2013) Developing and testing the nurse educator scale: a robust measure of students' intentions to pursue an educator role. *Journal of Nursing Education*, **52**, 6:323–9.

Allgaier A K, Pietsch K, Fruhe B, Sigl-Glockner J and Schulte-Korne G (2012) Screening for depression in adolescents: validity of the patient health questionnaire in pediatric care. *Depression and Anxiety*, **29**, 10:906–13.

Angel E, Craven R and Denson N (2012) The Nurses Self-Concept Instrument (NSCI): assessment of psychometric properties for Australian domestic and international student nurses. *International Journal of Nursing Studies*, **49**, 7:880–6.

Armstrong D and Ashworth M (2000) When questionnaire response rates do matter: a survey of general practitioners and their views of the NHS changes. *British Journal of General Practice*, **50**:479–80.

Barchard K A and Williams J (2008) Practical advice for conducting ethical online experiments and questionnaires for United States psychologists. *Behavior Research Methods*, **40**, 4:1111–28.

Bennell K L, Ahamed Y, Bryant C et al. (2012) A physiotherapist-delivered integrated exercise and pain coping skills training intervention for individuals with knee osteoarthritis: a randomised controlled trial protocol. *BMC Musculoskeletal Disorders*, **13**:129.

Bernhardsson S and Larsson M E H (2013) Measuring evidence-based practice in physical therapy: translation, adaptation, further development, validation, and reliability test of a questionnaire. *Physical Therapy*, **93**:819–832.

Bijur P E, Silver W and Gallagher E J (2001) Reliability of the visual analog scale for measurement of acute pain. *Academic Emergency Medicine*, **8**, 12:1153–7.

British Psychological Society (2007) Report of the Working Party on Conducting Research on the Internet: guidelines for ethical practice in psychological research online. Retrieved from http://www.bps.org.uk/sites/default/files/documents/conducting_research_on_the_internet-guidelines_for_ethical_practice_in_psychological_research_online.pdf (accessed 12 September 2013).

Broome M, Dougherty M C, Freda M C, Kearney M H and Baggs J G (2010) Ethical concerns of nursing reviewers: an international survey. *Nursing Ethics*, **17**, 6:741–8.

Brown J S L, Casey S J, Bishop A J, Prytys M, Whittinger N and Weinman J (2011) How black African and white British women perceive depression and help-seeking: a pilot vignette study. *International Journal of Social Psychiatry*, **57**:362–74.

Chan E A, Chung J W Y, Wong T K S and Yang J C S (2006) An evaluation of nursing practice models in the context of the severe acute respiratory syndrome epidemic in Hong Kong: a preliminary study example of videotaped vignettes. *Journal of Clinical Nursing*, **15**, 661–70.

Chipas A and McKenna D (2011) Stress and burnout in nurse anesthesia. *American Association of Nurse Anesthetists Journal*, **79**, 2:122–8.

Choi J and De Martinis J (2013) Nursing informatics competencies: assessment of undergraduate and graduate nursing students. *Journal of Clinical Nursing*, **22**, 13–14:1970–6.

Crichton N (2001) Information point: visual analogue scale. *Journal of Clinical Nursing*, **10**:706.

de Jong A E E, Bremer M, Schouten M, Tuinebreijer W E and Faber A W (2005) Reliability and validity of the pain observation scale for young children and the visual analogue scale in children with burns. *Burns*, **31**, 2:198–204.

de Melo Ghisi G L, Oh P, Thomas S and Benetti M (2013) Development and validation of an English version of the Coronary Artery Disease Education Questionnaire (CADE-Q). *European Journal of Preventive Cardiology*, **20**, 2:291–300.

Evans M, Robling M, Maggs Rapport F, Houston H, Kinnersley P and Wilkinson C (2002) It doesn't cost anything just to ask, does it? The ethics of questionnaire-based research. *Journal of Medical Ethics*, **28**, 1:41–4.

Festini F, Occhipinti V, Cocco M et al. (2009) Use of non-conventional nurses' attire in a paediatric hospital: a quasi-experimental study. *Journal of Clinical Nursing*, **18**, 7:1018–26.

Franzen K, Johansson J E, Karlsson J and Nilsson K. (2013) Validation of the Swedish version of the incontinence impact questionnaire and the urogenital distress inventory. *Acta Obstetricia et Gynecologica Scandinavica*, **92**, 5:555–61.

Gould D (1996) Using vignettes to collect data for nursing research studies: how valid are the findings? *Journal of Clinical Nursing*, **5**, 4:207–12.

Hakverdioğlu Yönt G, Korhan E A, Erdemir F and Müller-Staub M (2013) Nursing diagnoses determined by first year students: a vignette study. *International Journal of Nursing Knowledge*, 22 September, doi: 10.1111/2047-3095.12007. [Epub ahead of print].

Hawker G A, Mian S, Kendzerska T and French M (2011) Measures of adult pain arthritis. *Care and Research*, **63**, S11:S240–52.

Hellzén O, Kristiansen L and Norbergh K G (2003) Nurses' attitudes towards older residents with long-term schizophrenia. *Journal of Advanced Nursing*, **43**, 6:616–22.

Kutlu Y, Kucuk L and Yildiz Findik U (2012) Psychometric properties of the Turkish version of the Fraboni Scale of Ageism. Psychometric properties of the Turkish version of the Fraboni Scale of Ageism. *Nursing and Health Sciences*, **14**, 4:464–71.

Law G U, Rostill-Brookes H and Goodman D (2009) Public stigma in health and non-healthcare students: attributions, emotions and willingness to help with adolescent self-harm. *International Journal Nursing Studies*, **46**, 1:107–18.

Likert R (1932) *A Technique for the Measurement of Attitudes* (New York: Columbia University Press).

Long-Sutehall T, Willis H, Palmer R, Ugboma D, Addington-Hall J and Coombs M (2011) Negotiated dying: a grounded theory of how nurses shape withdrawal of treatment in hospital critical care units. *International Journal of Nursing Studies*, **48**, 12:1466–74.

Lydeard S (1991) The questionnaire as a research tool. *Family Practice*, **8**, 1:84–91.

Lynn P (2003) PEDAKSI: methodology for collecting data about survey non-respondents. *Quality and Quantity*, 37:239–61.

Mastaglia B, Toye C and Kristjanson L J (2003) Ensuring content validity in instrument development: challenges and innovative approaches. *Contemporary Nurse*, **14**:281–91.

McCorry N K, Scullion L, McMurray C M, Houghton R and Dempster M (2013) Content validity of the illness perceptions questionnaire – revised among people with type 2 diabetes: a think-aloud study. *Psychology and Health*, **28**, 6:675–85.

McKenna H P, Ashton S and Keeney S (2004) Barriers to evidence-based practice in primary care. *Journal of Advanced Nursing*, **45**, 2:178–89.

Mechanic D (1989) Medical sociology: some tensions among theory, method and substance. *Journal of Health and Social Behaviour*, **30**:147–60.

Osgood C E, Suci G J and Tannenbaum P H (1957) *The Measurement of Meaning* (Chicago: University of Illinois Press).

Paddam A, Barnes B and Langdon D (2010) Constructing vignettes to investigate anger in multiple sclerosis. *Nurse Researcher*, **17**:60–73.

Padden M L (2013) A pilot study to determine the validity and reliability of the level of reflection-on-action assessment. *Journal of Nursing*, **52**, 7:410–15.

Parahoo K (1993) Questionnaire: use, value and limitations. *Nurse Researcher*, **1**, 2:4–15.

Phan N Q, Blome C, Fritz F et al. (2012) Assessment of pruritus intensity: prospective study on validity and reliability of the visual analogue scale, numerical rating scale and verbal rating scale in 471 patients with chronic pruritus. *Acta Dermato-Venereologica*, **92**, 5:502–7.

Pritchard M (2010) Measuring anxiety in surgical patients using a visual analogue scale. *Nursing Standard*, **25**, 11:40–4.

Rahman N H and DeSilva T (2012) A randomized controlled trial of patient-controlled analgesia compared with boluses of analgesia for the control of acute traumatic pain in the emergency department. *Journal of Emergency Medicine*, **43**, 6:951–7.

Rahnama P, Montazeri A, Huseini H F, Kianbakht S and Naseri M (2012) Effect of *Zingiber officinale* R. rhizomes (ginger) on pain relief in primary dysmenorrhea: a placebo randomized trial. *BMC Complementary and Alternative Medicine*, **12**:92.

Redsell S A, Lennon M, Hastings A M and Fraser R C (2004) Devising and establishing the face and content validity of explicit criteria of consultation competence for UK secondary care nurses. *Nurse Education Today*, **24**, 180–7.

Schaeffer N C (1991) Hardly ever or constantly? Group comparisons using vague quantifiers. *Public Opinion Quarterly*, **55**:395–423.

Sechrist K and Pravikoff D (2001) *Semantic Differential Scale: CINAHL Information Systems* (Glendale, CA: CINAHL).

Sheikh A, Hurwitz B and Parker B (2001) Ethical and research dilemmas arising from a questionnaire study of psychological morbidity among general practice managers. *British Journal of General Practice*, **51**:32–5.

Sikorski C, Luppa M, Brähler E, König H-H and Riedel-Heller S G (2012) Obese children, adults and senior citizens in the eyes of the general public: results of a representative study on stigma and causation of obesity. *PLoS ONE*, **7**, 10:e46924.

Wahlberg AC, Cedersund E and Wredling R (2003) Telephone nurses' experience of problems with telephone advice in Sweden. *Journal of Advice Nursing*, **12**:37–45.

Waltz C, Strickland O L and Lenz E (2010) *Measurement in Nursing and Health Research*, 4th edn (New York: Springer).

Woo K (2000) A pilot study to examine the relationships of dyspnoea, physical activity and fatigue in patients with chronic obstructive pulmonary disease. *Journal of Clinical Nursing*, **9**:526–33.

Wynd C A, Schmidt B and Schaefer M A (2003) Two quantitative approaches for estimating content validity. *Western Journal of Nursing Research*, **25**, 5:508–18.

Interviews

> It is the province of knowledge to speak and it is the privilege of wisdom to listen.
>
> Oliver Wendell Holmes

Introduction

The beliefs, attitudes, experiences and perception of clients and staff are important for the organisation, delivery and evaluation of care and treatment. The interview has an important part to play in collecting data to inform the decisions and actions of health professionals, as well as in providing insights into how clients access and use health services and their experience of them.

In this chapter, we will discuss the use of interviews in clinical practice and in research, the different forms of research interviews and their advantages and disadvantages. We will also explore the ethical implications, as well as the validity and reliability, of different forms of interviewing. Finally, what you should look for when critiquing studies that use interviews will be suggested.

Interviews in clinical practice

In our everyday life, we engage in interactions that involve asking, and being asked, questions. We can say that we all are 'interviewers' and 'interviewees'. Verbal communication is the most effective means available to humans with which to convey our feelings, experiences, views and intentions. However, we do not normally call these verbal interactions interviews; most of the time they are merely casual conversations. Some of us have been interviewed for a job or a place on a course, or have watched others being interviewed on television. These interviews are different from casual conversations in that they have (or should have) a clearer agenda, often prepared in advance and with a specific purpose, and are limited in duration. Health professionals, too, carry out interviews for the purpose of obtaining information from clients that can be used to assess, plan, implement and evaluate care and treatment. Nurse–client interactions involve both formal interviewing and casual conversations throughout the time that the client is in contact with the professional. With clinical interviews, the aim is not only to obtain valuable information, but also to build trust between the professional and the client. Thus, a therapeutic relationship is initiated and developed.

Research interviews

A research interview, on the other hand, is a verbal interaction between one or more researchers and one or more respondents for the purpose of collecting valid and reliable data to answer particular research questions. In the clinical interview, the client is the raison d'être of the interview, while in a research interview, the interest in the respondent is as far as the interview goes. In some types of interview, the degree of interaction is greater than in others, but the researcher's aim is not to develop therapeutic relationships. The purpose of clinical interviews is to collect data to enhance the health of the client, while data collected in research interviews are to answer researchers' questions and may or may not ultimately be used to enhance client care.

Research interviews can be face to face (in the same room or by video-conferencing), via the internet (including Skype) and by telephone. Face-to-face interviews (individual or focus groups) will be discussed throughout this chapter. Although the internet is a medium frequently used to access available information, it is fast becoming a useful tool for researchers to obtain data from respondents from different parts of the country or of the world, in a simple and inexpensive way. However, this method may also exclude large sections of the population who do not have computers or access to the internet. Wienmann et al. (2012), who tested the feasibility of Skype in epidemiological research, concluded that 'Skype is not yet a feasible tool for data collection in Germany'. On the other hand, a survey of 'Skype: a tool for functional assessment in orthopaedic research' in Ireland showed the potential for this new technique in providing patients with more options for follow-up (Good et al., 2012).

The cultural, social, practical, ethical and methodological implications of Skype for clinical and research purposes are still unfolding. James and Busher (2006), reflecting on two of their studies using online interviewing, recognised 'the contribution that web-based approaches can make to research by allowing researchers to hold asynchronous conversations with participants, especially when they are distant from the researcher, and to generating reflective, descriptive data'. They conducted email-based semi-structured interviews 'to pursue a specific agenda that had been pre-selected by the researchers in order to gain a deeper understanding of the issues' in which they were interested. For a comparison of the advantages and disadvantages of face-to-face, telephone, e-mail and MSN messenger interviews, see Opdenakker (2006).

Telephone interviewing, on the other hand, has a long history. It is one of the most popular forms of collecting research data, especially in countries where the population is spread over wide geographical areas. Like online interviewing, it is less expensive and time-consuming than face-to-face interviewing. Its main disadvantage is that only those who are accessible via telephones can be interviewed. It is also difficult to ascertain who one is really speaking with.

Telephone interviews are suitable for quantitative and qualitative approaches. Jäckle et al. (2006) compared three types of quantitative interview: two interviewed face-to-face (one with showcards, one without) and the third by telephone. They found that 'telephone respondents were more likely to give socially desirable responses across a range of indicators'. Irvine (2010) explain that:

> Telephone interviews offer a range of potential advantages for qualitative research projects. Most obviously, they remove the need for travel, so reduce both time and cost. They also allow participants to remain more anonymous if desired, they may feel less emotionally intense or intrusive, and there may be physical safety advantages for both researcher and participants. However, the methodological literature has traditionally advised against using the telephone for qualitative interviews. The two main concerns that are raised relate to (i) implications for the social encounter and scope for achieving 'rapport' and (ii) the loss of visual or non-verbal cues which are thought to aid communication and convey more subtle layers of meaning.

See Irvine et al. (2010) for a comparison of semi-structured, face-to-face and telephone interviews. For examples of telephone interviews, see Hansen and Hunskaar (2011) and Daly et al. (2013).

Whatever the form of interviews, they can collect data inductively and deductively. They are used in surveys, case studies and experiments. The type of data collected also depends on how the interviews are structured and the degree of control that researchers or participants have over their content and process. Wengraf (2001) identifies four types of interview (on a continuum): 'unstructured', 'lightly structured', 'heavily structured' and 'fully structured'. Corbin and Morse (2003) describe three 'modes' of interviewing: 'unstructured', 'semi-structured' and 'quantitative/closed-ended'. There seems to be consensus in the literature that two types of interviews – 'structured' and 'unstructured' – are at the opposite ends of a spectrum. In between these positions are 'semi-structured' interviews, so called because researchers keep some control over the content and process of the interview. As we shall see later, the degree of researchers' control in semi-structured interviews can vary.

In structured interviews, the questions are structured, predetermined and standardised. They tend to collect quantifiable data. Unstructured interviews, on the other hand, are used mainly in qualitative studies to explore phenomena. The term 'unstructured' can be misleading, since in practice no research interview can be totally unstructured. Therefore, in this chapter, the term 'qualitative interview' will be used to describe interviews in which researchers ask broad questions and invite participants to express their feelings, opinions and perceptions on particular issues, events or experiences. The three types of interview – structured, qualitative and semi-structured – are described below.

Structured interviews

In the previous chapter, it was pointed out that questionnaires can be administered by researchers in person. This, in effect, is a structured interview. It involves the researcher asking all the questions as they are formulated in the questionnaire. Neither the wording nor the sequence of the questions can be altered. The questionnaire, in this case, is normally referred to as a standardised 'interview schedule'.

The presence of the researcher can be beneficial in many ways. If the researcher wants to prevent respondents from consulting other sources in answering the questionnaire (as is the case with knowledge questions), she can administer it in person. Face-to-face structured interviews can unwittingly help to boost the response rate as participants may feel 'obliged' to take part. The presence of the researcher may act as a pressure for them to participate. The main reason for the interviewer's presence, however, is to offer clarification and support, if needed. Respondents sometimes provide incomplete or inadequate responses or 'skip' questions altogether. Their non-verbal behaviour may also communicate their confusion or lack of understanding of certain questions. In such cases, the task of the researcher is to clarify terms without changing the meaning of the questions.

Probes such as 'In what way?', 'Can you give an example?' and 'Could you expand on this?' can be used to encourage respondents to think more seriously about the questions and provide more detail (where necessary) in the responses. The interviewer's task is to make sure that the respondent understands the question and that she, in turn, understands the answers. Another reason for structured interviews is for the interviewer to help those who have difficulty in reading questions or formulating written responses. By asking the questions and recording the answers, the interviewer also facilitates the research process since the meaning of what is said can be clarified on the spot and she does not have to decipher handwriting other than her own. In some cases, the interviewer codes the responses as they are offered.

The fewer the number of interventions by the interviewer, the more structured the interview is. Consistency in asking the questions as they appear on the schedule and in making the same information available to all respondents is the hallmark of structured interviews. The aim is to achieve standardisation.

As the purpose of the structured interview is to collect data from a predetermined and structured questionnaire, and the interviewer's role is to administer the questionnaire in the same way to all respondents without any alterations, the structured interview is a quantitative method of data collection. Structured interviews are particularly suitable for those who are ill, frail or too young to complete questionnaires. However, self-administered questionnaires may be more appropriate for data of an embarrassing or private nature, since the structured interview negates one of the main strengths of questionnaires – the potential for respondents to remain anonymous.

Validity and reliability of structured interviews

Since the questionnaire is the tool of data collection in structured interviews, it is subject to the same validity and reliability threats as the questionnaire. Equally, the same tests of validity and reliability can be carried out. The main advantage of the structured interview over the self-administered questionnaire is the opportunity provided to respondents to seek clarification. By helping them, where necessary, to understand the question, they are more able to give appropriate and relevant answers, thereby enhancing the validity of the instrument. In structured interviews, it is also possible for the researcher to observe non-verbal signs that alert her to occasions when respondents experience difficulties with the questionnaire.

Since all the questions are (ideally) asked in the same way, structured interviews have a high degree of reliability, but interviewers may have difficulty in ensuring that the amount and type of clarification they give to respondents is more or less uniform. When more than one interviewer is used in the same study, it is possible that some are more able than others to extract information from respondents. Since structured interviews seek to achieve a high degree of standardisation, these issues are pertinent to the reliability of the tool and can, to some extent, be resolved through interviewer training.

The presence of the interviewer can, on the other hand, introduce a number of biases. Respondents may be more inclined to give socially desirable answers or at least mould their responses to fit the occasion. The personal characteristics of the interviewers, such as gender, age, race, clothing, language and accent, can all affect the responses; there are numerous examples in the sociological literature of how personal characteristics can interfere with the collection of valid and reliable data (see Davis et al., 2010). Research Example 41 describes the use of structured interviews in one study.

Research example 41

Structured interviews

Factors contributing to the time taken to consult with symptoms of lung cancer *Smith et al. (2009)*

This study aimed to collect data on factors that are associated with the time people take to consult with symptoms of lung cancer, with a focus on those from rural and socially deprived areas.

A symptom checklist (based on Cancer Research UK lung cancer symptoms and Scottish Intercollegiate Guidelines Network guidelines) was used to collect data. Other data including knowledge of lung cancer symptoms, previous consulting behaviour, exposure to risk factors, family history of cancer and perception of self-risk of cancer as well as socioeconomic details were also collected.

Comments

1 This is a quantitative study. Therefore the questions had to be structured (hence the use of a checklist), standardised (all participants were asked exactly the same questions) and quantifiable (for statistical analyses such as univariate and *t*-tests to be carried out).

2   The authors explained that 'a total of 361 participants were recruited and completed quantitative interview surveys (all were face-to-face apart from two which were conducted by telephone)'. Large sample sizes are a feature of structured interviews (in contrast to qualitative ones), mainly because of the sample size required for statistical tests.

Qualitative interviews

A number of terms have been used to describe qualitative interviews. Among the most common are 'unstructured', 'in-depth', 'depth', 'informal', 'non-directive', 'focused', 'narrative' and 'open'. Sometimes a combination of these has been offered, such as 'unstructured non-directive interviews' (Reid and Taylor, 2007), 'unstructured narrative' (Nielsen et al., 2013), 'in-depth focused' (Copnell and Bruni (2006) and even 'in-depth semi-structured' (Mroz et al., 2013). Others, like Roberts et al. (2013), describe their method simply as 'qualitative interviews'. The array of terms reflects both the various ways in which qualitative interviews are carried out and the liberal use of terminologies in describing these methods. There may be subtle differences or more distinct differences between them. For example, narrative interviews (see, for example, Audulv, 2013) mainly involve 'story-telling', and researchers use strategies to enable participants to tell their stories. For a useful resource on different types of interviews, see the Economic and Social Data Service website (http://www.esds.ac.uk/qualidata/support/interviews/intro.asp).

The term 'unstructured' has become synonymous with 'qualitative'. Yet it is difficult to conduct a totally unstructured interview when one wants participants to focus on the topic under investigation. For example, in a study of 'pain in nursing home residents', Gran et al. (2010) found that:

> During the interview process, the residents often shifted their focus from pain to other issues, especially to topics related to their past such as where they lived, what they did, or what their lives were like. The interviewers spent the time listening to them, while at the same time refocusing their talk to their experiences of pain.

When researchers are unsure of the term to use to label their interviews, they should simply describe their methods as qualitative (if this is the case) and explain, in detail, the interview process. 'Qualitative interview' is a broad term used to denote a family of interviews that share the common purpose of studying phenomena from the perspective of the respondent. In its most unstructured form, the qualitative interview is like an everyday, informal conversation (although it rarely is!). The degree of structure and control, the process of interviewing as well as the content, can vary from interview to interview.

Structure and control

With structured interviews, the researcher must ask everyone the same questions in the same manner. A researcher wishing to explore, by means of a qualitative interview, a phenomenon such as students' experience of preparing for examinations may not have a list of questions or topics but may decide to let them talk about their experiences. This type of interview is known as 'non-directive' as the interviewer does not 'direct' interviewees to topics but allows them free expression. The task of the interviewer, in this case, is to facilitate the flow of information with as little interruption as possible. As topics are brought up by the students, the interviewer may focus on some rather than others. New topics or new perspectives on the same topics are often introduced as the interviews progress. Interviewers choose to have little control over the agenda in non-directive interviews.

This degree of control that interviewers have in qualitative interviews should not turn the interaction into a rigid question and answer session (as is the case in structured interviews) but should be as near as possible to normal conversations. The list of topics provides a guide to researchers on what they want respondents to talk about. It is not intended in any way to achieve uniformity or to prevent respondents from taking the initiative to let their perspectives be known.

The qualitative interview process

The process of qualitative interviews can also vary. As explained above, some researchers 'allow' respondents to talk without too many interruptions and facilitate the process by listening and probing as appropriate. In this type of interview, the researcher does not reveal her own values and experience. Other interviewers share their experiences with respondents and find that their 'disclosures' help to build a trust between themselves and the respondents in the same way that happens in everyday interactions. Not only do some people feel they have to divulge a little bit of themselves in order for others to be more forthcoming with their own disclosures, but also this type of 'give and take' brings people closer when they know that both of them have some experience of the same phenomenon.

Perry et al. (2004) discuss the issue of 'involvement-detachment' in their study of the 'life experiences of young lesbian, gay, and bisexual people'. They point out that 'interviews by definition, are interdependent relationships that involve interaction between the researcher and the participant' and that 'the nature and quality of the communication is in no small measure influenced by the nature and quality of the relationship developed during the interview'.

In practice, the interviewer–interviewee interaction in qualitative interviews differs from situation to situation, so researchers have to be flexible in their approaches. With structured interviews, although not all respondents take the same amount of time to answer all the questions, the duration of the interview is guided by the number of questions, and would not normally vary greatly between interviews in the same study. This is not the case with qualitative interviews. The latter are time-consuming because of the in-depth nature of the information required and the diminished control of the researcher over the interview agenda. They vary in length in the same study, because each interaction between the interviewer and interviewee is unique. They could last between 30 minutes and 2 hours. It is unlikely that any phenomenon could be explored in depth in less than half an hour. On the other hand, a 2-hour interview would tire researchers and respondents, and cast doubt on their ability to concentrate on the task at hand.

In quantitative research, once a structured interview has been carried out, the researcher does not normally go back to the respondents to ask for clarifications or to verify whether what was said was correctly understood by the interviewer. In qualitative research, the opportunity to go back to respondents exists and is often grasped. The reason for this is to continue the previous conversation, to find out whether people feel or think differently about the phenomenon on a different day, and to validate their responses.

Therefore, each unstructured interview is different in process from the next. The researcher's role can vary from a passive one to one in which the sharing of experiences between interviewer and respondent is a key strategy in obtaining data. The duration of interviews within the same study can vary, and researchers have the freedom to interview the same respondents more than once if they (and the respondents) so wish.

The content of qualitative interviews

Even with a list of topics, it is unlikely that every interview in the same study will cover strictly the same content. The aim of qualitative interviews is to know all possible ways in which respondents view or experience phenomena. As new perspectives are uncovered and new insights gained, the interviewer finds that earlier interviews are different in content from later ones. Qualitative interviews build on one another. The researcher accumulates perspective and experiences until a broad understanding of the phenomenon has been obtained. Reflecting on and analysing data between interviews are crucial in determining which questions to ask in the next interview and which direction the study is taking. And when saturation of data is reached (that is, no new perspectives emerge), the researcher may stop interviewing even if she had intended to do more interviews.

To sum up this section, we find that while the structure, process and content of structured interviews are characterised by consistency and standardisation, the key features of qualitative interviews are, in contrast, flexibility and versatility. These are reflected in the diversity of ways in which qualitative interviews are conducted.

Rigour of qualitative interviews

The concepts of reliability and validity belong to quantitative research and as such have been criticised as having little relevance to qualitative studies. This does not, however, mean that qualitative researchers are less rigorous in the way they collect, analyse and interpret data.

As already described, the term 'reliability' refers to the degree of consistency with which the instrument produces the same results if administered in the same circumstances. In qualitative interviews, no structured, predetermined or standardised tools are used. In their most structured form, qualitative interviews consist of a list of topics about which respondents are asked to talk. The qualitative interviewer is also a 'tool' of data collection. She sifts and analyses data in her mind during the interview, as well as transcribes and makes sense of the data thereafter. Each interview in the same study is a unique interaction and is not replicable. The same researcher would conduct the interview differently were it to happen again, and another researcher would also have conducted the interview differently. In the quantitative sense, it can be said that the reliability of qualitative data is difficult to establish. However, to qualitative researchers, reliability is secondary to getting to the core of the phenomena they investigate. As Deutscher (1966) explains:

> We concentrate on consistency without much concern with what it is we are being consistent about or whether we are consistently right or wrong. As a consequence we have been learning a great deal about how to pursue an incorrect cause with a maximum of precision.

Some qualitative researchers reject the concepts of reliability and validity and offer instead such terms as 'accuracy', 'truth' and 'credibility'. To ensure rigour, they adopt a number of strategies, including reflexivity and validation of data by the interviewees themselves.

Reflexivity is the continuous process of reflection by the researcher on her own values, preconceptions, behaviour or presence and those of the respondents, which can affect the interpretation of responses. According to Holloway and Fulbrook (2001), 'interviewers should be aware of their own mind set regarding the research topic, particularly when interview questions are being developed, because personal knowledge and experience inevitably shape them'. A researcher may also reflect on how the data she collects can be influenced by how she is perceived by the respondent. Larsson et al. (2003) describe how they tried to practise reflexivity in their study of the lived experiences of eating problems among patients with head and neck cancer:

> To ensure credibility, our own perspectives on having eating problems related to radiation therapy were identified and as far as possible 'set aside' prior to and throughout the data collection and data analysis. This was carried out through our self-awareness and critical reflection on our preconceptions of the phenomenon under study.

Reflexivity by the researcher is, however, not enough or easy to carry out. It is not always possible to stand back and examine the effect of one's preconceptions, especially if one is not always aware of what they are. This is why some researchers return to interviewees to find out whether or not they agree with the interpretation of the data. This data validation process by respondents is useful in providing the opportunity for clarification and for the researcher to recognise her own prejudices, if this is the case. Habjanic and Pajnkihar (2013), in their study of 'Family members' involvement in elder care provision in nursing homes' in Slovenia, explained how, after the interviews, participants were asked to review their transcribed exemplars and gave their confirmation that the written statements described their opinion.

Another way to validate the data is to ask other researchers to examine all or part of the transcripts. The common practice of tape-recording interviews and transcribing the data verbatim (word for word) allows others to have an insight into what transpired between the researcher and the respondents, and to compare their perception of it with that of the researcher. In their study, Habjanic and Pajnkihar (2013) explain how this was achieved:

> A further step assuring credibility was the involvement of an external researcher from the field of gerontology and institutional elder care during the process of content analysis. Categories formed by the researchers were confirmed by the external researcher, who also analysed all the interviews in full. Both authors and the external researcher were unanimous about the formation and content of the categories.

Qualitative researchers recognise the subjective component in the interviewing process and seek to utilise it in order to obtain meaningful data. Some believe that building trust between researcher and respondent is crucial in getting access to the latter's perception of the phenomenon. To do this, the interviewer has to bend and mould the interview method to suit the phenomenon. For example, some interviewers, as explained earlier, may share their experiences in order to encourage respondents to 'open up'. This inevitably makes the interview a very subjective and unique experience. To achieve a degree of objectivity, it is therefore necessary to resort to some of the strategies mentioned above. See Research Example 42 for an example of an unstructured qualitative interview in one study.

Unstructured interviews

Systematic ethnography of school-age children with bleeding disorders and other chronic illnesses: exploring children's perceptions of partnership roles in family-centred care of their chronic illness *Pritchard Kennedy (2012)*

This study investigated how children understand family-centred care and their inherent role in this approach. An ethnographic approach, involving unstructured interviews and document review, was used. The rationale for the use of unstructured interviews was based on the existence of a 'significant gap in our understanding given that school-age children are developing autonomy and need to learn how to make decisions about their health care'.

Research example 42

Unstructured interviews are based on the notion that the researcher wants to learn from the experience and knowledge of participants. In this study, Pritchard Kennedy (2012) explains that her 'role was explicitly defined as being that of the learner, and the child was regarded as the teacher and expert of their own experience'.

Informed consent was obtained from the parents while the children gave assent to be interviewed. The children were involved in the assent process and asked questions about the study. They were also informed about their right to terminate the interview at any time. To facilitate this process, the children 'had control of the audio-recorder, and were in charge of turning this off when they wished to end the interview'.

Pritchard Kennedy (2012, explained how data were recorded:

> Field notes were taken before and after each interview, with documentation as a reflective process on what was observed, significance and considerations for the next interview. Interviews were audio-recorded and transcribed for later analysis, along with documentation from the field notes.

To further ensure rigour, validation interviews with four children to confirm the findings were also carried out.

Semi-structured interviews

Sechrist and Pravikoff (2002) describe a semi-structured interview as a:

> verbal questioning of study participants using a combination of preset questions and follow-up probes. For example, researchers interested in post-operative pain control experiences may interview hospitalized patients using a preset list of questions but allowing opportunity for the participant to explain their answers by asking them to amplify responses.

The tool of data collection in semi-structured interviews is called an interview schedule. It differs from an interview guide in focused interviews in that the latter has broad areas or questions but allows the researcher the freedom to ask additional questions. However, in semi-structured interviews, respondents can formulate responses in their own words and are not faced by multiple-choice answers to choose from. Pathak and Intratat (2012), in their study of 'teacher perceptions of student collaboration' realised that prepared questions should be broad and limited. They had prepared only six questions and found that they really worked well as interviewees were allowed more freedom and flexibility to talk about their perceptions.

Semi-structured interviews have elements of quantitative and qualitative research. They are similar to structured interviews in that the number and types of question are the same for all respondents, although the actual wordings may be varied for the purpose of making sure that respondents understand the question. As with structured interviews, they emphasise the notion of standardisation; that is, respondents must be subjected to the same questions with minimal variations. In a semi-structured interview, the researcher is allowed some flexibility to 'probe'. The researcher is very much in control of the interview process, and the predetermined questions provide the structure to the interview.

Some semi-structured interviews have a mixture of closed and open-ended questions, while others may have only open-ended ones. This use of closed questions ensures a high degree of standardisation since all the responses fall within the categories offered by the researcher. Open-ended questions can be specific or broad, such as 'Can you list the items of food that you have stopped consuming since you have started to take medication X?' or 'Please give as many reasons as possible as to why you do not take medication Y.' On the other hand, broad open-ended questions such as 'Can you describe your feelings when you were first told that you have diabetes?' can prompt respondents to 'open up' and make it difficult for the researcher not only to probe cautiously and objectively, but also to offer the same amount and depth of probing to all respondents. Therefore, one can see how some semi-structured interviews are closer to quantitative and others to qualitative interviews.

By trying to keep standardisation and yet be flexible, the researcher uses a mixture of quantitative and qualitative methods, which purists may frown upon. Researchers conducting semi-structured interviews must recognise the tension between trying to have both standardisation and flexibility. Many qualitative researchers label their interviews as semi-structured when in fact they are focused qualitative interviews (with a list of broad questions to guide the interaction rather than constrain it).

In practice, it is questionable whether, in semi-structured interviews, researchers ask exactly the same number of questions of all respondents and try to maintain the same degree of objectivity with all of them. If this does happen, the semi-structured interview can be said to fit more into the quantitative approach. If the researcher departs from the list of questions she comes with and starts probing deeply, the interview can be said to be focused and thus qualitative. The degree of standardisation or flexibility can provide clues to how quantitative or qualitative a semi-structured interview is.

Semi-structured interviews are popular precisely because they can provide quantitative- and qualitative-type responses that allow comparisons between respondents in the same study and can be applicable to other similar settings. As with other methods, researchers must have a good rationale for using semi-structured interviews.

The validity of responses in semi-structured interviews is enhanced by the presence of the researcher, who can clarify the questions and seek clarification from the respondents. Because semi-structured interviews share elements of quantitative and qualitative interviews, they are subject to some of the same validity and reliability threats described earlier in this chapter. For further discussion of semi-structured interviews, see Adams (2010) and Bulpitt and Martin (2010). For an example of a semi-structured interview, see Research Example 43.

Semi-structured interviews

A qualitative interview study exploring pregnant women's and health professionals' attitudes to external cephalic version *Say et al. (2013)*

In this study, semi-structured interviews were conducted with a purposive sample of pregnant women with a breech presentation, and health professionals who manage breech presentation.

These researchers developed interview schedules by critically reviewing the literature and from their experience of developing decision support in other clinical situations. The questions were open-ended to avoid limiting discussion through prior categorisation or by structuring interviews around the researcher's ideas and assumptions.

Say et al. (2013) concluded that:

the use of semi-structured interviews to collect data enabled an in-depth exploration of attitudes that was not possible in previous cross sectional surveys, and the findings contribute to the limited evidence base on women's and clinicians' experiences of and beliefs about breech presentation.

Comments

In this study, the aim was to explore attitudes qualitatively. However, the authors also believed that validity was achieved because the interview schedules provided 'a standardised approach (although flexible in order to ensure responsiveness)'. Thus, one can see how these semi-structured interviews had both quantitative (a standardised list of questions) and qualitative (flexibility for participants' views to emerge) elements.

Focus groups

A focus group can be described as an interaction between one or more researchers and more than one respondent for the purpose of collecting research data. Kitzinger (1995) explains that 'the idea behind the focus group method is that group processes can help people to explore and clarify their views in ways that would be less easily accessible in a one to one interview'. The knowledge gain from focus groups is thus the outcome of this interchange and discussion of ideas. Interaction, the main ingredient of focus groups, takes place between the researcher (sometimes called a moderator or facilitator) and the participants, and between the participants themselves.

In selecting a focus group instead of individual interviews to explore participants' experience of a particular phenomenon, researchers want, specifically, to give them opportunities to share and discuss their ideas. It is an efficient way to obtain a broad understanding of phenomena from a variety of perspectives. For example, in a study of 'Drinking contexts and the legitimacy of alcohol use' in Denmark, Grønkjær et al. (2013) found that:

focus groups were very valuable in examining and revealing important influences on peoples' drinking. Individual interviews, for example, would not have provided such data content; rather as evidenced in the empirical examples, the interactions between participants functioned as a catalyst in gaining deeper insight into the participants' perceptions on alcohol use in different contexts.

The process of focus groups consists mainly of the interviewer asking a broad question and inviting the participants to volunteer answers, which in turn generates further questions. Sometimes, if the purpose is to evaluate a service or a programme, the interviewer may have a list of aspects or issues she wants them to focus on. Kitzinger and Barbour (1999) see the role of the interviewer as encouraging participants 'to talk to one another: asking questions, exchanging anecdotes, and commenting on each others' experiences and points of view'.

The purpose of focus group interviews differs from that of individual interviews. When researchers want different perspectives on a phenomenon, they can gather people who can offer such insight in one or two sessions. They provide examples for instant comparisons (of perceptions and experiences) and spontaneous comments and reflections that can contribute to an in-depth understanding of the phenomenon being studied. Purposive sampling may be used to group people known to have different views on the topic. However, researchers sometimes have to rely on volunteers, which may bias the findings.

Focus group interviews can follow or lead into individual interviews. Issues raised during these interviews can be pursued in more detail in the privacy of individual interviews. Alternatively, focus group interviews can be conducted in order to validate data previously collected in individual interviews. In the latter, respondents are asked their views or perceptions, free from group pressure. The interviewer can concentrate on one individual at a time and pursue the topic in greater depth. In focus group interviews, it is only possible to deal with general, and not personal, issues. For example, in a group interview, the researcher studying burnout may be able to find out what the respondents think generally of 'burnout' and may be interested in finding out whether people agree or disagree with its meaning. It is not a method to assess each individual's level of 'burnout'. The researcher can also answer general questions or attend to the concerns that participants may have in taking part in the study, thus allaying their anxieties.

Focus group interviews provide opportunities to brainstorm, sometimes for the purpose of generating items for a questionnaire. They can also be used to check question wordings and formats, and provide opportunities to 'pilot-test' an instrument. When focus group interviews are to be followed by individual interviews, the former can help to familiarise the interviewer with prospective or potential interviewees.

The major advantage of focus group interviews is that valuable data can be obtained quickly and cheaply. Some people are also more comfortable in voicing their opinions in the company of friends and colleagues than on their own, with an interviewer. Focus group interviews provide the opportunity for participants to reflect on, and react to, the opinions of others, with which they may disagree or of which they are unaware. Apart from the range of opinions that can potentially be obtained, underlying conflicts may be revealed that would otherwise have remained unknown to the researcher. Even when there is no heated discussion or disagreement, the sharing of experiences can provide valuable insight into phenomena.

Bloor et al. (2001) contend that 'focus groups have a much larger part to play as an ancillary method, alongside and complementing other methods' and that 'they are rarely an alternative to depth interviewing or surveys'. One must also be cautious when generalising from focus groups to the target population. The groups are rarely large enough or randomly selected to be representative of larger group. As a result of drop-outs (which are frequent), the original group composition and group dynamics intended by the researcher can be drastically altered.

In quantitative terms, the findings from focus groups are not, in themselves, generalisable. Consensus reached by participants is often a function of group dynamics, in particular group pressure, rather than reflecting what each individual thinks or believes. For example, simply because 7 out of 10 participants agreed that a service was beneficial does not mean that they would give the same answers in a private, face-to-face interview or in response to a questionnaire. The purpose of focus group interviews is to identify all the different views, no matter how little or how much they are supported in the group. These views can, thereafter, be tested more generally in a survey. According to Vicsek (2010):

> the strength of focus groups lies not in quantitative analysis or in making statistically probable generalisations but in the fact that focus groups can show some evaluations, approaches, and mechanisms that exist in the target population and they can provide a deep and differentiated characterization of these phenomena.

One of the major disadvantages of focus group interviews is that dominant personalities or factions can monopolise the discussion and express their views at the expense of others. Interactions can be both productive and inhibitive. The experiences and views of some participants can trigger reactions in others, thereby producing rich and varied perspectives with which to view phenomena. Group dynamics, in particular the personalities and status of some individuals, can inhibit others in participating fully and freely in the discussions. Some group members may be shy, unassertive or unable to articulate their views, so this type of interview requires group management as well as interviewing skills. The larger the group, the more difficult the task to manage it. Even if the interviewer is skilled, it is possible that the contribution of those who are frightened to voice their opinions will not be fully maximised.

Focus group interviews may not be suitable for the study of sensitive and personal issues and behaviours that do not conform to the norm. Klapowitz (2000), who compared data from focus groups with those from individual interviews, found that individual interviews were 18 times more likely to raise socially sensitive discussion topics than focus groups.

Recording data can also present difficulties. Taking notes when many people are talking at the same time is not feasible. Tape-recorders may record only those who are near to them, although video-recordings can be more effective as they are not only able to capture what is said, but can also reveal the group dynamics. The analysis of data from focus group interviews can also be daunting (Leung and Savithiri, 2009).

The process of focus group interviews varies, among other things, according to the number of participants, the skill of the researcher and the purpose of the interviews. If the purpose is to brainstorm, the process may be more flexible, with opportunities for spontaneous contribution. If the purpose is to seek respondents' views on a number of specific issues or if the researcher wants to validate findings from individual interviews, the agenda will dictate a more directive approach.

Focus group interviews are not replicable. The reliability and validity of the findings are difficult to ascertain on their own but can be compared with the findings of individual interviews or other methods, if used in the same study. Researchers have to reflect on the motives or reasons for what was said and by whom. They must also realise the potential effect of group pressure on the type of data they collect. The behaviour of participants in focus groups and in individual interviews can differ. There are examples in the literature of men showing more macho behaviours when in company of other men than when interviewed individually (Kitzinger, 1994; Wright, 1994). In a study of 'Men talking about Viagra', Rubin (2004) reported that 'men in group contexts talk about Viagra in ways that serve to project a masculine image' and that 'masculine image may be more important to men than their health'.

The interest in the behaviour of people when in groups is not new. In 1739, Hume, in *A Treatise of Human Nature*, wrote:

> Everyone has observed how much more dogs are animated when they hunt in a pack, than when they pursue their game apart. We might, perhaps, be at a loss to explain this phenomenon, if we had not experience of a similar in ourselves.

For more examples of focus groups in research, see Doody et al. (2013), Cresswell et al. (2013) and Turjamaa et al. (2013). For a comparison of focus groups, face-to-face and telephone interviews, see Frazier et al. (2010). Research Example 44 shows the use of focus group interviews.

Focus group interviews

Perceptions of plain and branded cigarette packaging among Norwegian youth and adults *Scheffels and Sæbø (2013)*

The aim of this study was 'to explore perceptions of different cigarette brands, the role of package design in communicating brand images, and how participants perceived cigarette packages when important design elements such as colors, symbols, logos, and branded fonts were removed'. According to the authors, 'a focus group approach was chosen because this approach is well suited to study how images and social understandings are articulated and negotiated in social situations'.

A sample of 16–50-year-olds participated in 11 focus groups. The composition of the groups varied in terms of age groups (16–21, 20–29 and 30–50 years). Participants included daily, occasional, former and non-smokers.

The interviews, which lasted between 90 and 120 minutes, followed a 'semi-structured interview guide that began with a general discussion of smoking and smoker identity, followed by questions about how brands are perceived and of the role of cigarette package design in perceptions of brand image and identity'.

Research example 44

Nominal group technique

One design that combines some aspects of focus group interviews and the Delphi technique (see Chapter 10) is the nominal group technique (NGT). Van de Ven and Delbecq (1972) define the NGT as 'a structured meeting which seeks to provide an orderly procedure for obtaining qualitative information from target groups who are most associated with a problem area'.

The purpose of the NGT is to seek the views of group participants on a particular topic and to seek a consensus or agreement by asking them to rank or rate their responses (Harvey and Holmes, 2012). For example, participants may be asked their views on how to ensure the efficiency of a particular service. Each participant's views would be noted and followed by voting rounds and discussions until the selected views had finally been ranked in order of importance.

The NGT differs from the focus group interview in that the format of the NGT is more structured. This is because the aim is to produce a ranked list of views or items. Each participant in a study using the NGT is asked to contribute his or her views to the discussion. In focus group interviews, some participants may be more vocal than others, and some may not participate at all. The researcher (or group facilitator) also uses group dynamics to encourage discussions that can be loosely structured. The NGT, on the other hand, uses discussion in order to seek agreement, not to encourage disagreements.

The NGT differs from the Delphi technique in that it brings participants face to face, while with the Delphi technique participants do not meet, and are surveyed at a distance. The purpose of the NGT is very similar to that of the Delphi technique. Therefore it is understandable that both techniques comprise a series of steps that consist mainly of seeking initial views from individuals followed by voting rounds until the researcher is satisfied with the final results.

To ensure that everyone in the group participates, the researcher usually asks them to write the answers to a specific question. Lengthy answers (as may be the case in focus group interviews) are not encouraged. Responses are listed on a board or flip chart. To facilitate the process, the researcher imposes a structure on the questions. For example, she may ask participants to write down five factors that contribute to their job satisfaction, rather than asking them broadly what contributes to job satisfaction. In the early part of the NGT process, the responses are listed but not discussed. Once a 'workable' list has been drawn up, discussion can begin in order to inform the voting, until finally (often after several rounds) a consensus is reached.

The advantage of the NGT is that it is a cheaper and quicker way than individual interviews to collect views. All participants have to contribute responses to the discussion since the researcher asks each one of them questions. Although this may give the impression that the views of each participant have equal weightings, one must take into account the group dynamics and the 'status' of participants in the sample. Anonymity and confidentially are also not guaranteed with the NGT since the process involves face-to-face interaction. As with other designs and methods, the NGT can be used not as a substitute for others, but for achieving the researchers' desired ends. Examples of the use of the NGT include studies by:

- Ives et al. (2013) 'Module evaluation: a comparison of standard evaluation with nominal group technique'.
- Pena et al. (2012) 'Nominal group technique: a brainstorming tool for identifying areas to improve pain management in hospitalized patients'.
- Uscher-Pines et al. (2010) 'Research priorities for syndromic surveillance systems response: consensus development using nominal group technique'.

For an example of using the NGT in a study, see Research Example 45.

A study using the Nominal Group Technique

The development of clinical competencies for use on a paediatric oncology nursing course using a nominal group technique *Gibson and Soanes (2000)*

In this study, Gibson and Soanes (2000) used the NGT in the initial phase of the development of clinical competencies. The NGT was used to gather data about their detailed practice. Data were collected from two groups: 'one with senior staff/ward sisters on a haematology/oncology unit', and one with course members of a paediatric oncology nursing course.

Comments

1 The reasons given for the choice of the NGT over other methods (such as the questionnaire, expert panels and the Delphi survey) were that the NGT could give 'quick results', was not 'too time-consuming', was 'cheap' and could resolve all their 'practical issues while also achieving consultation and consensus with a professional group'.

2 Gibson and Soanes (2000) follow the NGT steps proposed by Butterfield (1988).

These were:

- Introduce nominal group process to the group
- Silent generation of ideas in writing
- Round-robin listing ideas
- Discussion of ideas on a flip chart
- Rank ordering ideas
- Total rankings
- Discussion
- Conclusion.

3 Participants in each group were asked to identify the knowledge, decision-making skills and clinical attributes essential for successful performance as a paediatric oncology nurse.

One group generated 46 ideas and the other 66. Each group was subsequently asked to rank their top eight items. This process was useful in the development of competency statements and performance criteria.

Research example 45

Ethical implications of interviewing

Interviewing shares with experiments and postal questionnaires some of the ethical concerns discussed in previous chapters. Unlike the self-administered questionnaire, however, the researcher knows who she is talking to, and the respondent cannot therefore remain anonymous. The researcher has a moral obligation to keep the respondent anonymous from others, and the data collected must remain confidential. Anonymity and confidentiality are only two of the many ethical issues that researchers and others must consider if the rights of individuals are not to be compromised. The behaviour of the interviewer before, during and after the interview has the potential of harming respondents.

Before the interview

The issue of consent, especially in relation to patients as a captive population, has been discussed in earlier chapters. Even when people are interviewed in their own homes, they can still feel obliged to help health professionals, either because they are grateful for the services they have received or because they may require them later on. Interviewing as a method of data collection puts particular pressure on respondents to take part. The physical presence of researchers or the sound of their voice over the telephone has more 'weight' than a questionnaire through the letter box. Interviews are sometimes preferred precisely because they yield higher response rates than questionnaires.

To obtain consent, researchers must give as much information as possible to respondents to enable them to make up their minds. Among these may be people who are bereaved, depressed or recovering from a suicide attempt, an abortion or miscarriage, or have just been diagnosed as having a terminal illness. They constitute a vulnerable population who may not be in a position to fully comprehend and digest all the information given to them and may not be able to give proper informed consent. Many people who live alone crave someone to talk to. Many researchers have been surprised to find that they cannot leave because the respondent wants to carry on talking.

During the interview

The interview process itself is potentially harmful. Individuals have a right to privacy, which can be easily invaded once they have given consent. Therefore participants should be made aware that they can withdraw at any time during the interview. A 'skilful' interviewer can make the respondent reveal intimate details before the latter notices what is happening. Researchers must not use underhand tactics to achieve their ends. Qualitative interviews depend on in-depth probing and, as such, have the potential to violate the right to privacy.

Qualitative interviews operate on the basis that respondents will reveal their inner thoughts to the researcher (a stranger to them). However, in some cultures, it is offensive to probe into people's lives. Qualitative interviewers must pay particular attention to cultural norms in order to avoid violating the moral and ethical conduct of particular groups.

Interviews have the potential to reveal views, beliefs, attitudes and behaviours that can be damaging to respondents. In the course of the study, the researcher's view of the respondent may be confirmed or altered. This may not be very important if the respondent never comes into contact with the researcher again, but it has implications if, for example, the respondent is a student on a course in which the researcher is involved.

Interviews, especially qualitative ones, can arouse emotions and lead to catharsis. In one-to-one interviews, the researcher is in a position to observe overt or subtle changes in the verbal and non-verbal behaviours of the respondent, and may therefore respond to them. In focus group interviews, it is difficult for her to observe and respond to the distress of some individuals; a co-facilitator may, however, be able to help.

The interview process gives rise to a number of dilemmas that researchers have to face and which may cause themselves stress as well. Buckeldee (1994) gives an idea of her own feelings when exploring the feelings of her respondents (older carers). She describes the 'depth of sorrow and sadness', which she felt at times was 'overwhelming'. Respondents may tell researchers in confidence things that can become difficult to ignore and overlook. For example, a respondent may tell the interviewer of her intention of committing suicide or may describe the abuse of patients that she has recently witnessed. The researcher faces the dilemma of doing nothing about it or breaking the confidentiality. Nurse researchers often have to deal with the conflict between their roles as nurses and as researchers.

After the interview

What happens after the interview also has ethical implications. Should researchers care about their respondents when the interview is over? What responsibilities do researchers have towards respondents after the interview? What happens to the data after they have been collected is also important. There is the possibility that the views of respondents may be misrepresented. This is why some researchers go back to respondents for them to validate the researcher's interpretation of what was said. Since, usually, not all respondents are consulted in this exercise, could it be that interviewers go back to those who are more receptive and friendly, and avoid those who are perceived as unhelpful?

It has also been suggested that debriefing sessions are necessary to deal with some of the stresses that respondents face. Researchers also need such help to relieve some of their stresses as well. In focus group interviews, individuals may be distressed and frustrated if they feel that they have not been able, for whatever reason, to express their views. Researchers can help to allay some of these frustrations by talking to them individually afterwards. The safety of group members must also be of concern to the researcher. Some of the participants may be open to victimisation for the views they have offered. Researchers must be sensitive to these issues.

How interview data are reported can also have ethical implications. Alderson (2001) points to the possibility of qualitative reports causing distress to people 'who took part in the research by identifying them more readily than numerical quantitative reports are likely to do'.

Much of the potential harm to participants can be prevented by interviewers who are thoughtful, sensitive and alert to their discomfort, especially when this is not overtly manifested. Corbin and Morse (2003) emphasise the importance of the interviewer's skill in not provoking distress, in recognising signs of distress and in taking measures to diffuse it if necessary.

These are some of the main ethical issues in interviewing. In some cases, the worst possible scenarios have been described and, of course, they do not necessarily apply to all types of interview. They are discussed here for researchers and others to be alert and sensitive to the ethical implications of what could be seen as harmless activities, for which some researchers think (often wrongly) that no approval from an ethical committee is required. For a useful discussion on the ethical issues in the use of in-depth interviews, see Allmark et al. (2009).

Critiquing interviews

Critiquing or evaluating interviews is problematic, mainly because very often little information is provided on what takes place between the interviewer and the interviewee. No two interviews are the same. Researchers must therefore describe the interview process in some detail. For example, in structured interviews, although the list of questions is predetermined, structured and standardised, readers need to know whether the input of the interviewer (or interviewers) was the same across all the interviews and, if not, how this affects the data. In qualitative interviews, one can ask whether the researcher was more or less directive, whether she used disclosures to encourage respondents to talk, whether the same questions were asked of all of them or whether the researcher built upon issues raised in the previous interview. Answers to these questions can help to determine how much the topics discussed reflect the interviewer's or the respondents' perspective.

For semi-structured interviews, one can question the extent to which the prepared list of questions provided a loose or a rigid structure. For example, were respondents simply asked to provide answers to open-ended questions, or did the researcher follow up issues raised in these answers? This is to determine whether there was limited or ample scope for respondents to talk freely. In focus group interviews, the rationale for adopting this approach as opposed to personal interviews, as well as information about the size and relevant profile of the group and how the participants were recruited, must be provided. Readers can decide whether the group seemed too large for the interviewer to handle and, depending on the purpose of the group interview, whether or not the recruitment method was biased.

The duration of the interview is often an indication of whether or not it was rushed. While it is not possible to say with certainty that in a 2-hour interview respondents were able to talk freely, it is difficult to comprehend how a qualitative interview can last less than 30 minutes, especially when only one interview is carried out per respondent. It takes that length of time for the interviewer and interviewee to exchange 'civilities' and begin to engage in a conversation, let alone talk 'in depth' about anything.

As with other methods of data collection, researchers are better able than readers to reflect on whether their data can be taken at face value. Only they can tell whether their dress, appearance, accent, gender, race and other characteristics, or other events, had any bearings on the data collected.

Researchers must also explain how informed consent was obtained, access to respondents negotiated and respondents' privacy respected. They also have to report on where the interview took place and who else was present.

Measures taken for ensuring the validity and reliability of data must be fully explained. These should give an indication of the length to which the researchers have gone in order to ensure the credibility of their data. Finally, researchers should reflect on the limitations of their studies and indicate whether their findings can apply to other settings or whether they should be treated with caution.

Summary

The interview is one of the main methods of data collection and takes different forms. In structured interviews, the questions are pre-determined, standardised and highly structured, with only limited scope for clarification and elaboration.

Qualitative interviews are characterised by flexibility and versatility. The researcher can mould the interaction in order to obtain in-depth information about phenomena. Semi-structured interviews combine elements of both of these types: they give respondents some freedom to express themselves while answering a set number of questions. Finally, focus group interviews make use of group dynamics to obtain a variety of perspectives cheaply and quickly on the same phenomenon.

Each of these interviews has its value and limitations. We have discussed the strategies that researchers adopt to ensure that the data they collect are credible. They should describe the interview process in relevant detail to enable readers to evaluate these data.

Finally, interviews, whatever the type, have ethical implications that researchers must seriously consider. Respondents' human rights must always take precedence over any research consideration.

References

Adams E (2010) The joys and challenges of semi-structured interviewing. *Community Practitioner*, **83**,7:18–21.

Alderson P (2001) *On Doing Qualitative Research Linked to Ethical Healthcare*, Vol. I (London: Wellcome Trust).

Allmark P J, Boote J, Chambers E et al. (2009) Ethical issues in the use of in-depth interviews: literature review and discussion. *Research Ethics Review*, **5**, 2:48–54.

Audulv A (2013) The over time development of chronic illness self-management patterns: a longitudinal qualitative study. *BMC Public Health*, **13**:452.

Bloor M, Frankland J, Thomas M and Robson K (2001) *Focus Groups in Social Research* (London: Sage).

Buckeldee J (1994) Interviewing carers in their own homes. In: J Buckeldee and R McMahon (eds) *The Research Experience in Nursing* (London: Chapman & Hall).

Bulpitt H and Martin PJ (2010) Who am I and what am I doing? Becoming a qualitative research interviewer. *Nurse Researcher*, **17**, 3:7–16.

Butterfield P G (1988) Nominal group process as an instructional method with novice community health nursing students. *Public Health Nursing*, **5**:12–15.

Copnell B and Bruni N (2006) Breaking the silence: nurses' understandings of change in clinical practice. *Journal of Advanced Nursing*, **55**, 3:301–9.

Corbin J and Morse J (2003) The unstructured interactive interview: issues of reciprocity and risks when dealing with sensitive topics. *Qualitative Inquiry*, **9**, 3:335–54.

Cresswell K, Howe A, Steven A et al. (2013) Patient safety in healthcare preregistration educational curricula: multiple case study-based investigations of eight medicine, nursing, pharmacy and physiotherapy university courses. *British Medical Journal Quality and Safety* **22**:843–54.

Daly B, Arroll B, Sheridan N, Kenealy T and Scragg R (2013) Characteristics of nurses providing diabetes community and outpatient care in Auckland. *Journal of Primary Health Care*, **5**, 1:19–27.

Davis R E, Couper M P, Janz N K, Caldwell C H and Resnicow K (2010) Interviewer effects in public health. *Health Education Research*, **25**, 1:14–26.

Deutscher I (1966) Words and deeds: social science and social policy. *Social Problems*, **13**:233–54.

Doody O, Slevin E and Taggart L (2013) Focus group interviews in nursing research: part 1. *British Journal of Nursing*, **22**, 1:16–19.

Frazier L M, Miller V A, Horbelt D V, Delmore J E, Miller B E and Paschal A M (2010) Comparison of focus groups on cancer and employment conducted face to face or by telephone. *Qualitative Health Research*, **20**, 5:617–27.

Gibson F and Soanes L (2000) The development of clinical competencies for use on a paediatric oncology nursing course using a nominal group technique. *Journal of Clinical Nursing*, **9**:459–69.

Good D W, Lui D F, Leonard M, Morris S and McElwain JP (2012) Skype: a tool for functional assessment in orthopaedic research. *Journal of Telemedicine and Telecare*, **18**, 2:94–8.

Gran S V, Festva G L S and Landmark B T (2010) 'Alone with my pain – it can't be explained, it has to be experienced'. A Norwegian in-depth interview study of pain in nursing home residents. *International Journal of Older People Nursing*, **5**: 25–33.

Grønkjær M, Curtis T, De Crespigny C and Delmar C (2013) Drinking contexts and the legitimacy of alcohol use: findings from a focus group study on alcohol use in Denmark. *Scandinavian Journal of Public Health*, **41**, 3:221–9.

Habjanic A and Pajnkihar M (2013) Family members' involvement in elder care provision in nursing homes and their considerations about financial compensation: a qualitative study. *Archives of Gerontology and Geriatrics*, **56**, 3:425–31.

Hansen E H and Hunskaar S (2011) Understanding of and adherence to advice after telephone counselling by nurse: a survey among callers to a primary emergency out-of-hours service in Norway. *Scandinavian Journal of Trauma, Resuscitation and Emergency Medicine*, **19**:48.

Harvey N and Holmes C A (2012) Nominal group technique: an effective method for obtaining group consensus. *International Journal of Nursing Practice*, **18**, 2:188–94.

Holloway I and Fulbrook P (2001) Revisiting qualitative inquiry: interviewing in nursing and midwifery research … including commentary by C Bailey. *Nursing Times Research*, **6**, 1:539–51.

Hume D (1969) *A Treatise of Human Nature: Being an Attempt to Introduce the Experimental Method of Reasoning* (London: Pelican).

Irvine A (2010) Using phone interviews. Realities Toolkit #14. Social Policy Research Unit, University of York. Retrieved from http://eprints.ncrm.ac.uk/1576/1/14-toolkit-phone-interviews.pdf (accessed 7 September 2013).

Irvine A, Drew P and Sainsbury R (2010) Mode effects in qualitative interviews: a comparison of semi-structured face-to-face and telephone interviews using conversation analysis. *Research Works*, 2010–03, Social Policy Research Unit, University of York, York.

Ives J, Skelton J and Calvert M (2013) Module evaluation: a comparison of standard evaluation with nominal group technique. *Education for Primary Care*, **24**, 2:111–18.

Jäckle A, Roberts C and Lynn P (2006) *Telephone versus Face-to Face Interviewing: Mode Effects on Data Quality and Likely Causes. Report on Phase II of the ESS-Gallup Mixed Mode Methodology Project*. ISER Working Paper 2006-41 (Colchester: University of Essex).

James N and Busher H (2006) Credibility, authenticity and voice: dilemmas in online interviewing. *Qualitative Research*, **6**, 3:403–20.

Kitzinger J (1994) The methodology of focus groups: the importance of interaction between research participants. *Sociology of Health and Illness*, **16**:103–21.

Kitzinger J (1995) Introducing focus groups. *British Medical Journal*, **311**:299–302.

Kitzinger J and Barbour R E (1999) Introduction: the challenge and promise of focus groups. In: R S Barbour and J Kitzinger (eds) *Developing Focus Group Research: Politics, Theory and Practice* (London: Sage).

Klapowitz M D (2000) Statistical analysis of sensitive topics in group and individual interviews. *Quality and Quantity*, **34**:419–31.

Larsson M, Hedelin B and Athlin E (2003) Lived experiences of eating problems for patients with head and neck cancer during radiotherapy. *Journal of Clinical Nursing*, **12**:562–70.

Leung F-H and Savithiri R (2009) Spotlight on focus groups. *Canadian Family Physician*, **55**, 2: 218–19.

Mroz L W, Oliffe J L and Davison B J (2013) Masculinities and patient perspectives of communication about active surveillance for prostate cancer. *Health Psychology*, **32**, 1:83–90.

Nielsen M, Foster M, Henman P and Strong J (2013) 'Talk to us like we're people, not an X-ray': the experience of receiving care for chronic pain. *Australian Journal of Primary Health*, **19**, 2:138–43.

Opdenakker R (2006) Advantages and disadvantages of four interview techniques in qualitative research. *Forum: Qualitative Social Research*, **7**, 4:Art. 11.

Pathak A and Intratat C (2012) Use of semi-structured interviews to investigate teacher perceptions of student collaboration. *Malaysian Journal of ELT Research*, **8**, 1:1–10.

Pena A, Estrada C A, Soniat D, Taylor B and Burton M (2012) Nominal group technique: a brainstorming tool for identifying areas to improve pain management in hospitalized patients. *Journal of Hospital Medicine*, **7**, 5:416–20.

Perry C, Thurston M and Green K (2004) Involvement and detachment in researching sexuality: reflections on the process of semistructured interviewing. *Qualitative Health Research*, **14**, 1:135–48.

Pritchard Kennedy A (2012) Systematic ethnography of school-age children with bleeding disorders and other chronic illnesses: exploring children's perceptions of partnership roles in family-centred care of their chronic illness. *Child: Care Health and Development*, **38**, 6:863–9.

Reid B and Taylor J (2007) A feminist exploration of Traveller women's experiences of maternity care in the Republic of Ireland. *Midwifery*, **23**, 3:248–59.

Roberts D, Appleton L, Calman L et al. (2013) Protocol for a longitudinal qualitative interview study: maintaining psychological well-being in advanced cancer – what can we learn from patients' and carers' own coping strategies? *British Medical Journal Open* **3**:e003046.

Rubin R (2004) Men talking about Viagra: an exploratory study with focus groups. *Men and Masculinities*, **7**, 1:22–30.

Say R, Thomson R, Robson S and Exley C (2013) A qualitative interview study exploring pregnant women's and health professionals' attitudes to external cephalic version. *BMC Pregnancy and Childbirth*, **13**, 4:1–9.

Scheffels J and Sæbø G (2013) Perceptions of plain and branded cigarette packaging among Norwegian youth and adults: a focus group study. *Nicotine Tobacco Research*, **15**, 2: 450–6.

Sechrist K and Pravikoff D (2002) *CINAHL Information Systems* (Glendale, CA: CINAHL).

Smith S M, Campbell N C, MacLeod U et al. (2009) Factors contributing to the time taken to consult with symptoms of lung cancer: a cross-sectional study. *Thorax*, **64**:523–31.

Turjamaa R, Hartikainen S and Pietilä A-M (2013) Forgotten resources of older home care clients: focus group study in Finland. *Nursing and Health Sciences*, **15**, 3:333–9.

Uscher-Pines L, Babin SM, Farrell CL et al. (2010) Research priorities for syndromic surveillance systems response: consensus development using nominal group technique. *Journal of Public Health Management and Practice*, **16**, 6:529–34.

Van de Ven A H and Delbecq A L (1972) The nominal group as a research instrument for exploratory health studies. *American Journal of Public Health*, **69**:337–42.

Vicsek L (2010) Issues in the analysis of focus groups: generalisability, quantifiability, treatment of context and quotations. *Qualitative Report*, **15**, 1:122–41.

Weinmann T, Thomas S, Brilmayer S, Heinrich S and Radon K (2012) Testing Skype as an interview method in epidemiologic research: response and feasibility. *International Journal of Public Health*, **57**, 6:959–61.

Wengraf T (2001) *Qualitative Research Interviewing* (Thousand Oaks, CA: Sage).

Wright D (1994) Boys' thoughts and talk about sex in a working-class locality of Glasgow. *Sociological Review*, **42**:702–37.

18 Observations

Chapter

> **Opening thought**
>
> Where observation is concerned, chance favours only the prepared mind.
>
> Louis Pasteur

Introduction

In a practice-based profession such as nursing or midwifery, observation is perhaps the most important method of collecting information. As a research tool for the study of human behaviour, it is invaluable on its own or when used in conjunction with other methods. In this chapter, we will briefly explore the use, value and limitations of observation in nursing practice and nursing research. The main two types of observations (structured and unstructured) will be described and discussed. We will examine the ethical implications of using observation to collect data on people in general, and patients and nurses in particular. Finally, some suggestions will be made to facilitate those who undertake a critical reading of observational studies.

Observation and nursing practice

Researchers did not invent observation. Adler and Adler (1994) remind us that, 'for as long as people have been interested in studying the social and natural world around them, observation has served as the bedrock source of human knowledge'.

Although observation is part of daily life, some professionals, in particular nurses, need to be skilled at it. Without observation, effective nursing care is not possible. The process of nursing care, from assessment to evaluation, depends a great deal on precise and accurate observation. The ability to observe, although naturally possessed by some, can be developed with training. While observation is usually associated with sight, the other four senses (hearing, touch, smell and taste) are also involved. These senses vary in the extent to which they are used in nursing practice. Sight and hearing are understandably the most frequently used, although touch and smell provide valuable information as well.

Humans have also devised aids to increase their ability to observe. The most common ones include telescopes, microscopes and sound amplifiers. In nursing practice, thermometers, sphygmomanometers and stethoscopes are but some of a whole array of devices and equipment designed to make observations of body functions and changes as precise and accurate as possible, and to venture where normal human senses cannot reach.

To assess and monitor clients, nurses have to observe verbal and non-verbal signs. Many of the clients whom nurses treat are, however, either not able or not willing to speak. The ability to assess their conditions and attend to their needs depends greatly on the observational skills of nurses. Some client groups, such as people with a learning difficulty, have a higher incidence of communication impairment; they are especially dependent upon non-verbal communication and the accurate interpretation of their communication (Martin et al., 2010). There is also evidence that nurses use mainly eye gaze, head-nodding, and smiling to establish a good relationship with their patients (Roberts and Bucksey, 2007).

'Doing the obs' is a well-known expression in nursing that normally means recording the patient's temperature, pulse, respiration and blood pressure. Many of the observations carried out by nurses involve the use of more than one sense simultaneously. In 'taking' blood pressure, the nurse may use touch to find a vein, listen for the 'beats' and watch the movement of the 'needle' or 'mercury'. Apart from occasions when nurses are asked to 'observe' or 'special' a patient, or to carry out specific observations, they are, according to Peplau (1988), participant observers in most relationships in nursing. As she explains:

> This requires that she use herself as an instrument and as an object of observation at the same time that she is participating in the interaction between herself and a patient or a group. The more precise the nurse can become in the use of herself as an instrument for observation, the more she will be able to observe in relation to performances in the nursing process.

Nurses also use a large number of tools or instruments to record nursing activities, assess and monitor patients' condition.

Observation in nursing research

The purpose of observations in nursing practice differs from that in nursing research. Nurses use observations to collect information to attend to the needs of clients, while researchers conduct observations for the purpose of answering research questions. Many nursing observations, such as the monitoring of temperature, pulse and respiration or blood pressure require the utmost rigour and precision. However, many other observations are casual, accidental or haphazard. They are made, as Peplau (1988) described above, during everyday interactions between nurses and patients. Therefore observations are made as part of the process of care and are not necessarily the focus of interactions.

On the other hand, researchers' main purpose is not to deliver care but to observe. Therefore interactions are a means to an end, which is to collect research data. Adler and Adler (1994) explain how lay observations differ from research observations:

> What differentiates the observations of social scientists from those of everyday life actors is the former's systematic and purposive nature. Social science researchers study their surrounding regularly and repeatedly, with a curiosity spurred by theoretical questions about the nature of human action, interaction, and society.

As the nature of nurses' work requires them to observe all the time, a knowledge of how and why researchers carry out observations can enhance nurses' understanding of the complexity and implications of this method of collecting information. Some of the issues that will be raised in this chapter should, hopefully, help you to reflect on your own knowledge of, and skill in, observation. Like interviews, observations can be carried out in surveys, experiments and case studies. They are used in inductive, deductive, qualitative and quantitative research. They are more suited to some phenomena than others and can be used in conjunction with other methods such as questionnaires and interviews.

The need to choose the most appropriate method cannot, however, be overemphasised. Observations are particularly suited to the study of psychomotor activities and other non-verbal activities, while knowledge, attitudes and beliefs are better studied by questionnaires and interviews. Observations are most suited to studying the behaviour of patients and health professionals, in particular interactions, communication and performance. The observation of behaviour in its natural setting provides an insight into the context in which it occurs. Researchers have the opportunity to sample the physical, cultural, psychological and social environment in which the behaviour takes place.

Although observations on their own can tell us a lot about human behaviour, they can increase our understanding when used in combination with other methods such as interviews or document analysis. This is because, with observation, researchers can see and interpret behaviour but cannot have access to the meaning that participants give to their own behaviour. Researchers and practitioners interested in the link between knowledge, attitude and practice often find that there are discrepancies between these.

Self-reports (via questionnaires or interviews) are not always reliable. Bolster and Manias (2010), in their study of 'Person-centred interactions between nurses and patients during medication activities in an acute hospital setting', reported that there were discrepancies between what nurses said they did and what they actually did.

Some phenomena that have been studied by means of observation include: 'Clinical focus and public accountability in English NHS Trust Board meetings' (Endacott et al., 2013), 'Resident characteristics related to the lack of morning care provision in long-term care' (Simmons et al., 2013), 'evaluation of a drug monitoring system for ambulatory chronic disease patients' (Callen et al., 2013); and 'Nurse and patient characteristics associated with duration of nurse talk during patient encounters in ICU' (Nilsen et al., 2013).

Limitations of observations

Observation, as with other methods, has its own limitations and ethical implications (discussed in a later section). One of the main problems is the effect of the observer on the 'observed'. The awareness of being observed is likely to lead people to be self-conscious, and may influence them to behave in ways that they would not normally behave. In a classic study by Roethlisberger and Dickson (1939), in which they set out to find the effect of illumination levels on productivity at the Hawthorne plant of Western Electric in Chicago, they experimented with different levels of lighting over a period of two and a half years and found that no matter what the levels were, productivity continued to increase. Roethlisberger and Dickson concluded that the workers produced more mainly because they were being observed, rather than as a result of the different lighting. This type of observer effect is now known popularly as the 'Hawthorne effect'.

In an observation study of 'patient care in intensive care units', Turnock and Gibson (2001) queried whether the impact of their presence upon staff behaviour would have been different if they had been 'either true researchers or practitioners'. They described one incident which confirmed their suspicion that the observer's presence may have led to fewer nursing interventions than expected. To test this 'hypothesis', the observer changed position after 1 hour of observation. The same patient was observed for a second hour, but from a position much further away from the bed area. Once the new position had been taken up, several activities/interventions began to take place. Turnock and Gibson explained that 'this may have been a coincidence, but was more likely due to the influence of the observer's presence on staff behaviour'.

A number of strategies can be used to decrease the Hawthorne or reactivity effect. Bolster and Manias (2010) describe what they did to minimise the observer effect on participants' behaviour:

- meeting with the participants on two occasions prior to the commencement of data collection to enable participants to feel comfortable with the observer and the observation process;
- the use of unobtrusive positioning and avoidance of eye contact by the observer during the observation periods to ensure that participants were not distracted or prompted during their interactions;
- conducting observations over a 2-hour period, to allow time for the participants to become less aware of the researcher's presence.

While the effect of the observer's presence cannot be fully eliminated, researchers found that it is not always possible for people to change their normal behaviour and sustain it for long periods, especially when they are busy (Mulhall, 2003). This is supported by findings from the study by Qian et al. (2013) . They noticed that after a while, the observer's existence is 'ignored' (see Research Example 46 below). Some of the strategies to reduce this effect will be discussed later. Researchers are also best placed to know if their presence influenced the data they collected and must reflect on this. There is no perfect method, and some trade-off is often necessary for the collection of valid and reliable data. To some extent, the video can be used to reduce the observer's effect (this is discussed further on).

Another problem with observations is that they can be costly and impractical over long periods of time. For example, watching and waiting for aggressive behaviour to happen can be time-consuming. The researcher's ability to observe with precision can wane over time, as fatigue sets in. The difficulties of observing different aspects of the same phenomenon, which occur at the same time, and the ways in which researchers cope with these and other problems are discussed further in the next section.

Structured observation

A structured observation is one in which aspects of the phenomenon to be observed are decided in advanced (that is, predetermined). The phenomenon itself has be operationalised (see Chapter 9) before it can be broken down into observable *units* or *categories*. In their study of 'Clinical focus and public accountability in English NHS Trust Board meetings', Endacott et al. (2013) operationally defined the term 'clinical' as 'concerning the direct provision to patients of physical or psychological care or diagnoses (not the organization thereof)'. They then proceeded to develop a list of clinical and non-clinical categories as follows:

- Clinical: service design and standards
  - Clinical ethics
  - Clinical outcomes
  - Referral routes and volumes
- Activity levels
- Evidence-based care
- Non-clinical: the Board's internal processes and conduct
  - The National Health Service (NHS) national agenda
  - Finance
  - Organisational issues
  - Staffing
  - Patient feedback.

Some of these categories would still be difficult to interpret. For example, 'feedback' was categorised as clinical (such as complaints or feedback related to a specific incident) or non-clinical (for example, feedback regarding care organisation or specific methods of clinical care).

The reason for specifying aspects of the phenomenon in advance is mainly to find out if they are present, and if so, to what extent. The same type of data is required from each observation, thereby introducing standardisation into the process.

To carry out structured observation, a 'checklist' or 'schedule' is devised. This is similar to a questionnaire and can be highly or loosely structured. For example, in a study of touch in nurse–patient interactions, the observer could be asked to indicate the 'site' of touch without providing her with any categories of site. Alternatively, a number of sites (such as hand, arm, shoulder and so on) could be provided, and the observer could then select the appropriate category. This avoids the problem that may arise when different observers use different terms to describe the same site. A highly structured observation schedule leaves little for the observer to interpret other than to 'tick' the appropriate columns or boxes.

In structured observation, the phenomenon to be studied must be operationally defined. The categories or units depend on the particular definition that the researcher chooses. Whatever the definition, it must adequately represent the phenomenon, and it must be operationally feasible. This means that it must describe behaviours that can be observed. For example, in a study by Fuller and Conner (1995) of 'The effect of pain on infant behaviors', 'cries' and 'cry duration' were defined as follows:

> Cry duration. A single phonation with more than 3 seconds of silence preceding and following another phonation was defined as a cry. Phonations with less than 3 seconds separating each other were labelled subcries. A cry bout is a series of subcries separated by more than 3 seconds from a cry or second cry bout. The duration in seconds was measured for all cries, subcries, and cry bouts contained on each videotape.

Structured observations and structured interviews are similar in that both use predetermined, structured and standardised tools. The observer and interviewer also adopt a non-participative or non-interventionist stance. As with the administration of questionnaires, the observer stands 'outside' what is being observed and tries not to influence events or behaviours in any way. Turnock and Gibson (2001) explained how they 'experienced problems in maintaining a detached, researcher role' as non-participant observers. They were 'asked to keep an eye on the patient for a minute'. Turnock and Gibson (2001) also found it 'morally impossible to ignore the requests of patients not involved in the study'. Although researchers may not be able to keep a completely non-participant, detached stance when doing observations, they should be sensitive to the possible effects of such interactions on the data collected.

In structured observations, researchers seek to quantify specific aspects of the phenomena being observed. They usually want to find the presence or absence of a particular behaviour or characteristic, and the frequency or intensity with which it may happen. The underlying assumption in the use of structured observations is that researchers know what constitutes the behaviour or activity and only seek to discover to what extent they are present in the population under study.

Sampling in structured observation

It is not always feasible or possible to observe every behaviour or activity on a continuous basis. The prolonged observation of patients and nurses can cause them unnecessary stress. Therefore researchers resort to time sampling, where appropriate. Nurses are familiar with the concept of time sampling. Patients are monitored at set intervals, as in the case of a 4-hourly recording of temperature, pulse and respiration. In the same way, if patient activities are being observed, the researcher may decide to carry out observations during the first 15 minutes of each hour for the duration of the shift. This can be done if it is believed that these periods of 15 minutes are able to give an accurate and representative picture of activities over the whole shift.

In a study of 'pain assessment and management in hospitalised older people', Manias (2012) carried out observations during six periods: three between midnight and midday (at 3.30, 7.30 and 10.30 am), and three between midday and midnight (at 3.30, 6.30 and 10.30 pm). Each period lasted between 2 and 3 hours. These time samples were 'determined following discussions with nurses working in the units and covered change-of-shift and staff overlap times, night shift and pre-sleep planning routines, organisation of hygiene and toileting activities, and analgesic administration times' (Manias, 2012).

Intermittent observation, as in the case in time sampling, may not be appropriate in cases where the behaviour or activity happens rarely or unpredictably. For example, if a researcher wants to observe 'restless' behaviour among patients with dementia, continuous observation would be advisable. This can be achieved either by observing whole shifts or by dividing the day into, for example, 4-hourly sessions from 8.00 am to midnight. The researcher then carries out the 8.00 am to 12.00 midday observation on day one and the 12.00 midday to 4.00 pm session on day two. This is continued until all four sessions have been covered. In this way, data for the whole period between 8.00 am to midnight are obtained, although not in one day.

Alternatively, the researcher may want to observe communication behaviour during specific 'events' such as meal times or in discussion groups. In this case, these events become the focus of the study. However, not all meal times may be observed. The researcher may select a sample of meal times, for example lunch on Monday and Friday, dinner on Tuesday and Saturday, and breakfast on Wednesday and Sunday. Thus, a sample of meal times can be chosen to represent meal times in general in that particular ward. This is known as event sampling; the event becomes the sampling unit. In Simmons et al.'s (2013) study of 'morning care provision in long-term care', the events they sampled were 'transfer out of bed (time to get up), incontinence care (to include toileting assistance, use of bedpan or urinal, and changing of soiled under garments/bedclothes), and dressing (when to get dressed and what to wear)'.

Limitations of structured observations

Behaviours and activities happen simultaneously, and the observer may not be able to notice and record all of them. The position of the observer may be such that the behaviour may be outside her observation range or she may be obstructed, as in the case where a nurse is in the observer's line of vision and the patient cannot be observed. Some movements or changes may be so subtle or rapid that the researcher is unable to capture them. For example, eye contacts can be fleeting, or a facial expression can last a fraction of a second. As Lobo (1992) explains:

> If the behavior occurs very infrequently, it may be missed altogether because the length of the observation is not sufficient to capture the behavior. Or if the event is fleeting and the observation is over a long period of time, a fatigued observer may miss the event.
>
> In a busy environment, it is possible for the observer to be distracted, especially if she is concerned about what happens to other people. In continuous observation, fatigue may set in, leading to lack of concentration.

One of the major problems with structured observations is the difficulty of deciding which category or unit the observed behaviour or activity belongs to. Some categories are not adequately defined. In Endacott et al.'s (2013) study, the authors reported that their findings rested upon their broad definition of 'clinical'. Some categories require the observer to make more subjective judgements than others. In a study by Fader et al. (2003), in which the frequency and intensity of erythema (reddening of the skin) were observed, there were disagreements between observers relating to grade 0 ('no erythema') and grade 1 ('barely perceptible erythema'). It was acknowledged that 'these discrepancies could be real (i.e. the skin colour changed slightly during the lapsed time period) or as a result of error (because the degree of difference between the two grades was very slight and therefore difficult to accurately grade' (Fader et al., 2003).

Some of these problems can be reduced by providing adequate operational definitions, by piloting their observation schedule, by training observers and by making use of audio- and video-taping where possible, appropriate and ethical. Video-taping of behaviours and interactions would also offset some of these limitations, including observer fatigue. Video-recording has the advantage of providing continuous data over long periods of time. It can record more details than a human observer can. It has 'frame-by-frame', 'close-up' (useful for subtle movements) and 'play-back' facilities. Videotapes can be made available for other researchers to analyse the data.

The limitations of video-recordings are that they can be costly, unreliable (in cases of mechanical breakdown) and may present logistical problems, such as where to place the camera(s) in order to fully capture the action. Video-recording in the natural environment can be difficult if those being filmed are on the move rather than static. Cameras can also be intrusive and may influence the behaviour of people when they are being filmed. In a study of 'nursing report sessions and interdisciplinary team meetings' in a psychiatric unit, Latvala et al. (2000) used video-taping as a method of data collection. They found that some nurses 'changed their habits and presented their ideal selves' when being taped.

A number of ethical issues should be considered when video-recording is used in research studies. Participants must not feel under pressure to take part, and must be free to withdraw after viewing the tapes. Researchers have the responsibility to keep the tapes in a safe place and destroy them when data have been analysed. For examples of studies using video-recordings, see 'Nurse and patient characteristics associated with duration of nurse talk during patient encounters in ICU' (Nilsen et al., 2013) and 'Evaluating health visitor assessments of mother-infant interactions' (Appleton et al., 2013).

Validity and reliability of structured observation

The reliability and validity of structured observations depend on the reliability and validity of the observation tool and on the ability of the observer to make precise observations of behaviours or events (Waltz et al., 2010). For structured observations to have validity, the observer must observe what she is supposed to observe. Observation schedules can be assessed for content validity in the same way as for questionnaires (see Chapter16). The operational definition of the phenomenon must be clear and precise, and the categories or units must represent the phenomenon. To ensure content validity, the observation schedule can be given to a panel of experts for review.

The observer's presence can also affect the validity of the data. As mentioned earlier, the observer's effect can be reduced when those observed 'get used' to the presence of the observer. Sometimes the observer spends little time in the setting prior to the observation, and therefore has little or no opportunity for 'settling in'. The personal attributes – such as gender, sex, race, dress or manner – of the observer may influence how people behave when they are observed. Researchers must be sensitive to this possibility and make allowance for this when they analyse and interpret the data.

When a number of people witness an accident, it is unlikely that their individual accounts of the event will be entirely consistent, even if it happened just 5 minutes earlier. Police officers are familiar with instances when witnesses give different descriptions of the same burglary or assault. Research observers are not immune to such inconsistencies. The observation schedule, the instructions to observers and the opportunity to record behaviours as they happen facilitate the observation process. However, observers are human and can be influenced by a number of factors, including their own assumptions and prejudices, that can distort their perception, or they may simply make mistakes.

Reliability in structured observations refers to the consistency with which the observer matches a behaviour or activity with the same unit or category on the observation schedule and records it in the same way each time it happens. Intra-observer reliability is the consistency with which one observer records the same behaviours in the same way on different occasions. One way to achieve a high degree of intra-rater reliability is for the researcher to rate several video-recordings of the behaviour to be observed and to rate them on different occasions and compare the ratings. In this way, the observer can learn whether or not she is consistent, and refine her observation skills and/or the observation schedule.

Observations in the same study are often carried out by two or more observers. It is important that they observe, interpret and record the same behaviour or activity in the same way. Inter-observer or inter-rater reliability can be monitored by asking two or more observers to record the same behaviours, and their findings are then analysed. A correlation coefficient (r) of 1.00 indicates total agreement and thereby excellent reliability, while a score of below 0.60 (an agreement in 6 instances out of 10) is of doubtful reliability. However, each study may set its own acceptable levels of reliability depending on the type of phenomenon. The more difficult the phenomenon is to observe, the less likely it is to achieve a score close to 1.00.

There is normally a consensus in the research literature on what constitutes an acceptable level of reliability depending on the complexity of the observational task. A high level of agreement between two or more observers usually means that they have consistently recognised and recorded the same behaviour in the same way. However, they could also be consistently wrong. When observations do not match, observers must discuss their perception of the particular behaviours or activities in dispute and arrive at an agreed interpretation of it. In their observational study, Simmons et al. (2013) explain how inter-rater reliability was ensured:

> Research staff observers (n = 5) were trained prior to data collection in [long term care] facilities using real care situations until inter-rater reliability was achieved at a kappa level of .80 or higher for each observation-based coding element. The project coordinator and research geriatric nurse practitioner continued to conduct interrater reliability checks twice per month with each observer to prevent observer drift during the 3 months of data collection. Most relevant to the current study as the primary outcome measure, the kappa value for whether care was provided ranged from .94 to 1.0 (n = 140, p < .001) across the three care areas.

The validity and reliability of structured observations depend mainly on how the observation schedule is constructed and used. For an example of a study using structured observation, see Research Example 46.

Structured observation

The work pattern of personal care workers in two Australian nursing homes: a time–motion study *Qian et al. (2012)*

In this time–motion, observational study in two Australian nursing homes, 'a pre-defined classification of activities' was used to develop an observation schedule or checklist to record the activities of personal health workers. The checklist comprised 58 activities, grouped in the following eight categories: 'direct care, indirect care, infection control, documentation, transit, staff break, oral communication and other activities not included in the previous categories'.

Observations were conducted by a single observer. However, to ensure the reliability of the observation process, a second, experienced observer jointly recorded four nurses' activities for a period of 4 hours. The recordings were compared and discussed. A high inter-rater reliability (over 95 per cent) was achieved.

The authors mentioned that there may have been a Hawthorne effect, in that the participants may have changed their behaviour when being observed. However, they found that these workers were very busy focusing on their job and soon ignored the existence of the observer.

Research example 46

Unstructured observation

The French novelist Maupassant, in a preface to *Pierre and Jean* in 1887, wrote:

> In everything there is an unexplored element because we are prone by habit to use our eyes only in combination with the memory of what others before us have thought about the thing we are looking at. The most significant thing contains some little unknown element. We must find it.

According to Kirk and Miller (1986):

> In science, as in life, dramatic new discoveries must almost by definition be accidental ('serendipitous'). Indeed, they occur only in consequence of some kind of mistake.

They relate how radioactivity was discovered when Henri Becquerel 'tossed the uranium salts into a drawer with his photographic materials and knocked off work'. Alexander Fleming also found that 'some kind of mold got into his staphylococcus culture and ruined the bacteria', thus accidentally discovering penicillin (Kirk and Miller, 1986).

Although the ability to understand what happens is based on prior knowledge, these examples also show the need to study phenomena with fresh eyes and an open mind. By adopting a deductive approach, researchers collect data to test what is already known. The categories to be observed are formulated in advance, based on previous knowledge. Alternatively, researchers can observe phenomena without any predetermined categories and allow these to emerge from the data collected.

When we observe people's behaviour on buses, we do not have categories to 'tick'. Instead we record and analyse mentally what we watch. We may notice that some people sit by themselves rather than join others, younger people sit at the back, some sit comfortably while others sit on the edge of their seat, and some people read while others meditate or talk to others. We will, in fact, have carried out 'unstructured' observations.

In unstructured observation, the researcher does not start with any predetermined categories, but instead constructs them while she observes or after all the observations have been made. Unstructured observations therefore adopt an inductive approach and are described as qualitative or naturalistic observations. They are appropriate in cases where little is known about the phenomenon. The knowledge gained can be used afterwards to construct categories for structured observations. In the above example, a researcher can thereafter try to see whether people on buses in fact behave as described above. To do this, she has to construct an observation schedule containing the various behaviours mentioned above and record their presence or absence and their frequency.

Unstructured observations are also undertaken when researchers believe a wholistic view of the phenomenon (that is, behaviour in context) can be obtained. Manias (2012) explains why she chose naturalistic observation in her study of pain assessment and management in hospitalised older people. As she explained:

The assumptions of the author of this paper are that nurses' and older patients' experiences in hospital are socially organised. As such it is important to examine how these experiences unfold in actual practice, and of how the broader social relations have shaped these experiences. Her [The researcher's] interest in the research topic extends beyond the symptom of pain experienced by older patients – it involves considering older patients' nuances of how pain affects them and the way they function, the underlying organisational and environmental context, and the competing responsibilities confronting nurses as they assess and manage pain in older patients.

In structured observations, the boundaries of what is to be observed are set prior to data collection. Observers are expected to collect only information required in the schedule or checklist. Each observation session lasts for about the same amount of time, and the researcher also carries out the same observation for each and every session.

Unstructured observations, however, are less standardised and more flexible. Each observation session is treated as a unique event, and no two sessions are considered to be the same. What is learnt in the first session can be built upon in the later sessions, as is the case with qualitative interviews. In everyday life, we learn by accumulating 'facts' that are confirmed or rejected as we come across the same event time and again. This 'cumulative' process of confirmation and validation is adopted by researchers as they move from one observation to the next. Barber-Parker (2002), in her study of patient teaching, used the data from the initial observations to generate questions that were explored in later observations.

The purpose of an unstructured observation is to arrive at as complete an understanding of the phenomenon as possible. For this to happen, researchers must be flexible enough to make the most of the observation situation and should not feel constrained to observe only the categories decided in advance. They must also be flexible in the duration of each observation session.

Unlike the case in structured observations, no specific research questions, objectives or hypotheses are set at the beginning of unstructured observations. Researchers decide during the observation what to focus on. The initial observations are usually 'unfocussed and general in scope', and later when observers become more familiar in the settings their attention may be more focused (Adler and Adler, 1994). According to Mulhall (2003), researchers 'may have some ideas as to what to observe', but these 'may change over time as they gather data and gain experience in the particular setting'.

When structured observations are conducted, researchers make recordings on the schedule or enter the data directly into a portable computer. These 'tools' are essential; without them no observation can take place, in the same way that one cannot conduct a survey without a questionnaire or a checklist. In unstructured observations, researchers take notes in a variety of ways. As explained before, in a qualitative study the researcher is herself a tool of data collection and analysis during the process of data collection. This is sometimes supplemented by note-taking in one form or other. These notes can range from scribbles to extensive descriptions and tape-recordings. Notes are usually taken as inconspicuously as possible so as not to disturb the normal flow of events. Barber-Parker (2002) describes how, in her study, only brief notes were taken in the presence of others, but 'planned time alone to create detailed notes, including quotes, context and personal thoughts' was incorporated. Whatever the practice adopted for taking notes, it should not interfere with the flow of the observation, inhibit participants in behaving in their normal ways or raise suspicions about the actions and motives of the observer.

The analysis of data collected by unstructured observations is similar to that for qualitative interviews. There are many examples in the literature of the analysis of unstructured observation data (see, for example, Barber-Parker, 2002; Skovdahl et al., 2003; Endacott et al., 2013; Manias et al., 2014). Barber-Parker (2002) gave a summary account of the process of data analysis in her study of patient teaching:

> Through repeated reading of the notes, the investigator identified the who, what, where, when, why and how of teaching activities. Incentives and barriers for patient teaching were searched for in the data and a third category emerged, that of facilitators for patient teaching. The critical attributes (items that appeared repetitively) of teaching activities were identified and the investigator created a precise operational definition of patient teaching for this setting. The entire analysis remained concrete and well grounded in the data.

If observations are carried out as part of an ethnographic or grounded theory study, the data are analysed using the framework of these approaches.

Observational data are not more 'factual' than other types of data (from interviews, questionnaires, documents or records). They are the interpretations of researchers, and as such must be treated with the same caution as other data. The problem of the observer's effect is also as real in unstructured as it is in structured observation. To offset this limitation, researchers have to use strategies to 'blend in' with the environment and reflect on the effect of their presence.

Validity and reliability of unstructured observations

By not seeing behaviours and activities through the lens of predetermined categories, it is possible to some extent to observe a phenomenon 'as it is'. The purpose of unstructured observations is to seek as many different ways in which the phenomenon manifests itself. As explained earlier, each observation builds on the previous one by providing data that contribute towards an in-depth understanding of the phenomenon.

The flexibility of unstructured observations allows the researcher to search for the 'truth' whenever she can find it. This means that she can observe for longer or shorter periods in some sessions if the data are considered valuable. Thus, the validity of unstructured observations is increased. The selectivity bias present in this type of observation is one of the main limitations. As explained earlier, there is little doubt that different researchers are likely to collect different data while observing the same phenomenon.

It is not possible for others to replicate unstructured observational studies. However, their data can be compared with those collected by different methods and in similar settings. The validity and reliability of unstructured observations will be further discussed in the next section.

So far, observation methods have been presented in the form of two ideal types: structured and unstructured. While this may be helpful for the purpose of teaching and learning, they do not adequately describe what happens in practice. Mulhall (2003), for example, emphasises that 'the label 'unstructured' is misleading'. As with unstructured interviews, unstructured observations are not totally without structure or focus. The process of unstructured observation, in any particular study, rarely remains the same. It is likely that observers, as they become interested in some ideas, events or issues, impose more structure on the observations than they do at the start of a study. Examples were given earlier of how researchers making 'structured' observations could not remain totally detached but were instead drawn into interaction by the participants.

Observations can also vary in terms of the degree of structure imposed by the researcher. This has led some researchers to label their observations as semi-structured (see, for example, Drach-Zahavy and Dagan, 2002; Kawai et al., 2010) in the same way that this label is applied to interviews. It is more helpful, as Turnock and Gibson (2001) suggest, 'to describe the role of the observer rather than struggle to identify the "correct" theoretical label'. According to them, readers can make their own judgement about the validity and reliability of the study if they are able 'to follow the decision making trail'. For an example of a study using unstructured observation, see Research Example 47.

Participation in observation

Observers can adopt a detached role or can participate fully in the activities that they observe. In between these two stances, there are a number of positions that observers can occupy. Gold (1958) suggested the following four roles: 'the complete participant, the participant-as-observer, the observer-as-participant and the complete observer'. Adler and Adler (1994) describe the complete observer role as:

> researchers who are fundamentally removed from their settings. Their observations may occur from the outside, with observers being neither seen nor noticed. Contemporary varieties of this role might include the videotaping, audiotaping, or photographing noninteractive observer. This role most closely approximates the traditional ideal of the 'objective' observer.

The complete participant role is described as one in which the researcher is one of the participants in the activities or events that are observed without, however, revealing that in fact she is also carrying out research observations while being part of the group. This covert role has serious ethical implications that will be discussed later. The rationale on which this covert, total participative role is based is that observers can never fully avoid the effect of their presence. They believe that, by revealing their role as researchers, they are not observing what would have normally happened if they had not been present, and thereby do not collect valid data.

The other two roles, participant-as-observer and observer-as-participant, are similar. The former reflects a more participative role, and the latter a more research role. Gold's classifications (which are four points on a continuum with complete participant at one end and complete observer at the other) are ideal types; in practice, these four roles may be more problematic than one might think. For example, although researchers may be overt about their role, how much they reveal can affect the data. Some observers ask permission to observe but do not reveal the exact nature of their study. Nurse researchers may also conceal the fact (or do not volunteer the information) that they are trained nurses. Making others aware that one is a researcher is not enough to remove the charge of 'covert' research.

Research example 47

Unstructured observations

Observation of pain assessment and management – the complexities of clinical practice *Manias et al. (2002)*

This observational study investigated 'nurse–patient interactions associated with pain assessment, and management' in a surgical unit. Twelve field observations were carried out by one non-participant observer. A portable audio-recorder was used to record all the observations 'and to allow for rapid descriptions of actions'. Nurses were also asked to clarify decisions and the context in which they were made. Four major themes were identified after the data had been transcribed and analysed.

Comments

1 Observation was selected as a method because of the authors' perceived limitations of self-reports (in interviews) as the latter may 'differ from what occurs in actual clinical practice'. They explained that 'observational studies may provide a more effective means of describing some of the complex issues that influence pain assessment and management'.

2 According to Manias et al. (2002), previous observation studies of pain in clinical settings 'focused on issues that were preconceived prior to data collection'. This study, using unstructured observations, allowed the themes to emerge out of the data. The observer did not use a predetermined and structured observational schedule to record what was happening.

3 Each observation period lasted 2 hours, and various observation times were selected to 'cover' the whole spectrum of activities that occurred over a 24-hour period.

4 All nurses in the unit and each patient involved in the observation 'were invited to consent to participate in the data collection process and to allow their medical records to be accessed for relevant demographic information'.

5 The authors concluded that the observational method was 'invaluable for exploring work demands in clinical areas, levels of accountability surrounding pain assessment and management, and the complexity of competing demands between nurses, doctors and patients'.

The nature of participation differs from observer to observer even when they adopt a participant-as-observer role. For example, a trained nurse's participation in this role will differ from that of a non-nurse. Her participation in nursing care and access to information would be different from that of, for example, a sociologist.

Participant observation is the choice method in ethnographic studies. To get a glimpse of people's feelings and behaviour, ethnographers not only have to be present where the action is, but also, as much as possible, have be part of their environment and become an insider. The purpose of participating is to try to see things from the subjects' point of view and to understand how (and why) they behave in their social and cultural groups. The participant observer aims to perceive and feel things in the same way as the participants do. See Chapter 14 for more explanation of participant observation in ethnography.

Ethical implications of observation

The ethical principles outlined in Chapter 6 are all relevant to observation as a research method. In this section, we will examine the specific ethical implications of conducting observations.

Research observation, whether overt or covert, is a visual intrusion into other people's privacy. Obtaining informed consent to enter the private world of others does not give researchers the right to treat the data as they wish. When informed consent is given, the observer has the duty to respect the privacy of the participants (including those who happen to walk in when the observations are in progress) and to keep the confidentiality of the information collected. Obtaining informed consent from everyone in the setting where the study is carried out can be problematic. Visitors and other professionals can drop in and out. It is not practical to inform each and every one of the purpose of the study and to seek informed consent from them.

Another issue is the right of participants to withdraw from the study. This may cause considerable inconvenience if participants, after seeing the tape-recording, decide they do not want the data to be used. The right of patients to withdraw should be respected even if it means that the study is not completed.

With all the best intention and goodwill, it is not always possible to maintain confidentiality. Reporting observation data carries some threats to anonymity and confidentiality. Since observation studies are usually carried out in one or two settings, it is sometimes possible for readers to identify the setting and some of the personalities in them. Researchers must continue to respect participants' rights and ensure that there is no breach of confidence even well after the data have been collected.

Compared with other methods of data collection, observational studies may create more dilemmas for researchers regarding whether or not they should intervene when patient safety is compromised. As a rule, participants' well-being and safety should take precedence over research objectives. However, deciding what constitutes 'threats' to participants' well-being and safety is not always as straightforward as it seems. There is also the question of whether to report malpractices and unsafe practices. This can lead to the investigation and suspension of the very people who granted access in the first place.

Covert observation brings with it particular ethical implications. Three main, not mutually exclusive, reasons are given to support this type of observation. First, some researchers believe that the only way to obtain valid data is not to let partici- pants know they are being observed. In this way, it is possible to observe things 'as they are' normally, unaffected by the observer's presence. Second, access to research sites may be denied by gatekeepers for various reasons. For example, the owners of a private nursing home may not want a researcher to 'pry' around. Third, there are those who believe that research is a political act and that the results benefit some people at the expense of others, especially the more deprived and vulnerable groups such as people with mental illness or a learning difficulty and older people in insti- tutions. Those who carry out covert research may believe that although the rights of some participants are infringed, the findings will benefit a larger number of people in similar situation as theirs.

Covert observations are often discussed in terms of 'either/or'. However, even when participants are made fully aware that they are being observed, it is impossible to give everyone concerned all the details of a project. Sometimes what researchers focus on in the later part of a project was not foreseen at the beginning of the project. There are also cases where a semi-covert approach is used. In a study by Turnock and Gibson (2001) on patient care in an intensive care setting, the authors 'employed a degree of cover by not informing staff about which particular aspects of their activity were being observed'. Therefore it is possible to be 'open' by inform- ing participants about the 'broad' focus and 'covert' by not revealing the 'specific' focus. Participants would have to be debriefed afterwards and given the right to withdraw. Researchers must balance 'harm' and 'benefits' when taking a decision to use a degree of concealment. Research ethics committees will consider the argu- ments and advise accordingly.

According to the British Sociological Association (2002), there are serious ethical issues in the use of covert research methods, although there may be situations when this 'may be justified', such as when access is denied by 'powerful and secretive interests'. The British Sociological Association also states that 'in such studies it is important to safeguard the anonymity of research participants'.

Researchers undertaking covert research may also experience a 'backlash' that could affect their career. For a fuller discussion of the practical, ethical and legal implications of covert research, see Johnson (1992), Clarke (1996), McKenzie (2009) and Petticrew et al. (2007).

Critiquing observation

To evaluate data from structured observations, readers need to know exactly what phenomenon was observed and how it was defined. Researchers must also provide adequate information on how the observations were carried out. This includes information relating to how the research tool was constructed and comments on its content validity. If an observation checklist is provided, you can attempt to assess its face validity. Researchers must also explain how intra- and inter-reliability were achieved, and what other steps were taken to ensure the validity and reliability of the instrument.

The context in which the observations are conducted and the strategies designed to reduce the observer effect need to be explained; the sampling of periods to be observed must be justified. For example, is 1 hour's observation every 4 hours appropriate for a study of ward teaching? If the observations take place at 9.00 am, 1.00 pm, 5.00 pm and 9.00 pm, it is likely that the last three sessions may not be appropriate as they could be the times that staff are at lunch, on a coffee break and handing over to the next shift, respectively.

The observer is also in a position to explain whether or not difficulties were experienced when observing certain behaviour or events. If this was the case, she must discuss how this might have affected the collection of valid and reliable data. For unstructured observations, researchers must provide information on the type of observation and their degree of involvement with the participants. The thought processes and the actions of the observer during the observation must be conveyed for readers to have an idea of what happened. Information on how the participants were recruited and the reasons for their selection, as well as a description of the setting, must also be provided. Finally, the measures taken to ensure rigour and respect for people's rights (which applies to structured observations as well) should be described in detail.

Summary

Observations provide useful information for clinical and research purposes. They are particularly suited to the study of verbal and non-verbal behaviour. They are used in qualitative and quantitative studies, and in both experimental and non-experimental designs. As a quantitative tool, observation can be structured, predetermined and standardised. Researchers know in advance the data required and use an observation schedule or checklist, constructed prior to the collection of data. Qualitative researchers prefer not to be influenced by prior knowledge and instead allow phenomena to unfold before their eyes. From the data collected, they aim to formulate themes, conceptual models, hypotheses and theories. The degree of researcher participation with the people, and in the setting where the observations take place, varies according to the aims of the study. Each type of observation has its value, limitations and ethical implications. As with other research methods, the challenge to researchers is to find ways to collect useful data without infringing people's rights.

References

Adler P A and Adler P (1994) Observational techniques. In: N K Denzin and Y S Lincoln (eds) *Handbook of Qualitative Research* (Newbury Park, CA: Sage).

Appleton J V, Harris M, Oates J and Kelly C (2013) Evaluating health visitor assessments of mother-infant interactions: a mixed methods study. *International Journal of Nursing Studies*, **50**:5–15.

Barber-Parker E D (2002) Integrating patient teaching into bedside patient care: a participant-observation study of hospital nurses. *Patient Education and Counselling*, **48**:107–13.

Bolster D and Manias E (2010) Person-centred interactions between nurses and patients during medication activities in an acute hospital setting: qualitative observation and interview study. *International Journal of Nursing Studies*, **47**, 2:154–65.

British Sociological Association (2002) Statement of ethical practice for the British Sociological Association. Retrieved from http://www.britsoc.co.uk/about/equality/statement-of-ethical-practice.aspx (accessed 5 September 2013).

Callen J, Hordern A, Gibson K, Li L, Hains I M and Westbrook J I (2013) Can technology change the work of nurses? Evaluation of a drug monitoring system for ambulatory chronic disease patients. *International Journal of Medical Informatics*, **82**, 3:159–67.

Clarke L (1996) Covert participant observation in a secure forensic unit. *Nursing Times*, **92**, 48:37–40.

Drach-Zahavy A and Dagan E (2002) From caring to managing and beyond: an examination of the head nurse's role. *Journal of Advanced Nursing*, **38**,1:19–28.

Endacott R, Sheaff R, Jones R and Woodward V (2013) Clinical focus and public accountability in English NHS Trust Board meetings. *Journal of Health Services Research and Policy*, **18**, 1:13–20.

Fader M, Clarke-O'Neill S, Cook D et al. (2003) Management of night-time urinary incontinence in residential settings for older people: an investigation into the effects of different pad changing regimes on skin health. *Journal of Clinical Nursing*, **12**:374–86.

Fuller B F and Conner D A (1995) The effect of pain on infant behaviors. *Clinical Nursing Research*, **4**, 3:253–73.

Gold R L (1958) Roles in sociological field observations. *Social Forces*, **36**:217–23.

Johnson M (1992) A silent conspiracy? Some ethical issues of participant observation in nursing research. *International Journal of Nursing Studies*, **29**, 2:213–23.

Kawai M, Namba K, Yato Y, Negayama K, Sogon S and Yamamoto H (2010) Developmental trends in mother-infant interaction from 4-months to 42-months: using an observation technique. *Journal of Epidemiology*, **20**, Suppl. 2:S427–34.

Kirk J and Miller M L (1986) *Reliability and Validity in Qualitative Research* (Newbury Park, CA: Sage).

Latvala E, Vuokila-Oikkonen P and Janhonen S (2000) Videotaped recording as a method of participant observation in psychiatric nursing research. *Journal of Advanced Nursing*, **31**, 5:1252–7.

Lobo M L (1992) Observation: a valuable data collection strategy for research with children. *Journal of Paediatric Nursing*, **7**, 5:320–8.

Manias E (2012) Complexities of pain assessment and management in hospitalised older people: a qualitative observation and interview study. *International Journal of Nursing Studies*, **49**, 10:1243–54.

Manias E, Botti M and Bucknall T (2002) Observation of pain assessment and management – the complexities of clinical practice. *Journal of Clinical Nursing*, **11**:724–33.

Manias E, Kinney S, Cranswick N and Williams A (2014) Medication errors in hospitalised children. *Journal of Paediatrics and Child Health*, **50**:71–7.

Martin A-M, O'Connor-Fenelon M and Lyons R (2010) Non-verbal communication between nurses and people with an intellectual disability: a review of the literature. *Journal of Intellectual Disabilities*, **14**, 4: 303–14.

McKenzie J S (2009) 'You don't know how lucky you are to be here!': reflections on covert practices in an overt participant observation study. *Sociological Research Online*, **14**, 2:1–12.

Mulhall A (2003) In the field: notes on observation in qualitative research. *Journal of Advanced Nursing*, **41**, 3:306–13.

Nilsen M L, Sereika S and Happ M B (2013) Nurse and patient characteristics associated with duration of nurse talk during patient encounters in ICU. *Heart Lung*, **42**, 1:5–12.

Peplau H E (1988) *Interpersonal Relations in Nursing*, 2nd edn (London: Macmillan Education).

Petticrew M, Semple S, Hilton S et al. (2007) Covert observation in practice: lessons from the evaluation of the prohibition of smoking in public places in Scotland. *BMC Public Health*, **7**:204.

Qian S-Y, Yu P, Zhang Z-Y, Hailey D M, Davy P J and Nelson M I (2012) The work pattern of personal care workers in two Australian nursing homes: a time-motion study. *BMC Health Services Research*, **12**:305.

Roberts L and Bucksey S J (2007) Communicating with patients: what happens in practice? *Physical Therapy*, **87**:586–94.

Roethlisberger F J and Dickson W J (1939) *Management and the Worker* (Cambridge, MA: Harvard University Press).

Simmons S F, Durkin D W, Rahman A N, Choi L, Beuscher L and Schnelle J F (2013) Resident characteristics related to the lack of morning care provision in long-term care. *Gerontologist*, **53**, 1:151–61.

Skovdahl K, Kihlgren A L and Kihlgren M (2003) Dementia and aggressiveness: video recording morning care from different care units. *Journal of Clinical Nursing*, **12**:888–98.

Turnock G and Gibson V (2001) Validity in action research: a discussion on theoretical and practice issues encountered whilst using observation to collect data. *Journal of Advanced Nursing*, **36**, 3:471–7.

Waltz C, Strickland O L and Lenz E (2010) *Measurement in Nursing and Health Research*, 4th edn (New York: Springer).

19

Making Sense of Data

Opening thought ▶ Statistics are no substitute for judgement.

Henry Clay

Introduction

Collecting data is a crucial part of the research process, but data in themselves do not answer research questions or support or reject hypotheses. Researchers have to make sense of them before presenting them to readers in ways that they, in turn, can understand. In this chapter, some of the common methods of data analysis and presentation in quantitative and qualitative studies are examined. A brief outline of some of the descriptive and inferential statistics in quantitative analysis is given. Finally, some of the ways in which researchers make sense of, and report, qualitative data are described.

What does making sense of data mean?

In Chapter 2, it was explained that data means all the information collected during the process of research for the purpose of answering questions, testing hypotheses or exploring a phenomenon. In the course of a study, a large amount of data are collected. All the individual bits of information from questionnaires, interviews or observations are known as 'raw' or 'crude' data. In themselves, crude data do not immediately make sense. The answers to research questions do not 'jump out' of the pile of questionnaires; they have to be 'teased out' or analysed, a process called data analysis.

The analysis of data in quantitative studies tends to take place after all the data have been collected. However, it is not an afterthought but an integrated part of the research design. The level of research (descriptive, correlational or experimental), the research questions, objectives or hypotheses and the type of data collected determine which type of analysis is required. Those who have left decisions about data analysis to the end phase of a research project have learnt that this can be a serious mistake.

In qualitative research, data analysis begins during the data collection phase. The researcher processes the information, looks for patterns during the interview or observation and selects themes to pursue. Data analysis continues between interviews and after all the data have been collected. In the first part of this chapter, we will focus mainly on data analysis in quantitative studies.

Quantitative data analysis

In Chapter 3, it was explained that the purpose of quantitative research is to measure phenomena. Some of these can be measured more accurately and easily than others. For example, we can measure participants' weight with more precision than we can measure their satisfaction with nursing care. For measurement to take place, there must be numbers. Some measures are already in the form of numbers. For example, weight is expressed in grams and height in centimetres. Others have to be converted into numbers if they are to be analysed quantitatively. For example, if public health nurses are asked to rate the degree of importance of research to their practice according to whether this is 'high', 'moderate' or 'low', these categories would be allocated numbers to reflect their order of importance.

Quantitative analysis can only be carried out with numbers, but in some cases numbers have no intrinsic worth: they have to be given meaning by those using them. For example, number 1 can mean 'first' or 'most important' or it can be the lowest value on a scale of 1 to 10. To make sense of numbers, they are given a value, usually according to a scale. For example, when respondents are asked to rate, in order of importance, their sources of health information on a scale of 1 to 10, the researcher must specify whether 1 is the most important or the least important.

Levels of measurement

To measure, one needs a scale. As explained earlier, not all phenomena are readily amenable to measurement, nor can they all be measured with the same degree of precision. The scales devised to measure them also differ in their degree of precision. Mathematicians have classified scales into a hierarchy of four levels. The lowest is nominal, followed by the ordinal, interval and ratio.

Nominal scale

Some of the variables with which quantitative researchers deal cannot in themselves be measured, although some aspects of them can. For example, being male cannot be measured against being female, although their weight, height and attitudes can be measured and compared. In the same way, when a researcher asks respondents to state their professional qualifications, she cannot measure and compare adult nursing with mental health nursing; for example, it would be arbitrary and controversial to assign more value to one qualification than to the other.

However, these variables (gender or qualifications) are given a number for the purpose of quantitative analysis. When researchers code their questionnaires for manual or computer analysis, they may assign numbers as follows:

Adult nursing	1
Mental health nursing	2
Care of people with a learning disability	3
Children's nursing	4

Although the scale is numbered 1 to 4, the numbers in this case have no value: 4 does not mean twice as good or as many as 2. It is simply a way of labelling or coding the variable 'nursing specialty'. This type of scale is known as 'nominal'. The *Oxford Dictionary* describes 'nominal' as 'existing in name only, not real or actual'. The numbers on a nominal scale are therefore in name only and do not have any real worth or value: they serve only to distinguish one category from another.

Ordinal scale

Sometimes respondents are asked to state whether or not they are satisfied with the care or treatment they receive, using a scale similar to the one below:

Very satisfied
Satisfied
Neither satisfied nor dissatisfied
Dissatisfied
Very dissatisfied

The ranking of these categories from 'very satisfied' to 'very dissatisfied' implies a hierarchy or ordering of satisfaction. In coding responses from this type of question, the researcher may allocate numbers as follows:

Very satisfied	5
Satisfied	4
Neither satisfied nor dissatisfied	3
Dissatisfied	2
Very dissatisfied	1

While those responses allocated a number of 5 denote a higher satisfaction than those with a 4, there is no equal distance implied between the numbers. Those who are satisfied (4) are not twice as satisfied as those who are dissatisfied (2), only more satisfied. The ordinal scale is different from a nominal scale in that the numbers signify the order or hierarchy of these variables. The higher numbers indicate that the respondents have more of the property (in this case, satisfaction) than do the lower numbers, but the scale cannot specify by how much.

Interval scale

An interval scale is a more precise ordinal scale. In it, the distances between the numbers on the scale are known. A thermometer is an example of an interval scale; the degrees are numbered in such a way that the distance between 5 degrees and 10 degrees is the same as between 75 degrees and 80 degrees. In this example, the centigrade or Fahrenheit thermometers have no absolute zero, since there are degrees below zero. Zero degrees centigrade does not mean 'nil' temperature. Twenty degrees is warmer than 10 degrees, but it does not mean that it is twice as warm: it means that it is 10 degrees warmer.

Ratio scale

A ratio scale is an interval scale with an absolute zero. For example, rulers and weighing scales have an absolute zero. A zero on a ruler means no length and 20 cm is twice as long as 10 cm. Therefore, the numbers on a ratio scale tell us not only the amount by which they differ (that is, by 10 cm) but also by how many times (twice as long or four times as heavy).

The distinction between these four levels is usually made because there is a view that 'the level of measurement specifies the type of statistical operations that can be properly used' (Waltz et al., 2010). The choice of statistical techniques should also relate to the research question asked. We will pursue this theme later in this chapter.

To sum up, the purpose of quantitative research is to measure, and measurements are carried out by scales consisting of numbers. There are different levels of measurement and different levels of scale. The meaning of the numbers differs from scale to scale: numbers can be used as labels, as indicating order or rank, or can have values.

Statistical levels

How data are analysed and presented depends on the types of question that the researchers ask. In Chapter 10, three levels of quantitative research were identified – descriptive, correlational and experimental. The types of question that can be asked depend on these levels.

There are two types of descriptive question that are usually asked. The first refers to the sample, especially its demographic characteristics (for example, how many respondents are there in the sample?, what is their age and gender distribution?). The second type refers to their responses (for example, how many respondents indicated a preference for primary nursing rather than team nursing?, what were the scores of respondents on the 'assessment of pain scale'?).

At the correlational level, researchers are mainly interested in finding answers to two types of question: whether there is a relationship between variables (for example, between educational background and compliance with treatment) and whether there are differences between groups (for example, whether there is a difference between male and female nurses' attitudes to nursing research).

At the experimental level, the main question asked is whether changes in one or more independent variables actually cause changes in one or more dependent variables (for example, does an educational programme cause an increase in patients' knowledge of diabetes?).

Descriptive statistical analysis is carried out to answer descriptive questions, while correlational and causal relationships are explored by the use of inferential statistics.

Descriptive statistics

Statistics has a language and logic of its own. If you were asked to describe a car to someone who has not seen it, you could convey a picture of it by referring to its colour, size, make, engine capacity, age and number of doors. These main features are essential to adequately describe the car. Similarly, when researchers describe data, they normally report the main features, which can give an idea of what the data consist of without the need to see the crude data.

To describe quantitative data, researchers use terminologies for which there are agreed meanings. Some layman's terms, such as 'average' or 'majority', are vague and may not have the same meaning for everyone. Statisticians have devised terms that describe the essential features of data, and have explained precisely what they mean. The three main features that researchers use to describe and summarise data are:

- frequency
- central tendency
- dispersion.

Frequency

The most basic analysis of quantitative data involves counting the number of times a value appears in the data. Samples are described in terms of frequency. For example, in a study of 'Smoking initiation and personal characteristics of secondary students in Hong Kong', Tang and Loke (2013) reported that:

> There were 361 (56.1%) male and 283 (43.9%) female secondary students. A total of 125 (19.4%) reported that they had tried smoking, and 25 (3.9%) reported that they were regular smokers.

This extract shows that frequency can be reported in terms of both percentages and absolute numbers.

It is sometimes difficult to compare absolute numbers. If 20 out of 60 male students and 12 out of 48 female students prefer lectures to seminars, the difference between these numbers is not immediately obvious since the sizes of the groups they belong to are not similar. When converted to proportions or percentages, however, they can make more sense. A proportion is calculated by dividing the number of units (people, events, and so on) within the larger group that has a particular characteristic by the total number of units. In the above example, the number of male students who prefer lectures (the number of units within the larger group) is 20. The total population of the male group (the larger group) is 60. The proportion of male student nurses who prefer lectures is therefore:

$$\frac{20 \text{ (number who prefer lectures to seminars)}}{60 \text{ (total number of units)}} = \frac{1}{3}$$

and for female students

$$\frac{12}{48} = \frac{1}{4}$$

Thus, by converting these numbers into proportions, it is possible to see that proportionately more male than female students prefer lectures.

Percentages also facilitate comparisons. A percentage is a proportion multiplied by 100. In the above example, the percentage of male students is:

$\frac{1}{3} \times 100 = 33.3$ per cent

Frequencies are commonly reported in the form of tables, bar charts and pie charts. An example of data reported in tabular form (Table 19.1) comes from a study by Ussher et al. (2013), entitled 'Information needs associated with changes to sexual wellbeing after breast cancer'. In this table, the authors give a frequency distribution of responses in absolute numbers and in percentages.

Tables facilitate the presentation of large amounts of data in a concise way. To report the data from the above table in the text would require many sentences, which would have to be read a number of times to be fully comprehensible and digestible. A quick glance at Table 19.1 not only gives the frequency of the different responses, but also enables instant comparisons between items in the health index.

Diagrammatic presentations of data are designed to attract the readers' attention and give a sense of proportion; this is important if the purpose is to compare data. A bar chart is one type of diagram used for this purpose. An example of a bar chart (Fig. 19.1) comes from a study by Röndahl et al. (2004) on nurses' attitudes towards lesbians and gay men. The bar chart shows the number of nurses who held negative, neutral or positive attitudes. At a glance, it is possible to clearly see that most nurses in this study held positive attitudes towards lesbians and gay men. The sense of proportion is conveyed graphically by the relative height of the bars. Some bar charts can have multiple bars, and they can be presented sideways as well.

Pie charts, although less popular and less versatile than bar charts, are also used to convey the sense of proportion in data. Unlike bar charts, the numbers must be converted into proportions or percentages before the pie chart can be constructed, although absolute numbers can additionally be included. An example of a pie chart (Fig. 19.2) is taken from a study by Gudmundsdottir et al. (2004). The segments show the number and proportion of respondents in each nursing specialty.

Table 19.1 Satisfaction with information obtained about sexual well-being (N = 790)

Information content	Obtained information, % (N)	Satisfied (%)	Neither (%)	Not satisfied (%)
Effects of cancer treatments on sexual well-being	59.4 (470)	52.4	28.7	12.4
Changes to my body	56.5 (447)	56.5	26.4	8.5
Breast reconstruction	45.9 (363)	61.0	18.9	9.6
Body image and appearance	38.3 (303)	51.4	31.8	9.8
Sexual functioning	34.5 (273)	50.0	33.3	10.1
Information about partners	25.8 (204)	55.2	27.8	7.5
Where to go for support	20.7 (164)	53.7	22.9	14.9
Relationship communication	19.6 (155)	48.9	29.8	11.2
How to talk about sex and intimacy	19.5 (154)	47.4	30.4	12.4
Fertility	11.4 (90)	53.2	23.4	15.3
Sex aids and products	10.2 (81)	44.4	35.2	12.0
Contraception	7.7 (61)	52.4	28.0	12.2
Sexual well-being for same sex couples	2.7 (21)	33.3	38.1	28.6

Source: Ussher et al. (2013, p. 331). Reproduced with kind permission from John Wiley and Sons Ltd.

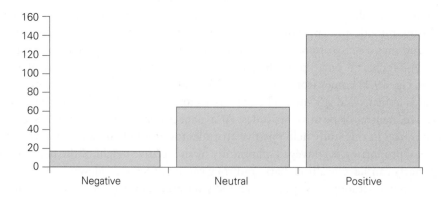

Figure 19.1 Categorisation of scores on the Attitudes towards Homosexuality Scale
Source: Röndahl et al. (2004). Reproduced with kind permission from John Wiley and Sons Ltd.

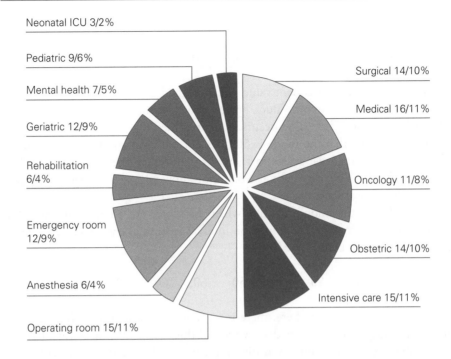

Figure 19.2   Number and proportion of respondents by nursing specialty (*n* = 140)

Source: Gudmundsdottir et al. (2004). Reproduced with kind permission from John Wiley and Sons Ltd.

Bar charts and pie charts have an advantage over textual reporting in that they can present large amounts of data in a concise and visual form. They must, however, be clearly labelled and, where appropriate, properly shaded, as shading often fades in the process of photocopying. Tables, bar charts and pie charts must not be overloaded with data and should require little effort on the part of readers to understand them.

Central tendency

To make sense of information, we use such concepts as 'average', 'typical' or 'common'. We may ask, 'How many people, on average, are admitted to the accident and emergency department of the local hospital on a Saturday night' or 'What is the "typical" injury or illness with which they attend the accident and emergency department?' In effect, in statistical terms, we are looking for the central tendency rather than for extreme cases. The statistical measures of central tendency are the mode, median and mean. To explain these terms, we will use Example A.

Suppose 10 patients on a medical ward were administered a 'satisfaction with nursing care scale' and the scores (from 0 to a possible 100) for each patient (represented here by the letters A to J) were as follows:

Example A

A	B	C	D	E	F	G	H	I	J
50	40	60	50	70	40	20	50	90	60

The *mode* is the most frequent value. It can be used on any scale of measurement and is unaffected by extreme values. In the above example, the value '50' occurs three times and no other value occurs as many times. Therefore the mode is 50. However, knowing that the mode is 50 does not tell us anything about the other scores (if we did not have access to them, as is normally the case). The mode is therefore of little value, especially if we do not know what percentage of respondents had this typical score.

The *median* is the midpoint value when the scores are arranged in ascending order, as shown below. It can be used on interval or ordinal level data and, like the mode, is unaffected by extreme values.

20	40	40	50	50	50	60	60	70	90

Since there are 10 scores here, there is no one single midpoint. The average of the two middle values is the median, which in this case is 50 (this is calculated by adding the two middle values and dividing the total by 2). Fifty per cent of the values fall below and 50 per cent above the midpoint. By knowing that the median is 50, we also know that half of the respondents scored below, and half above, 50.

The *mean* is the arithmetic average of a set of values and can be used on interval or ratio-level data. It is calculated by adding all the scores and dividing by the number of responses. The total score in the above example is 530 and the number of responses is 10. Therefore the mean is:

$$\frac{530}{10} = 53$$

Unlike the mode and the median, the mean is actually determined by a calculation that takes into account all the other scores and can thus be distorted by a single extreme score in one direction. If one score is greatly increased or reduced, it may not affect the mode or median, but it will change the mean. For example, if the score of patient 'J' were 90 instead of 60, the mode and the median would remain 50 while the mean would increase to 56.

The limitations of the mode, median and mean can be demonstrated by Example B, showing the satisfaction scores of the same 10 patients:

Example B

A	B	C	D	E	F	G	H	I	J
20	30	20	30	40	70	90	90	90	90

The mode is 90
The median is (40 + 70)/2 = 55
The mean is 570/10 = 57

The mode in this case gives the impression that patients scored very high, yet only 40 per cent did. The median indicates that five patients scored less than 55, but it fails to show that some patients scored very low and others very high. The mean of 57 is deceptive as it suggests that the level of satisfaction of these 10 patients is medium (57), yet as the crude scores show, none of them had medium-level satisfaction.

What these measures of central tendency do not tell us is how the scores vary. In Example A, the scores bunched around 50 (with only two extreme scores – 20 and 90) and the mean was 53. In Example B, there were four very low and four very high scores, and the mean was 57. We may conclude that the patients in Example B were more satisfied with the care they received (mean 57) than the patients in Example A (mean 53), yet only one patient scored below 40 in Example A, while four patients in Example B did.

Dispersion

Central tendency measures are, therefore, not enough to make sense of the data. We need to know the variance of the scores (that is, how they vary). The three measures which can describe variance are the:

- range
- interquartile range
- standard deviation.

The *range* is the easiest way to measure the variation in a set of data. This is simply the difference between the highest and lowest values in a data set. In Example B, the range would be:

90 – 20 = 70

The problem with using the range is that it uses only two values in the dataset and ignores all other scores in the distribution. Thus, it can be easily affected by extreme scores and is considered to be an unreliable measure of variability.

The *interquartile range* gives a better description of variation in the data. If you recall, the median is the score that divides a distribution exactly in half. Using the same technique, scores in a distribution can be divided into four equal parts using quartiles. The first or lower quartile (Q1) is the midpoint between the lowest value and the median (second quartile, Q2), and the upper quartile (third quartile, Q3) is the midpoint between the highest value and the median. We can refer to Example A to show the lower and upper quartiles. The scores (arranged in ascending order) of the ten patients were as follows.

		Q1		median (Q2)			Q3		
		↓		↓			↓		
G	B	F	A	D	H	C	J	E	I
20	40	40	50	50	50	60	60	70	90

The median is 50. This was obtained by arranging the scores in ascending order and selecting the midpoint score. As the number of values is even (10), there are two midpoint scores: 50 and 50. The median lies between them, as shown above.

The lower quartile (Q1) is calculated by finding the midpoint of the scores below the median. There are five scores and the midpoint is 40. Similarly, the upper quartile (Q3) is the midpoint of the five scores above the median, in this case 60.

The interquartile range is the distance between the first quartile and the third quartile. In the above example the interquartile range is 20.

$$Q3 - Q1 = 60 - 40 = 20$$

The semi-interquartile range is half the difference between the upper and lower quartiles. It provides a descriptive measure of the 'typical' distance of scores from the median.

$$\text{Semi-interquartile range} = \frac{Q3 - Q1}{2} = \frac{60 - 40}{2} = 10$$

The measure most widely used for describing the spread of a distribution is the *standard deviation* (SD). The SD is a 'kind of average deviation of the observations from the mean' (Moore, 1985) and takes into account all values in the distribution. The SD is always reported in conjunction with the mean.

If the scores are homogenous, there is little or no deviation from the mean, and therefore the SD is zero or close to zero. The larger the SD, the more the scores deviate from the mean. This deviation from the mean can be positive or negative. If the mean of 19 scores is 65 and the SD is 1.75, this means that the scores are closely bunched around 65. If, on the other hand, the mean is 65 and the SD is 30.5, many of the individual scores are far from the mean. In general, almost 70 per cent of all scores in a distribution fall within 1 SD of the mean.

Frequency, central tendency and dispersion are the main measures of descriptive statistics. Together, they can convey the main features of the data, although the most commonly reported ones are frequency, mean and SD.

Finally, the term 'normal distribution' needs to be explained. In a normal distribution, most of the scores cluster around the mean, and the extreme scores are few and are more or less equally distributed above and below the mean. This is illustrated in Fig. 19.3 and is referred to as a 'bell-shape' distribution. A normal distribution has the following characteristics: 34 per cent of all scores fall between the mean and 1 SD on either side of the mean; similarly, 28 per cent of all scores fall between 1 SD and 2 SD from the mean, as in Fig. 19.3.

The 'normal distribution' is crucial in statistics because many statistical techniques were developed on the assumption that scores were bell-shaped or normal. As explained later on, some statistical tests can only be performed if the distribution is normal, although techniques may generally be applied to data that are only roughly bell-shaped without losing too much accuracy.

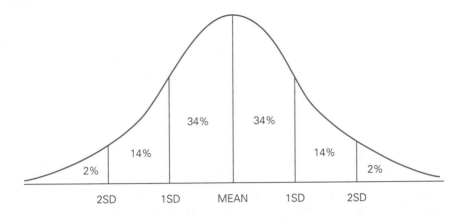

Figure 19.3   A normal distribution curve

Inferential statistics

Researchers using quantitative approaches such as surveys and experiments seek to find relationships between variables and, where possible, to establish the exact nature of these relationships, with the aim of making predictions. They also seek to generalise the findings from their samples to equivalent populations. To do so, they resort to inferential statistics.

To find out whether there are relationships between variables, researchers formulate hypotheses. A null hypothesis (H0) states that there is no actual relationship between variables, whereas a research (or alternative) hypothesis (H1) predicts some relationship between the variables. Data are collected to accept or reject the null or alternative hypothesis.

Errors are sometimes made in the testing of hypotheses, and two possibilities are presented here. A type I error happens when a statistically significant relationship is reported, in the study sample, between two variables (for example, educational attainment and the practice of breast self-examination) when, in fact, no such relationship exists in the population. A type I error can result in the researchers making a false report of a treatment effect. A type II error occurs when no such relationship is found in the sample when, in fact, it exists in the population. In this case, the researcher could conclude that a treatment had no effect when in fact it did (Fig. 19.4).

		Actual situation	
		No effect H0 true	Effect exists H0 false
Researcher's decision	Reject H0	Type I error	Decision correct
	Retain H0	Decision correct	Type II error

Figure 19.4   Testing of hypotheses

To establish statistical significance, researchers can select from a number of tests, some of which will be described later. The results from these tests will signify whether or not there are relationships between variables. However, there is always a probability that the results were obtained by chance. You have perhaps seen the following:

$p > 0.05$

The symbol > denotes 'greater than' and the letter 'p' is used to denote the probability of a chance occurrence. The figures and decimal points (for example, 0.05) are the levels set by researchers above which they will accept the null hypothesis and conclude that there is no relationship between the variables. Researchers can use several levels of probability, but 0.05 is a standard level, above which no researcher should claim significance for the result.

Selecting a test

The choice of statistical tests depends on, among other things, sample size and sampling method (that is, random or not), on the level of measurement (nominal, ordinal and so on) and on whether the variables to be measured in the sample are normally distributed in the population. For parametric tests, the variable has to be normally distributed, while for non-parametric tests no such assumption is made. Munro et al. (1986) explain:

> The main difference between these two classes of techniques is the assumptions about the population data that must be made before the parametric tests can be applied. For t-tests and analysis of variance (ANOVA), for example, it is assumed that the variable under study is normally distributed in the population and that the variance is the same at different levels of the variable. The nonparametric techniques have relatively few assumptions that must be met before they can be used.

In this section, we will take a brief look at some of the commonly used tests in nursing research, namely the Pearson product moment correlation coefficient, t-test and chi-square (or chi-squared) test.

The Pearson product moment correlation coefficient

The Pearson product moment correlation coefficient is the 'most usual method by which the relationship between two variables is quantified' (Munro et al., 1986) and relates to parametric data. Correlation coefficients (represented by the letter r) can be positive or negative. They vary between +1 (a perfect positive relationship) and −1 (a perfect negative or inverse relationship). Published statistical tables can be used to interpret the significance of the correlation coefficient, but Fink (1995) suggests the following interpretation:

0 to +0.25 (or −0.25) = little or no relationship
+0.26 to +0.50 (or −0.26 to −0.50) = a fair degree of relationship
+0.51 to +0.75 (or −0.51 to −0.75) = a moderate to good relationship
over +0.75 (or −0.75) = a very good to excellent relationship.

An example of the use of Pearson' correlation comes from a study, comparing two scales for measuring nursing workload, by Carmona-Monge et al. (2013). As the authors explain:

> In order to analyse the existing relationship between both scales, Pearson's correlation was calculated for the individual measurements obtained through the NAS [Nursing Activities Score] and NEMS [Nine Equivalents of Nursing Manpower Use] scales (r=.672; R 2 =.452), as well as for the daily workload measured in the unit through the NAS and NEMS (r=.932; R 2 =.868), both of which were statistically significant (p<.001).

The *t*-test

The *t*-test is a parametric test to compare the means of two samples, for example the mean knowledge scores of one group of patients who were given verbal information about their illness compared with that of another group who were given written information.

According to DePoy and Gitlin (1994), the '*t*-test must be calculated with interval level data and should be selected only if the researcher believes that the assumptions for the use of parametric statistics have not been violated'. As they explain: 'The *t*-test yields a *t* value that is reported as $t = \times$, $p = 0.05$ where $\times$ is the calculated *t* value and *p* is the level of significance set by the researcher. There are several variations of the *t*-test.'

To find whether a *t* value is statistically significant, it has to be compared with the critical value of *t* reported in statistical tables. This critical value is the level the *t* value must equal or exceed to be deemed statistically significant. Tables of critical values are readily available, but we assume that most researchers will now be using appropriate computer software to calculate statistical values and tell you if they are statistically significant. The level of the critical value is determined by the significance level set by the researcher and the degrees of freedom (df). Both of these values need to be known and are always reported alongside the *t* value. It is beyond the scope of this book to explain what degrees of freedom are. What is important to know is how they are calculated and how to use them. The df in a *t*-test for independent groups is calculated by summating the number of subjects in each group together and subtracting two.

An example of the use of a *t*-test is from a study by Reyes et al. (2013) comparing 'beginning and graduating nursing students' cultural competence'. They reported that 'Independent t-test findings demonstrated that perceptions of cultural diversity were significantly higher in the graduating nursing student group as compared with beginning nursing students (t=−3.233, df=97, p=.002)'.

The chi-square test for independence

The chi-square test for independence (χ^2) can be used to test whether or not there is a relationship between two variables and is normally used with non-parametric data. For example, 100 smokers attended anti-smoking sessions and only 60 stopped smoking after a month, while in another group of 80 smokers who received no sessions, 20 stopped smoking (Table 19.2) The χ^2 statistic is used to test if the differences are statistically significant (that is, whether attendance at an anti-smoking session enabled more people to stop smoking). The χ^2 statistic for the example in Table 19.2 is calculated (by computer software) to be 20.52.

The df is calculated by subtracting 1 from the number of rows and multiplying this by the number of columns minus 1. This can be expressed as:

$$(R - 1) \times (C - 1)$$

where R = rows and C = columns.

In the example in Table 19.2, there are two columns and two rows. Therefore df is $(2 - 1) \times (2 - 1) = 1$. Once the df value and the p value (a level set by the researcher) are known, it is possible to compare the calculated χ^2 value with the critical value of χ^2 from the appropriate statistical table. The calculated χ^2 value must equal or exceed the critical value to be deemed statistically significant.

Table 19.2   Effect of anti-smoking sessions

	Stopped smoking	Did not stop	Total
Number attending a session	60	40	100
Number not attending a session	20	60	80
Total	80	100	180

McCleary and Brown (2003) used the χ^2 test in their study investigating barriers to paediatric nurses' research utilisation. They reported:

> while just under half of the paediatric nurses reported that their feeling incapable of evaluating the quality of the research was a barrier (47.8%), they were less likely to report this barrier than nurses in the US sample (69.9%, $\chi^2 = 21.9$, d.f. 1, $p < 0.001$) or the UK sample (59.3%, $\chi^2 = 7.4$, d.f. 1, $p < 0.01$).

For the above example, McCleary and Brown (2003) reported their results to be statistically significant because the values of their χ^2 statistics were greater than the critical values of χ^2 using the appropriate df and probability level.

It is beyond the scope of this book to explain how these tests are carried out or to discuss other tests. If you are in doubt about statistical data, you should consult a statistician or a statistics text. Useful references include:

- Scott and Mazhindu (2005) *Statistics for Health Care Professionals.*
- McCrum-Gardner (2008) 'Which is the correct statistical test to use?'
- Plichta and Garzon (2009) *Statistics for Nursing and Allied Health.*
- Waltz et al. (2010) *Measurement in Nursing Research and Health Research.*

Qualitative data analysis

Quantitative research is described as objective partly because it is believed that the research process, including data analysis, can be replicated. If the crude data are made available to other researchers, it is possible for them to carry out the same statistical tests and obtain the same results. It is also possible to carry out other tests or challenge the original tests. Qualitative data analysis is to some extent subjective, although researchers have developed strategies to allow others to follow and validate their actions. Different researchers analysing the same sets of data may not produce the same findings.

In quantitative research, data analysis starts once all the data have been collected. In qualitative research, data analysis takes place during data collection and thereafter. The researcher processes the data as they are received and makes judgements relating to aspects of the phenomenon to pursue. For example, as she carries out more and more interviews, she has to remember some of what was said in previous interviews. She analyses and synthesises the information while talking to the respondents. However, once all the data have been collected, she will systematically analyse the data in order to make sense of what participants said or what she observed. Therefore one of the main features of qualitative data analysis is that data collection and analysis are carried out both concurrently and after data collection has been completed.

Textual data analysis

Qualitative researchers record their data in a number of ways. The term 'field notes' is frequently used to refer to data kept by researchers prior to, during and after their interaction with their participants. Audiotape-recordings are commonly used to record the interviews 'verbatim' (word by word). These are normally transcribed and analysed thereafter. Other methods of data recording include memos, videos and diaries in which researchers (and sometimes participants) keep notes of their thoughts, their ideas, the chronology of events, patterns or trends. Field notes, transcripts, memos, diaries, letters, leaflets and case notes all constitute the 'texts' that qualitative researchers analyse.

Types of data analysis

There are different types of data analysis in qualitative research depending on how structured the questions are. Different approaches are used for the analysis of data from open-ended questions (in questionnaires), semi-structured interviews, documents and unstructured interviews or observations.

Open-ended questions can be specific or broad. An example of a specific, open-ended item from a questionnaire is: 'Please list the sources of information that you access regarding sexual health'. A researcher analysing the data will list as many sources as provided by respondents and their frequency of access. This is no different from quantitative analysis. In fact, it is likely that researchers will seek to find correlations between 'sources of information' and other demographic variables such as education or gender. A broad open-ended item could be: 'Briefly explain how you felt when you were told of the diagnosis'. The responses are likely to be in the form of a description of the respondent's feelings, experiences and whatever they think they should tell the researcher. In this case, researchers will have to sort, decipher and interpret the responses. Therefore the broader the question, the more complex the data analysis is. The same applies to the analysis of data from semi-structured interviews. The questions guide the search for answers.

Any text can be subjected to quantitative or qualitative analysis or a mixture of the two. An example of the quantitative analysis of qualitative data comes from Klapowitz (2000). He carried out a study to test the null hypothesis that participants in focus groups raise sensitive issues as frequently as those in individual interviews. Klapowitz compared data from 12 focus groups and 19 individual interviews. The study investigated participants' use, understanding and perceptions of their 'shared mangrove ecosystem'. 'Sensitive issues' were defined as 'mention' of relevant 'conflicts' or 'complaints'. He then counted the number of times that conflicts and complaints were mentioned. Using a chi-square test, he concluded that individual interviews were 'more likely to raise socially sensitive discussion topics than focus groups'. This study demonstrates the use of numbers and frequencies in qualitative research. The quantitative treatment of qualitative data, and vice versa, demonstrates the value of going beyond the quantitative–qualitative divide in pursuit of answers to our research questions.

The qualitative analysis of data from unstructured interviews and observations is a process that is rarely described in detail. It is a lonely journey that many researchers undertake and for which, often, they receive little training. There are a number of textbooks (see, for example, Gibbs, 2002; Miles et al., 2013) that have taken up the challenge of preparing researchers for this task. Although each textbook or guideline has its own number of steps or procedures that researchers can follow, the purpose of analysing qualitative data is the same. Researchers have to 'unravel' and make sense of the phenomena they are investigating.

The process of qualitative data analysis

Data analysis in phenomenology, grounded theory and ethnography has been described in their respective chapters. There are also 'generic' or 'thematic' qualitative data analysis. The term 'generic' refers to different types of qualitative data analysis in studies that are not based on any particular approach. In their introduction to their book *Applied Thematic Analysis*, Guest et al. (2012) suggest that good data analysis combines appropriate elements and techniques from across traditions and epistemological perspectives. According to Braun and Clarke (2006), although thematic analysis is a common practice in qualitative research, it is rarely acknowledged. They offered their own example and version of thematic analysis, which consists of the following six steps: familiarising yourself with your data, generating initial codes, searching for themes, reviewing themes, defining and naming themes, and producing the report.

The 'framework approach', developed from large-scale social policy research in the 1980s (Ritchie and Lewis, 2003), is becoming increasing popular in medical, health and nursing research (Smith and Firth, 2011; Gale et al., 2013). Gale et al. (2013) summarise the method thus:

> The Framework Method sits within a broad family of analysis methods often termed thematic analysis or qualitative content analysis. These approaches identify commonalities and differences in qualitative data, before focusing on relationships between different parts of the data, thereby seeking to draw descriptive and/or explanatory conclusions clustered around themes.

For an example of the use of the framework approach, see Ward et al. (2013). The Joanna Briggs Institute Thematic Analysis Program is another tool for 'researchers and practitioners in fields such as health, social sciences and humanities, to assist in the analysis of qualitative research data' (Joanna Briggs Institute, 2013).

Drawing from these and other frameworks, one can summarise the process of analysis of data from unstructured interviews and observations in the following three stages. To start the process of data analysis, researchers have to 'open up' or break the data into as many parts or categories as they can identify. This is followed by grouping some of these parts together into manageable themes based on their similarities. The final part of the process is to put the themes together in order to describe the 'whole'. Thus, one can say that there are three levels of analysis: basic, intermediate and higher. These levels are neither distinct nor linear. They facilitate a process that began during data collection. Researchers continually move forwards and backwards between these levels or stages, until a comprehensive understanding of the phenomenon as a 'whole' is ready to be reported.

Below is a hypothetical example to illustrate these three levels of analysis. Suppose a researcher carries out in-depth interviews about nurses' perceptions of obstacles to, and facilitators of, research utilisation in their practice. Once the transcripts are available, she reads them and begins to 'open up' the data by noting all the parts she comes across. These may include:

- Skills to appraise research
- Time to make changes to practice
- Managers' support
- Permission to introduce change
- Resources
- Funding to go to conferences
- Time to read and update
- Good leadership
- Support to attend courses
- An organisation that recognises and rewards initiative
- Autonomy to make changes
- IT skills
- Understanding of research

This list is, however, likely to be much longer. Already, by comparing these individual parts, the researcher can begin to group them. For example, 'support to attend courses' can be put together with 'funding to go to conferences'. She may decide to have a category called 'support', which has sub-categories such as support for courses, support for conferences, support to undertake a research project and so on. This exercise is repeated with other categories such as 'time', 'training', 'education' or 'attitudes to research'.

At the next level, all the categories can be further grouped into themes. For example, the researcher may find that a number of categories, such as education, training and attitudes, have something in common in that they are related to characteristics of nurses. She could label these 'personal' factors. In the same way, she may group the others into themes such as 'research', 'organisation' and 'settings'. At this level, researchers engage in intellectual activities such as identifying, defining, delineating, differentiating and comparing the categories or concepts that emerge. By this process, categories and sub-categories are formed before they are grouped into a number of themes.

At the third level of analysis, the researcher begins to explain how the themes are interrelated. For example, is one of these themes more important than the others? How does the 'organisation' create a 'setting' that encourages 'personal development'? How does leadership influence research utilisation? The researcher has to constantly read the scripts and look for relationships, links, patterns, transitions, stages, phases, preconditions or outcomes in the data. This is when a number of techniques, such as mapping, constructing networks (of relationships between concepts) or using diagrams are useful in helping researchers to keep control of the large number of categories and themes in order to make sense of the data. In presenting and discussing the findings, researchers often make selective use of direct quotes from respondents.

Codes, themes and categories

The terms 'codes', 'categories' and 'themes' are sometimes used interchangeably in the literature. Coloured highlighter pens are sometimes used to differentiate between categories, the purpose of different colours being only to group categories that have similar meanings. Numbers, colours and verbal descriptions are commonly used for coding purposes. Because a word is used as a code, it becomes a variable rather than a representation of a variable. For example, if 'support' is used as a code, it has a meaning of its own, similar to a category.

Weber (1983) describes a category as a 'group of words which have similar meanings and/or connotations'. Perhaps one should add 'group of statements' or 'phrases' as well. He describes 'theme' as a cluster of words with different meanings or connotations that, taken together, refer to some theme or issue.

Computer-assisted qualitative data analysis

Computer packages for the analysis of quantitative data are an established feature. In contrast, researchers have been slow in using qualitative data analysis software, despite their availability for almost two decades. There has recently been a noticeable increase in their use, perhaps partly because they offer more features and because there are more opportunities for acquiring the skills to use them. Wiedemann (2013) notes that social scientists have not readily embraced the new technology for qualitative data analysis:

> Since computer technology became available widespread at universities during the second half of the last century, social science and humanities researchers used it for analyzing huge amounts of textual data. Surprisingly, after 60 years of experience with computer-assisted automatic text analysis and an amazing development in information technology, this is still not a common approach in the social sciences.

The new computer-assisted qualitative data analysis (CAQDAS) software offers more possibilities to manipulate data than before, as the makers of NVivo (QSR International, 2013) claim:

> With NVivo you can deeply analyze your data using powerful search, query and visualization tools. Uncover subtle connections, add your insights and ideas as you work, rigorously justify findings, and effortlessly share your work.

A wide range of software programs has been developed over the years. These include Ethnograph, HyperQual, HyperRESEARCH, Hypersoft, QualPro, ATLAS.ti, NUD*IST and NVivo. They differ in the functions they offer, and new versions of these programs come on to the market quite regularly. The earlier packages operated more as an indexing system, while the later ones, responding to the needs of qualitative researchers, are designed to facilitate theory-building. For a discussion of the potential of NVivo in facilitating qualitative data analysis, see Welsh (2002). For a text on the use of NVivo, see Bazeley and Jackson (2013). Bergin (2011) offers some insight into the use of NVivo8. In a grounded theory study of 'psychiatric nurses' responses to clients who were sexualizing the nurse-client encounter', Higgins et al. (2009) used NUD*IST 4 to help with the analysis of their data. Lee and Jin (2013), on the other hand, made use of ATLAS.ti 5.0 in their grounded theory study of 'older Korean cancer survivors' depression and coping'.

The main advantage of using CAQDAS is that it helps researchers to manage large amounts of data, which can be indexed, coded, stored and retrieved. Manual data analysis can be overwhelming and time-consuming. The more recent software versions facilitate conceptual mapping and networking. QSR International (2013) describes what such software can do:

> With purpose built tools for classifying, sorting and arranging information, qualitative research software gives you more time to analyze your materials, identify themes, glean insight and develop meaningful conclusions.

And cannot do:

> Computers are useful for administrative functions and at arranging and sorting data. What computers can't do is think like a qualitative researcher. But the fact that computers don't think is not a limitation at all; in fact, it leaves the researcher doing what they most want to do – the thinking.

In the UK, the Economic and Social Research Council has funded the CAQDAS Networking Project (http://caqdas.soc.surrey.ac.uk/), which provides 'practical support, training and information in the use of a range of software programs which have been designed to assist qualitative data analysis'.

Ensuring rigour in data analysis

Researchers report a number of strategies that they use to ensure rigour in the analysis of qualitative data. One of their first tasks is to make sure that the transcription of audiotapes is an accurate version of what was said during the interviews. Transcribing is an arduous task and is often carried out by secretaries with little experience of research. Accents, the 'pace' of speech, tone and other speech mannerisms can all affect this process. Some transcripts contain paralanguage as well (for example, 'uums', 'aahs', pauses, half-words or silences). When transcribing and translating (in cases where the interview is in a different language from the one being used in transcription) happens at the same time, more than one translator is often required to ensure inter-translator reliability.

Expert validation is the process whereby one or more 'experts' (in the methodology and/or the subject matter) are called upon to 'verify' the findings. This is usually done by giving all the scripts to the experts and letting them analyse the data. The findings can thereafter be compared. More often, the researcher will make a sample of scripts and the themes extracted available to the expert for confirmation (or discussion thereafter in cases of different interpretations).

Expert validation has been the subject of much discussion (see, for example, Sandelowski, 1998; Cutcliffe and McKenna, 1999, 2004). The problems with expert validation relate to a number of issues including the definition of 'expert' and the different analytical processes that more experienced researchers (compared with less experienced ones) use. Additionally, researchers' decisions during data analysis are not easy to articulate as they are often made at a subconscious level (Cutcliffe and McKenna, 2004). Sandelowski (1998) questions whether experts, 'no matter how impressive their credentials', are 'in any position to certify as valid the findings in studies in which they played no part'. One of the main differences in quantitative and qualitative data analysis is that, in the latter, the process of analysis starts with the very first opportunity of data collection. This process is even more difficult to articulate and convey to others. Sandelowski (1998) concludes that 'no outsider-expert can confer the validity stamp of approval on a project, but they can provide expert criticism of a project'.

Some researchers (see, for example, Hantikainen, 2001) ask some of their participants 'to verify the interpretations made of their descriptions for validation of the findings'. This is known as 'participant validation' or 'member checking'. There are also a number of contentious issues with this practice, including the difficulties, and cost, of going back to all the participants or deciding who to sample, in case this is not possible. Disagreements between participants may not be easy to resolve. Sandelowski (1998) points out that 'participants may not understand an interpretation intended for an audience of researchers'. For some insight into the challenges and implications of the process of member checking interview, see Koelsch (2013).

Issues of rigour in qualitative research will be discussed further in the next chapter.

In this chapter, the purpose and process of quantitative and qualitative data analysis were described. In quantitative studies, descriptive and inferential statistics help researchers and readers to make sense of the data. The main measures in descriptive statistics are frequency, central tendency and dispersion. Inferential statistics help researchers to determine whether relationships exist between variables, and whether there are differences between groups.

In qualitative research, the process of data analysis is laborious and ongoing. It starts during data collection and continues after the field notes and/or tapes have been transcribed. Researchers have also developed ways of allowing others to understand their thinking processes and actions. The purpose of qualitative analysis is ultimately to gain insights into phenomena. The themes, patterns and categories generated can lead to the development of hypotheses and theories.

Summary

References

Bazeley P and Jackson K (2013) *Qualitative Data Analysis with NVIVO*, 2nd edn (Thousand Oaks, CA: Sage).

Bergin M (2011) NVivo 8 and consistency in data analysis: reflecting on the use of a qualitative data analysis program. *Nurse Researcher*, **18**, 3:6–12.

Braun V and Clarke V (2006) Using thematic analysis in psychology. *Qualitative Research in Psychology*, **3**, 2:77–101.

Carmona-Monge F J, Rollán Rodríguez G M, Quirós Herranz C, García Gómez S and Marín-Morales D (2013) Evaluation of the nursing workload through the nine equivalents for nursing manpower use scale and the nursing activities score: a prospective correlation study. *Intensive and Critical Care Nursing*, **29**, 4:228–33.

Cutcliffe J R and McKenna H P (1999) Establishing the credibility of qualitative research findings: the plot thickens. *Journal of Advanced Nursing*, **30**:374–80.

Cutcliffe J R and McKenna H P (2004) Expert qualitative researchers and the use of audit trawls. *Journal of Advanced Nursing*, **45**, 2:126–33.

DePoy E and Gitlin L N (1994) *Introduction to Research* (St Louis, MO: C V Mosby).

Fink A (1995) *How to Analyse Survey Data* (Thousand Oaks, CA: Sage).

Gale N K, Cameron E, Rashid S and Redwood S (2013) Using the framework method for the analysis of qualitative data in multi-disciplinary health research. *BMC Medical Research Methodology*, **13**:117.

Gibbs R G (2002) *Qualitative Data Analysis: Explorations with Nvivo* (Philadelphia: Open University Press).

Gudmundsdottir E, Delaney C, Thoroddsen A and Karlsson T (2004) Translation and validation of the nursing outcomes classification labels and definitions for acute care nursing in Iceland. *Journal of Advanced Nursing*, **46**, 3:292–302.

Guest G, MacQueen K M and Namey E E (2012) *Applied Thematic Analysis* (Los Angeles: Sage).

Hantikainen V (2001) Nursing staff perceptions of the behaviour of older nursing home residents and decision making on restraint use: a qualitative interpretative study. *Journal of Clinical Nursing*, **10**:246–56.

Higgins A, Barker P and Begley C M (2009) Clients with mental health problems who sexualize the nurse-client encounter: the nursing discourse. *Journal of Advanced Nursing*, **65**, 3:616–24.

Joanna Briggs Institute (2013) Thematic Analysis Program. Retrieved from http://joannabriggs.org/jbi-tap.html (accessed 15 October 2014).

Klapowitz M D (2000) Statistical analysis of sensitive topics in group and individual interviews. *Quality and Quantity*, **34**:419–31.

Koelsch L E (2013) Reconceptualizing the member check interview. *International Journal of Qualitative Methods*, **12**:168–79.

Lee H Y and Jin S W (2013) Older Korean cancer survivors' depression and coping: directions toward culturally competent interventions. *Journal of Psychosocial Oncology*, **31**, 4:357–76.

McCleary L and Brown G T (2003) Barriers to paediatric nurses' research utilization. *Journal of Advanced Nursing*, **42**, 4:364–72.

McCrum-Gardner E (2008) Which is the correct statistical test to use? *British Journal of Oral and Maxillofacial Surgery*, **46**:38–41.

Miles M B, Huberman A M and Saldaña J (2013) *Qualitative Data Analysis: A Methods Sourcebook*, 3rd edn (Thousand Oaks, CA: Sage).

Moore D S (1985) *Statistics: Concepts and Controversies*, 2nd edn (New York: W H Freedman).

Munro B H, Visintainer M A and Page E B (1986) *Statistical Methods for Health Care Research* (Philadelphia: J B Lippincott).

Plichta S B and Garzon L S (2009) *Statistics for Nursing and Allied Health*. Philadelphia: Lippincott Williams & Wilkins.

QSR International (2013) NVivo. Retrieved from http://www.qsrinternational.com/products_nvivo.aspx (accessed 6 October 2013).

Reyes H, Hadley L and Davenport D (2013) A comparative analysis of cultural competence in beginning and graduating nursing students. *ISRN Nursing*, 23 May:Art. 929764.

Ritchie J and Lewis J (eds) (2003) *Qualitative Research Practice: A Guide for Social Science Students and Researchers*. London: Sage.

Röndahl G, Innala S and Carlsson M (2004) Nurses' attitudes towards lesbians and gay men. *Journal of Advanced Nursing*, **47**, 4:386–92.

Sandelowski M (1998) The call to experts in qualitative research. *Research in Nursing and Health*, **21**:467–71.

Scott I and Mazhindu D (2005) *Statistics for Health Care Professionals: An Introduction* (London: Sage).

Smith J and Firth J (2011) Qualitative data analysis: the framework approach. *Nurse Researcher*, **18**, 2:52–62.

Tang S M and Loke A Y (2013) Smoking initiation and personal characteristics of secondary students in Hong Kong. *Journal of Advanced Nursing*, **69**, 7:1595–606.

Ussher J M, Perz J and Gilbert E (2013) Information needs associated with changes to sexual wellbeing after breast cancer. *Journal of Advanced Nursing*, **69**, 2:327–37.

Waltz C F, Strickland O L and Lenz E R (2010) *Measurement in Nursing Research and Health Research* (New York: Springer).

Ward D J, Furber C, Tierney S and Swallow V (2013) Using framework analysis in nursing research: a worked example. *Journal of Advanced Nursing*, **6**, 9:2423–31.

Weber R P (1983) Measurement models for content analysis. *Quality and Quantity*, **17**:127–49.

Welsh E (2002) Dealing with data: using NVivo in the qualitative data analysis process. *Forum: Qualitative Social Research*, **3**, 2:Art. 26.

Wiedemann G (2013) Opening up to big data: computer-assisted analysis of textual data in social sciences. *Forum: Qualitative Social Research*, **14**, 2:Art. 23.

Evaluating Research Studies

Introduction

The previous chapters have described, explained and discussed the basic concepts and the research process in qualitative and quantitative research. Issues relating to the validity and reliability of methods and findings have been extensively covered. Where appropriate, suggestions have been made on how to critique particular aspects of research studies.

This chapter provides a structure for the evaluation of research studies and a summary of the relevant questions to ask. Sources of bias and some of the common practices in the reporting of research are identified. In addition, the role of researchers in facilitating evaluation will be raised.

Critiquing skills

The terms 'critique', 'appraise' and 'evaluate' will be used interchangeably here to mean making a value judgement on what is reported. By now, readers should have the necessary knowledge and comprehension to begin to read research studies critically. In particular, they should be able to describe the aim of the research, its methodology and findings.

However, description is only the first step towards evaluation. The latter requires a judgement on the part of the reader of the actions and interpretations of the researcher. This can be done mainly by weighing what was done against accepted practice by researchers, although new and unconventional approaches should be considered on their own merit. For example, there is consensus among researchers that if, in quantitative studies, samples are not randomly selected, the findings cannot be generalised to the target population. Therefore, if a researcher states that her findings can be generalised when the sample is one of convenience, the reader can question the validity of this claim. Although individual readers may critique a study differently, the criteria they use during their evaluation must be objective. One cannot state that a literature review is inappropriate or inadequate without giving reasons to explain why. The task of critiquing is a challenging one and can only be acquired through practice.

Although nurses are expected to implement research findings in their practice, it is unsafe to base their decision on one single study, however good it is. Reviewing studies with a view to using them in practice must also be done by experienced practitioners and researchers. The Cochrane Collaboration (http://www.cochrane.org/), the Centre for Review and Dissemination (http://www.york.ac.uk/inst/crd/index.htm) and the Joanna Briggs Institute (http://joannabriggs.org/) are three of the many organisations that carry out reviews to facilitate health practitioners in using research findings.

One may question whether all nurses should possess the skills to critically appraise research studies, particularly since this requires an in-depth knowledge of a wide range of research methodologies. The answer to this question lies in the purpose of the exercise. Nurses need to have a questioning attitude and the skills to critically read the relevant literature, including research studies. Although they may not be expert in research, they should be able to know, appraise and keep up to date with what is written in their particular field of work. They should be able to distinguish between opinionated, one-sided arguments and poor research on the one hand, and well-balanced arguments or good research on the other. Guidelines for policy and practice based on evidence should be developed by experienced researchers and practitioners after a systematic review and appraisal of the literature. They may sometimes require the help of more experienced colleagues to understand or interpret what researchers report.

A structure for evaluating quantitative studies

Individuals may approach the evaluation of a study in different ways. Beginners sometimes prefer to be guided through the process. A step-by-step guide is provided here for this purpose. Only a summary of the main questions to ask is included, as the relevant chapters already have a section on critiquing; readers are strongly advised to consult these for more details. The following headings (based on the format in which quantitative studies are most often reported) provide a structure for the evaluation of research articles:

- Title of article
- Abstract
- Literature review
- Methodology
- Results
- Discussion and interpretation
- Conclusions.

Title of article

The title should draw readers' attention to the precise area of study and make reference to the population from whom data were collected. For example, the title 'Comparison of the experiences of having a sick baby in a neonatal intensive care unit among mothers with or without the right of abode in Hong Kong' (Yam and Kan, 2004) makes clear the phenomenon being investigated (experiences of mothers having a sick baby in a neonatal unit) and the population (mothers with or without right of abode). This title also suggests that the purpose of the study is to 'compare' experiences.

Too much information in the title can make it long and inelegant. For example, the title below (from Chen et al., 2013) is very informative, but some of the details could perhaps be confined to the abstract.

> Effects of adjunctive metformin on metabolic traits in nondiabetic clozapine-treated patients with schizophrenia and the effect of metformin discontinuation on body weight: a 24-week, randomized, double-blind, placebo-controlled study.

Titles can also be misleading or confusing.

Abstract

An abstract is a short summary of a study (the number of words normally being stipulated by the journal). The purpose of an abstract is to give readers enough information for them to decide whether or not the article is of interest to them. The abstract should state briefly the background and aim of the study, the design, including the method(s), sample(s) and sampling, and the main findings. This information is essential as it describes what the study is about, how it was carried out and what was found. The importance of succinct and brief summaries has increased since the advent of online databases. The information contained in abstracts helps readers to decide whether or not they should access the whole article. Readers should not ask too much from an abstract as details are provided in the rest of the article.

Literature review

Readers may want to know why the current study is important, what research, if any, has previously been carried out and what the study will contribute. The four functions of a literature review described in Chapter 7 can be used as a framework for evaluation. In particular, the following questions may be asked:

- Is a rationale provided? If so, what is it? How convincing are the reasons? Does the author support it with evidence such as research findings, statistical data and, to a lesser extent, expert opinion?
- Does the author provide a critical overview of similar research that has been carried out?
- Are the relevant concepts and issues dealt with adequately?

- Is there a conceptual framework? How does the author use it?
- Is there a reliance on primary or secondary sources? Are the references dated?
- Is it likely that there may be more recent material? Has the author been selective in her review of the literature?

The title, abstract and literature review have little bearing on the reliability and validity of the findings. Readers are advised not to spend too much time critiquing them. The methodology of the study determines the quality of the research and, as such, deserves the most attention.

At the end of the literature review, the research question(s) (or aims and objectives or hypotheses) should be clearly stated.

Methodology

Questions to ask of the methodology include:

- Are the research questions, objectives or hypotheses clearly stated?
- What is the design of the study? Is the design the most appropriate for the phenomenon under study? If, for example, the researcher uses a cross-sectional design to study the difficulties that mothers face breastfeeding in the first 6 months, is a longitudinal design more appropriate? What are the limitations of a cross-sectional design for this study (see Chapter 10)?
- Does the study use a quantitative, qualitative or mixed methods approach? Is a rationale given for the choice?
- Are the operational definitions adequate? The criteria of clarity, precision, validity, reliability and consensus (see Chapter 9) can be used for this purpose.
- What are the methods of data collection? Are any instruments (questionnaires, interviews or observation schedules) used in this study? Are they constructed for the purpose of the current study? Do they have face, content or other forms of validity? How was this achieved? Where do the items in the instruments come from?
- Is the instrument reliable? Was a test–retest or a split-half test, if appropriate, carried out (see Chapter 16)?
- Was the instrument borrowed? What are its established validity and reliability? How extensively has it been used in other similar studies?
- If the borrowed instrument has been modified for the purpose of the current study, what changes have been made? How do they affect the validity and reliability of the original instrument? What measures have been taken to ensure the validity and reliability of the modified instrument?

One important aspect of methodology that researchers sometimes omit to report in detail is the sampling method. It is not unusual to find that a random sample is used without any explanation of how the participants were selected and what the target population was. Although such terms as 'systematic', 'stratified' or 'random' have specific meanings, they are not in themselves self-explanatory. The questions to ask are:

- Who were selected? From what population were they selected? What was the precise method of selection? What implications does the sampling method have for generalisability of the findings?
- What was the response rate? What implications does the non-response rate have for the findings?

In addition to the above aspects of methodology, researchers must describe the steps taken to ensure that the rights of individuals were respected, and whether approval from an ethical committee, where appropriate, was obtained. They must also explain how access to the study population was obtained as this may have implications for the data.

Remember that the author is restricted by word limits, but if the lack of information affects your understanding of the study, it is a good indication that the information should have been provided.

Results

The method of data analysis must be described and justified. Researchers are often selective in their presentation of results. Readers should refer back to the questions or hypotheses set at the start of the study to find out whether they are addressed in the results section. Tables and figures must also make sense. The way in which some results are presented can be misleading. Stevens et al. (1993) give the following example:

> when an author writes that sixty per cent of respondents state that they drink alcohol because of stress, it must be explained that they were asked to choose from a list of reasons provided by the researcher. By not stating the format of the question, i.e. whether it was an open or a multiple-choice one, it is difficult for the reader to put the responses in context.

Beginners may find it difficult to understand statistical tests and jargon. A good journal referee should query mistakes or inconsistencies in the analysis. If you are in doubt about some of the calculations, you should, if possible, consult someone who knows about statistics. What is more important is for the author to explain what the results mean.

Discussion and interpretation

Results can be presented on their own or with discussion and interpretation. Whatever the choice of presentation, it is important that results are explained, discussed and interpreted. One of the first tasks of a critical reader is to find out if the research questions, objectives or hypotheses set at the start of the study have been addressed, and, if not, reasons should be provided. Researchers sometimes only discuss results in which they are interested and/or which support their particular views. As far as possible all results, positive or negative, should be discussed. To contribute to the pool of knowledge, results should be compared with findings from other studies, and when these are different, possible explanations should be offered.

It is not enough to report that the results are statistically significant; researchers must also explain the clinical significance of the results or identify why the results are not (perhaps on their own) clinically significant. It may be that the results of the study show that, with the new treatment, people are cured of their illness more quickly. However, their degree of discomfort with the new treatment may be greater than with the usual one.

The discussion and interpretation of data often reflect the subjective opinion of researchers. To evaluate this aspect of a study, one can ask:

- Can you follow the steps leading to the conclusions?
- Are there any gaps in the development of the arguments?
- How consistent are the arguments?
- Is the author contradicting him- or herself?
- Do the arguments make sense according to your experience?
- Does your experience lead you to see different meanings in the data?
- Overall, do you agree with the findings and/or the interpretation of the author?

Conclusions

Readers must first ask whether the conclusions are based on the research findings of the present study. Researchers are often in favour of certain policies or practices, and they peddle them in the form of recommendations even when the findings of their studies are not conclusive. The recommendations must also be practical, feasible and well thought out. In fact, researchers should be expected to discuss the limitations of their recommendations rather than simply state them.

Validity and reliability in quantitative studies

In quantitative studies, 'validity' and 'reliability' are two of the most important concepts used by researchers to evaluate the rigour with which they are carried out. These concepts have been described in previous chapters. Therefore, in evaluating these studies, readers must look for measures taken to produce valid and reliable results. These include strategies to avoid bias and to enhance objectivity.

Biases represent the greatest threat to the reliability and validity of data. To ensure rigour, researchers must avoid bias or, if this is not possible, account for it. The main sources of bias are:

- the respondents;
- the researchers;
- the methods of data collection;
- the environment;
- the phenomenon.

Respondents' motivation, perception, social class affiliation, personal and collective agendas or even communication skills (or lack of), among others, can bias the results. Similarly, researchers' own prejudices, values, beliefs or lack of research skills, and other factors, can affect the collection, analysis and presentation of data. Questionnaires may contain leading or ambiguous questions, and interview and observation schedules may not be valid or reliable. The environment can also influence the findings. Captive populations (such as patients in hospitals) may yield different data from if they were studied in their own homes. In experimental studies, data contamination can occur when subjects in the control group share information with those in the experimental group, especially when both are on the same ward. Finally, the phenomenon may not reveal itself in its usual form on days when it is studied. For example, if the researcher sets out to observe aggression among patients, it may not necessarily occur in the way it normally does while the researcher is present. These and other sources of bias are extensively discussed in this book. The few examples given above are only a reminder to readers.

In quantitative studies, the quality of the tools determines the validity and reliability of the findings, provided sources of bias are controlled. Quantitative researchers are also expected to remain detached (objective) from the respondents and the environment in which the data are collected. Therefore as long as the tools are valid and reliable, they are administered in an objective way and the data/analysis techniques are appropriate, the quality of the findings is assured. The main task of critical readers is to make a judgement on the extent to which this is achieved. The second task is to find out how 'generalisable' the findings are. This is assessed by examining the sampling technique, and the size and characteristics of the sample.

Evaluating qualitative studies

We can use the same headings as above for evaluating qualitative studies since they are commonly reported in the same way as quantitative ones. The questions to be asked about the abstract and title are also the same.

Purpose, aim or research questions

Qualitative researchers seek to 'explore' phenomena from the perspectives of the participants. They may not know what precise questions to ask in advance of the data collection. They must, however, make clear what the area of enquiry is, and what they are focusing on. Readers can, thereafter, assess whether the aim is achieved.

Literature review

There are different views about whether the literature should be reviewed before a qualitative study is carried out. This was dealt with in Chapter 7. When a qualitative study is reported in a journal, readers need to be introduced to the rationale and background of the study, in particular to the gaps that it seeks to fill. Therefore this section should demonstrate the particular contribution the study makes in terms of adding to current knowledge in that field. When a different methodology (from that in previous studies) is proposed, the rationale for its use should be stated. The author should also explain how the aim of the study evolved.

Methodology

The research process must be detailed as much as possible for readers to understand the decisions for the actions taken and the rationale on which they are based. Articles are limited in length, depending on the type of journal in which they are published. This should not be an excuse for omitting vital information, which often takes only a few words to describe.

One aspect of the methodology that is often not well described is the sampling strategy and the profile of the participants. In Webb's (2004) analysis of all papers published in the *Journal of Advanced Nursing* in 2002, she found that 'the type of sample was rarely stated'. When the sampling is described as 'purposive' and no other information provided, it is assumed that the term is self-explanatory.

Purposive sampling means that the researcher carefully selects the participants on the basis of the varied experience they may bring to the study. Readers need to know why and how particular participants were selected, and how 'varied' they were. Samples are chosen from a target population, yet in many studies there is little or no information about this. Information on samples is vital for readers to assess whether the study is relevant to their 'clinical' population. Theoretical sampling is another term that requires description and explanation (see Chapters 13 and 15).

The methods of data collection (such as interviews or observations) should be described in such a way that readers have a 'feel' of what happened. Researchers often report only the broad question they are asking, and leave readers in the dark about the interactions and the context in which the interviews or observations took place. Readers need to know what degree of control the researcher or the participants had over the interview agenda.

Readers should also look for the researcher's awareness of the ethical implications of the study and how these were dealt with.

Findings

This is often a difficult section to evaluate since qualitative researchers report their 'findings' in a variety of ways. Sandelowski and Barroso (2002), in a review of qualitative studies of women with HIV infection, found that it was difficult to find the findings. There were often 'lengthy description and many quotes, but virtually no interpretation of data'. This is similar to a quantitative researcher presenting readers with their SPSS software print-outs. Researchers in qualitative studies should go beyond the raw data and provide answers to the research questions. For readers to critically appraise the findings of a qualitative study, these must be presented clearly and succinctly. If themes are presented, readers must look for an explanation of how they were developed out of the data. Participants' experience of a phenomenon is not fragmented into themes. Therefore a good study should show the interconnections between these themes (Sandelowski and Barroso, 2002).

Discussion

The questions to ask when evaluating this section are the same as those detailed earlier for quantitative studies. This section should put the findings in the context of previous knowledge, in particular existing theories. It should explore the extent to which the findings are new.

Recommendations for policy and practice

Readers should look at the match between the findings and the recommendations. One way to do this is to examine each recommendation and look for the findings that support it. A good study should also make realistic and feasible recommendations. It is easy to say that a particular service or intervention should be made available to everyone. However, the resource and other implications should also be taken into consideration.

Increasingly, there is pressure on researchers to take the dissemination of findings more seriously. This is a requirement of funding organisations. Researchers should, therefore, be expected to suggest ways in which their findings can be used.

Ensuring rigour in qualitative studies

Researchers are still grappling with what constitutes rigour in qualitative research. As explained earlier, 'validity' and 'reliability' in quantitative studies refer to the tools of data collection and analysis. Valid and reliable findings depend on the degree of objectivity with which the tools are administered and on the extent to which sources of bias can be controlled. However, in qualitative studies, the tools of data collection are not predetermined, structured and standardised. There may not be a 'visible' tool to test for validity and reliability. There can be differences in the content and wordings from one interview or observation to another. The researcher is also an instrument of data collection and analysis.

The notion of objectivity is also redundant in qualitative studies since the researchers interact with the participants, and together they co-create the data produced. Therefore, far from attempting to remain 'detached', qualitative researchers aim to 'enter' the world of participants by getting close to them. Instead of 'controlling' the factors in the environment that may affect the results, qualitative researchers aim to find out how the context in which people live can influence their perceptions, experience or behaviour. Rejecting validity, reliability, objectivity and bias as conceptualised in quantitative studies, qualitative researchers have offered 'parallel' terms such as 'credibility', 'auditability', 'transferability', 'fittingness' and 'confirmability'. Credibility refers to the 'truth, value or believability of the findings' (Dreher, 1994). Auditability relates to the detail provided in the report to allow others 'to follow the methods and conclusions of the original researcher' (Streubert and Carpenter, 1999). Transferability or fittingness is the extent to which the findings of a qualitative study can be of use to other populations or settings similar to those in the study. Confirmability depends on participants and other 'experts' agreeing with the researcher's interpretation.

Despite the use of different terms, one can detect some notions of validity, reliability and generalisability as used in quantitative studies. To some extent, this is inevitable since researchers want their findings to reflect 'truthfully' the phenomenon they study, and to contribute to knowledge that is useful to others.

To ensure rigour, qualitative researchers have proposed a number of strategies such as the audit trail, reflexivity and validation by experts and/or participants. The term 'audit trail' was first described by Lincoln and Guba (1985), based on the work of Halpern (1983). Wolf (2003) explains the purpose of audit trail:

> Qualitative investigators use the audit trail to establish the rigor of a study by providing the details of data analysis and some of the decisions that led to the findings. The audit trail is also called the confirmability audit; it attests to the interpretations of the researcher. This record provides evidence that recorded raw data have gone through a process of analysis, reduction, and synthesis. It helps the peer reviewer or auditor to trace the textual sources of data back to the interpretations and the reverse.

Cutcliffe and McKenna (2004), after discussing the difficulties and implications of providing an audit trail, suggest that 'the absence of audit trails does not necessarily challenge the credibility of qualitative findings'. Auditing all the actions and decisions of qualitative researchers is an impossible task. However, where possible, researchers should give details and rationales for some of the key decisions taken. According to Koch (2004), 'an audit trail can be a creative way to shape the text, if signposts are offered along the way, readers can decide whether a piece of work is credible or not'. For an example of the use of audit trail, see Davies and Howell's (2012) qualitative study of 'clinical decision making in low back pain'.

There is a lot written about 'reflexivity' in the literature (see, for example, Cutcliffe, 2003; Carolan, 2004; Pellatt, 2004; Clancy, 2013). If one takes the view that the researcher's presence, characteristics (including values and beliefs) and interpretations have an effect on the participants and the environment, and vice versa, then reflexivity is the process of making this transparent. Drawing upon other authors' work, Sandelowski and Barroso (2002) describe reflexivity as:

> the ability to reflect inward toward oneself as an inquirer; outward to the cultural, historical, linguistic, political, and other forces that shape everything about inquiry; and, in between researcher and participant to the social interaction they share.

Describing the process of reflexivity can be taken too far in some studies. Researchers should tell us more about their findings than about what they learnt about themselves (Sandelowski and Barroso, 2002).

According to Cutcliffe (2003), 'there appears to be a clear perception among methodological researchers that the purpose of reflexivity, at least in part, is to enhance the credibility of the findings by accounting for researcher values, beliefs, knowledge, and biases'. Reflexivity is important as it gives researchers the opportunity to account for their influence on the research process. There are examples in the literature of researchers describing their background (such as the fact that they are nurses) or political beliefs (for example, feminism), expecting readers to read 'between the lines'. They should give examples of how their background affects the way they view phenomena, and how it helped or hindered their understanding of what was happening. Within the context of a journal article, researchers are constrained by word limits to provide meaningful reflexive accounts. Cutcliffe (2003) is sceptical about the ability of researchers to engage in reflexivity mainly because they are not always totally conscious of their cognitive processes, and because they draw on 'tacit' knowledge and intuition in their interpretation of phenomena. These processes do not lend themselves to detailed descriptions.

Newton et al. (2012) conducted a systematic critical appraisal of qualitative research into the individual's experience of chronic low back pain. They reported that they did not find a single article that provided evidence of good reflexive practice. At best, some articles offered a few lines which suggested that reflexivity had been considered, while in some articles there was simply no evidence of reflexivity (Newton et al., 2012).

With the increase in popularity of mixed methods studies, the issue of rigour in those studies needs to be considered as well. For a discussion on this topic, see Walker et al. (2013).

When reading a study, it is important to know the actions and decisions taken by the researchers and the rationale for them. It is helpful when they are self-critical and aware of the different influences on the data collected. Discussing their interpretations with participants, experts or others may help them to interpret data in unexpected ways. Thus, thus audit or decision trail, reflexivity and validation by others are indications that the study was thoughtfully carried out. They can help readers to understand the findings better than if these issues had not been explained and discussed. Ultimately, the real value of the findings of a qualitative study rests upon its contribution to knowledge and how this knowledge is used thereafter. Its credibility and usefulness should stand the test of time. No doubt, in time, the findings will be built upon, adapted or rejected.

Omission and exaggeration

There are two types of omission – deliberate and unintentional. Deliberate omission is an attempt to deceive. Most omissions, however, are not intentional. Some of the common omissions identified in the earlier chapters include sampling methods, the description of 'usual care' in control groups and the precise method of randomisation in randomised controlled trials. In qualitative studies, researchers often omit descriptions of the process of data collection, as well as the rationale for their method of sampling. Researchers are sometimes so familiar with their studies that they assume that readers also are. Jargon and specialist terminologies, when not frequently used in the literature, must be avoided or explained. The lack of information about a study may lead readers to make their own assumptions. Readers sometimes assume what the author means when the meaning is obscure. It is better to keep an open mind than to make assumptions. The assistance of colleagues, fellow students and lecturers may be helpful in clarifying ambiguities.

Researchers are also prone to exaggeration in their reporting. They often put their own 'spin' on the significance of their findings. For example, it is not unusual for one researcher to report '45 per cent of the population' as 'almost half the population' and another as 'less than half the population'.

The role of researchers in facilitating evaluation

It is the researchers' responsibility to present data clearly and in sufficient detail for others to understand how the research was carried out. Equally important are the researcher's own reflection on and evaluation of the study and its findings. Unfortunately, some researchers treat their findings as sacred and fail to be critical of them. If researchers were expected to include a section in their papers in which they attempted to falsify their own findings, readers would be better informed. In any case, researchers, as mentioned before, should be required to offer other plausible explanations for their findings. After all, it is they who know the circumstances in which the data were collected, and are therefore in a position to identify possible sources of bias and error. They are also in possession of the raw data.

While the research enterprise is about asking questions, we must realise that we cannot always find answers to them. However, in the process of enquiry, we come to learn more about ourselves and others, and about the means by which we study people. We are, therefore, the richer for it. Very often, researchers and readers learn more from the process of research than from the findings. But we must not forget that the aim of research is to provide answers to the research question.

Journal editors and referees, too, have an important part to play in making sure that articles are written and presented in a form that informs rather than confuses readers. There is perhaps a case for some referees to be given training in evaluating research; some of them are clinical experts but have little research experience.

Finally, there is much to learn when reading research studies. The task of evaluation should be approached with an open and inquiring mind. As Parahoo and Reid (1988) conclude:

> Critical reading of research helps to develop a research imagination. With practice, the individual's sense of enquiry will be heightened as his or her disposition to passive acceptance of the written and spoken word diminishes. Healthy scepticism rather than negative, cynical attitudes will transform a fault finding activity into a learning experience which can only lead to the development of research-mindedness.

Frameworks and checklists for evaluation

Beginners sometimes need some guidance on how to approach the huge task of critically appraising a study. Different authors have produced models, checklists or frameworks designed to help this process. For example, Evans and Shreve (2000) propose the ASK ('applicability, science and knowledge') model for practitioners 'to quickly review and grasp the potential clinical significance of a journal study'. Others have offered guidelines to assess particular types of studies. A number of frameworks and checklists to evaluate qualitative research have been also developed. Three popular and useful frameworks are:

- Joanna Briggs Institute Qualitative Assessment and Review Instrument (JBI QARI) (see Joanna Briggs Institute, 2011).
- Spencer et al. (2003) *Quality in Qualitative Evaluation: A Framework for Assessing Research Evidence*.
- Critical Appraisal Skills Programme (2014) 'Ten questions to help you make sense of qualitative research'.

The Critical Appraisal Skills Programme and the Joanna Briggs Institute also provide checklists for quantitative designs. Other useful articles discussing the quality of qualitative research include Hammersley (2007), Tracy (2010) and Seers and Toye (2012).

These checklists, frameworks and assessment tools can guide readers in the task of critically appraising research studies. However, training and practice in appraisal are still required.

In this chapter, the purpose of critiquing or evaluating research studies is outlined. The main aspects of quantitative and qualitative studies to look for in a review have been discussed. Issues and strategies relating to rigour have been examined. The role of researchers in facilitating evaluation has also been emphasised. Finally, references to checklists and frameworks for critical appraised have been provided.

This book, as a whole, provides the necessary knowledge and insight to enable nurses and others to read, understand and critique research studies. It is hoped that, by putting research in perspective, readers will realise the value, potential and limitations of research in contributing to the advancement of knowledge.

Summary

References

Carolan M (2004) Reflexivity: a personal journey during data collection. *Nurse Researcher*, **10**, 3:7–14.

Chen C H, Huang M C, Kao C F et al. (2013) Effects of adjunctive metformin on metabolic traits in nondiabetic clozapine-treated patients with schizophrenia and the effect of metformin discontinuation on body weight: a 24-week, randomized, double-blind, placebo-controlled study. *Journal of Clinical Psychiatry*, **74**, 5:e424–30.

Clancy M (2013) Is reflexivity the key to minimising problems of interpretation in phenomenological research? *Nurse Researcher*, **20**, 6:12–6.

Critical Appraisal Skills Programme (2014) Ten questions to help you make sense of qualitative research. Retrieved from http://www.casp-uk.net/wp-content/uploads/2011/11/CASP-Qualitative-Research-Checklist-31.05.13.pdf (accessed 14 January 2014).

Cutcliffe J R (2003) Re-considering reflexivity in the case for intellectual entrepreneurship. *Qualitative Health Research*, **13**:136–48.

Cutcliffe J R and McKenna H P (2004) Expert qualitative researchers and the use of audit trails. *Journal of Advanced Nursing*, **45**, 2:126–33.

Davies C and Howell D (2012) A qualitative study: clinical decision making in low back pain. *Physiotherapy Theory and Practice*, **28**, 2:95–107.

Dreher M (1994) Qualitative research methods from the reviewer's perspective. In: J M Morse (ed.) *Critical Issues in Qualitative Research Methods* (Thousand Oaks, CA: Sage).

Evans J C and Shreve W S (2000) The ASK model: a bare bones approach to critique of nursing research for use in practice. *Journal of Trauma Nursing*, **7**, 4:83–91.

Halpern E S (1983) Auditing naturalistic inquiries: the development and application of a model. Indiana University (USA), unpublished doctoral dissertation.

Hammersley M (2007) The issue of quality in qualitative research. *International Journal of Research and Method in Education*, **30**, 3:287–305.

Joanna Briggs Institute (2011) Reviewers' manual. Retrieved from http://joannabriggs.org/assets/docs/sumari/ReviewersManual-2011.pdf (accessed 1 February 2014).

Koch T (2004) Expert researchers and audit trails. *Journal of Advanced Nursing*, **45**, 2:134–5.

Lincoln Y S and Guba E G (1985) *Naturalistic Inquiry* (Newbury Park, CA: Sage).

Newton B J, Rothlingova Z, Gutteridge R, LeMarchand K and Raphael J H (2012) No room for reflexivity? Critical reflections following a systematic review of qualitative research. *Journal of Health Psychology*, **17**, 6:866–85.

Parahoo K and Reid N (1988) Critical reading of research. *Nursing Times*, **84**, 43:69–72.

Pellatt G (2004) Ethnography and reflexivity: emotions and feelings in fieldwork. *Nurse Researcher*, **10**, 3:28–37.

Sandelowski M and Barroso J (2002) Finding the findings in qualitative studies. *Journal of Nursing Scholarship*, **34**, 3:213–19.

Seers K and Toye F (2012) What is quality in qualitative health research? *Evidence Based Nursing*, **15**:1 .

Spencer L, Richie J, Lewis J and Dillon L (2003) *Quality in Qualitative Evaluation: A Framework for Assessing Research Evidence – A Quality Framework* (London: National Centre for Social Research).

Stevens P M J, Schade A L, Chalk B and Slevin O D'A (1993) *Understanding Research* (Edinburgh: Campion Press).

Streubert H J and Carpenter D R (1999) *Qualitative Research in Nursing: Advancing the Humanistic Imperative*, 2nd edn (Philadelphia: Lippincott).

Tracy S J (2010) Qualitative quality: eight 'big-tent' criteria for excellent qualitative research. *Qualitative Inquiry*, **16**, 10:837–51.

Walker S, Read S and Priest H (2013) Use of reflexivity in a mixed-methods study. *Nurse Researcher*, **20**, 3:38–43.

Webb C (2004) Editor's note: Analysis of papers in JAN in 2002. *Journal of Advanced Nursing*, **45**, 3:229–31.

Wolf Z R (2003) Exploring the audit trail for qualitative investigations. *Nurse Educator*, **28**, 4:175–8.

Yam B M C and Kan S (2004) Comparison of the experiences of having a sick baby in a neonatal intensive care unit among mothers with or without the right of abode in Hong Kong. *Journal of Clinical Nursing*, **3**, 1:118–19.

Evidence-based Practice

Introduction

The evidence-based practice movement that gathered momentum in the early 1990s has implications for the way in which health, social and other services are organised and delivered. In this chapter, we will trace the factors that led to its emergence worldwide. The meaning, objectives and benefits of evidence-based practice and the barriers to its implementation in nursing practice will also be explored.

Justifying practice

Suppose you are treating a wound using a particular dressing and your patient asks: 'Does it work?', 'How does it work?', 'Are there other treatments available?', 'Why did you decide that this is the best treatment for me?' Would you also know what effects this intervention has on patients or what their views are on this treatment? When did you last read about the treatment of wound care? How often do you update your knowledge regarding your practice? Is there any research study, or better still a systematic review, of treatments for this particular type of wound care? Do you have the knowledge and skills to access, select and appraise a review? Are there guidelines on the treatment of wound care from your hospital or your professional organisation? How were these guidelines developed or adapted? Are they based on research? Do you follow these guidelines? Does your organisation have a written policy on wound care? Does your clinical environment have the facilities (online access to databases and training opportunities) to enable you to access and use relevant literature in your practice?

These are some of the questions that the evidence-based practice movement have sought to stimulate. No doubt, many practitioners are aware of these issues and are well able to justify their practice on sound evidence. Many others, however, are unaware of what, and if, evidence exists on which to base their practice. They would find it hard to explain why they use particular interventions, other than that it has always been done in this way.

The evidence-based practice movement places particular emphasis on the use of evidence, in particular research findings, in clinical decision-making. It is a reaction to what was seen as an overreliance on experience and intuition, and to the lack of knowledge of the effectiveness of interventions.

Rationale for evidence-based practice

The context that gave rise to the evidence-based practice movement in the UK includes the increasing cost of healthcare, a glut of research, the variation in healthcare and unnecessary interventions.

The cost of healthcare worldwide continues to rise. In the UK alone, the net expenditure of the National Health Service (NHS) increased from over £49 billion in 2001/2002 to £104 billion in 2011/2012 (NHS Confederation, 2013). It is believed that a more efficient use of resources can help to keep down the cost of NHS spending.

Health research spending also continues to rise as well. In 1998, £435 million was spent on research and development in the NHS (Millar, 1998); this rose to nearly £1 billion in 2012 (Department of Health, 2013). Charities and drug companies, in particular, spend large amounts of money on research. The Wellcome Trust alone spends £600 million a year 'to support the brightest scientists with the best ideas' to carry out research (Wellcome Trust, 2013).

Global health research funding rose by an average US $7 billion annually from nearly US $85 billion in 1998 to US $105.9 billion in 2001. This in turn led to significantly more research and more publications. Fraser and Dunstan (2010), referring to the 'avalanche' of information, explain that 'there are now 25400 journals in science, technology and medicine and their number is increasing by 3.5% a year'. They also pointed out that these journals published 1.5 million articles in 2009 and that PubMed cites more than 20 million papers (Fraser and Dunstan, 2010). The CINAHL (Cumulative Index to Nursing and Allied Health Literature) is a database of 3,075 nursing and allied health journals (EBSCO, 2013). The question is how to harness this vast amount of knowledge in order to improve people's lives. Evidence-based practice is currently the framework that is recommended to practitioners and policy-makers to achieve this goal.

Unintended variations in clinical practice and unnecessary practices can cause harm and cost money. Although anecdotal observations point to numerous variations in practices between healthcare professionals and between hospitals, there is a lack of systematic data to gauge the extent of the problem in nursing. Creedon et al. (2008) carried out a study of the compliance of healthcare workers (nurses, student nurses, doctors, medical students, healthcare assistants, radiotherapists, porters and technicians) with hand hygiene guidelines in four hospitals in Ireland.

They reported variations in compliance rates among the healthcare staff as well as between hospitals. Doctors and medical students had the highest rate of non-compliance (41%) compared with nurses and nursing students (28% and 21%, respectively). The variation in non-compliance between hospitals varied from 24% to 44% (Creedon et al., 2008).

The term 'postcode lottery' is used to describe inequalities in access to the provision, treatment and outcome of healthcare services. Variations in the availability of cancer drugs and life expectancy in different parts of the UK are well publicised. However, these variations are not confined to any one country. For example, Graverholt et al. (2013) reported a more than nine-fold variation in annual hospitalisation rates among nursing home residents in one municipality in Norway. New et al. (2010) also reported practice variations in the transfer of premature infants from incubators to open cots between metropolitan and rural areas of Australia and New Zealand.

Some variations in clinical practice can be enduring. Lavery (1995) surveyed skin care following radiotherapy in 48 radiotherapy units in the UK. The results showed that skin care practices were highly variable and included a range of products such as talcum powder, steroids, simple creams, aloe vera and calamine (Lavery, 1995). Sixteen years later, Harris et al. (2011) carried out a survey of radiotherapy skin care in 54 radiotherapy departments and reported that 'products and their use for skin conditions varied and some outdated and unfounded practices were still being used which did not always reflect current evidence'.

Justifying one's practice on evidence and conforming to evidence-based guidelines are ways in which these unwarranted variations can be reduced. Evidence-based practice is also expected to wean out unnecessary practices and interventions such as the blanket prescription of antibiotics and unnecessary caesarean sections. The American Academy of Family Physicians recently released a list of 10 tests and procedures that both doctors and patients should carefully consider and openly discuss in order to reduce unnecessary or harmful treatments. The list includes, among others, imaging for low back pain within the first 3 weeks, the routine prescription of antibiotics for sinusitis and routine elective inductions of labour between 39 weeks and 41 weeks (American Academy of Family Physicians, 2013). Unnecessary practices may be benign or harmful; in both cases, they are costly. Systematic reviews of the effectiveness of interventions are crucial in promoting policy and practice based on evidence.

With considerable resources spent on research, it is not surprising that attention has turned to the benefits that research brings to people's lives. The World Health Organization has emphasised the importance of knowledge production leading to health gain and of estimating the economic value of health research (Pang et al., 2003). The emphasis on 'value for money' in the 1980s and 1990s has now shifted to a 'return on investment' for funding allocated to research (Parahoo, 2011). The term 'research impact' has been introduced to reflect this emphasis on the benefits that research brings, or should bring, to society. In health terms, research is expected to impact on the quality of life and general well-being of the population so that people can continue to lead healthy and productive lives.

What is evidence-based practice?

The term 'evidence-based practice' is derived from definitions of evidence-based medicine. The Evidence-Based Medicine Working Group (1992) describes evidence-based medicine as the process of de-emphasising intuition, unsystematic clinical experience and pathophysiologic rationale as sufficient grounds for clinical decision-making and stresses the examination of evidence from clinical research. Later, the McMaster University Evidence-Based Medicine Group (1996) offered this more comprehensive and workable definition:

> the collection, interpretation, and integration of valid, important and applicable patient-reported, clinician-observed, and research-derived evidence. The best available evidence, moderated by patient circumstances and preferences, is applied to improve the quality of clinical judgements and facilitate cost-effective health care.

The most quoted definition of evidence-based medicine comes from Sackett et al. (1996). It is described as:

> the conscientious, explicit and judicious use of current based evidence in making decisions about the care of individual patients. The practice of evidence based medicine means integrating individual clinical expertise with the best available external clinical evidence from systematic research.

Sackett et al. (1996) went on to add that evidence-based medicine involves the 'thoughtful identification and compassionate use of individual patients' predicaments, rights, and preferences in making clinical decisions about their care'.

Clinical decisions also takes place in the context of what is legally and ethically acceptable and financially feasible. For example, if a particular drug is the most effective one for a certain condition, it is not always possible to prescribe it if it costs more than the health service could afford. In reality, compromises sometimes have to be made. Figure 21.1 shows the components and context of evidence-based decisions (based on the above definitions).

A number of other professions have coined their own phrases, such as 'evidence-based nursing', 'evidence-based occupational therapy', 'evidence-based public health', 'evidence-based policy' or 'evidence-based dentistry'. Others have offered their own versions of evidence-based practice (Gerrish and Clayton, 1998; Goode and Piedalue, 1999; Ingersoll, 2000). 'Evidence-based practice' will be used in this chapter as a generic term to describe all decisions and actions that are based on the best available evidence, taking into account clinical expertise and patients' wishes. Where appropriate, terms such as 'evidence-based medicine' or 'evidence-based nursing' will be used to refer to the use of evidence in these professions. Evidence-based nursing will be discussed in a later section.

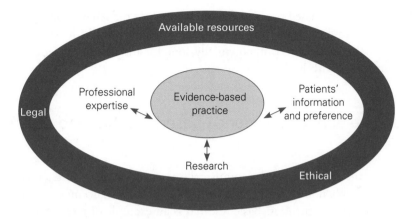

Figure 21.1 Components and context of evidence-based practice (expanded from Sackett et al., 1996)

Steps in evidence-based practice

The main steps of evidence-based practice involve the formulation of a clear question related to policy or practice, the search for relevant research studies, the appraisal of selected studies (based on their quality), the analysis and the synthesis of the findings of these studies, the dissemination of the results and the implementation of the evidence. At the heart of evidence-based practice lies the systematic review (see Chapter 7).

However, evidence-based practice is more than systematic reviews; it involves the use of evidence, clinical expertise and patients' views to make clinical decisions. The implementation of evidence can take place when a clinician looks for the evidence (often the result of a systematic review) and uses it to determine which treatment a particular patient will receive. Clinical guidelines, based on research evidence, have also been developed to facilitate the use of evidence in practice.

Objectives of evidence-based practice

The main objective of evidence-based practice is to increase awareness of the effectiveness of the decisions and actions of practitioners, educators and policy-makers. In the health service, it is designed to improve decision-making and achieve clinical effectiveness by enabling clinicians to use the most effective interventions, thereby reducing waste and eliminating unnecessary practices. With the dissemination of the best evidence to the widest imaginable audience with the use of information technology, it is expected that variations in the provision of services and in patients' outcomes will be reduced. The development and use of clinical guidelines based on evidence can also help to achieve this objective.

Finally, evidence-based practice also aims to reduce the reliance on expert knowledge and increase the transparency of decision-making. With the evidence in the public domain, lay persons can, potentially, look for and use the evidence to inform their discussions with health professionals.

Difference between evidence-based practice and research utilisation

Research is the systematic and rigorous collection and analysis of data to describe and/or explain phenomena. It aims to contribute to the advancement of knowledge, often in the form of theories. Basic research is an example of research that may or may not have direct or immediate use in clinical practice. Applied research, as the term suggests, has direct application to the area being studied as, for example, when the benefits of two clinical interventions are compared. Therefore while research can answer questions directly related to clinical practice, its scope is broader than evidence-based practice. Researchers can make recommendations, but these may or may not be implemented by clinicians.

Estabrooks et al. (2003) identified three types of research utilisation: instrumental/direct, conceptual/indirect and symbolic/persuasive. Squires et al. (2011) explain what these terms mean in the literature:

> Instrumental utilization refers to the concrete application of specific knowledge to practice; conceptual utilization refers to a change in thinking, but not necessarily behaviour, in response to research findings; and persuasive utilization refers to the use of certain knowledge to persuade others regarding a predetermined position.

When the term evidence-based practice is used, it normally means the direct use of research in one's practice. 'Knowledge transfer' is another term that is now used as a strategy to bridge the research–practice gap. The Research Councils UK (2013) describe knowledge transfer as the process through which 'knowledge and ideas move between the knowledge source to potential users of that knowledge'.

The question that is often asked is why practitioners do not use research findings. The focus is on findings. These findings may or may not have direct application to one's practice. Evidence-based practice, on the other hand, starts with a clinical question (for example, which of the two types of treatment currently in use is more effective in treating a particular condition, in certain type of patients?). The focus is, therefore, on practice-relevant questions.

The practitioner looks for available evidence (in the form of a systematic review of studies already carried out) or sets in motion the process of producing the evidence (through primary research). The findings from the review or research study are then applied to practice. Therefore evidence-based practice starts with questioning practice and ends with using the evidence in practice. If the loop is not completed, evidence-based practice does not occur. Therefore evidence-based practice and research are interdependent.

Types and levels of evidence

The evidence-based practice movement uses the following hierarchy of study designs for studies of effectiveness (Centre for Reviews and Dissemination, 2008):

1 Randomised controlled trials (RCTs)
   – Parallel group trials
   – Randomised crossover trials
   – Cluster randomised trials
2 Quasi-experimental studies
   – Non-randomised controlled studies
   – Before-and-after studies
   – Interrupted time series
3 Observational studies
   – Cohort studies
   – Case-control studies
   – Case series.

The RCT is considered the 'gold standard' in producing evidence of effectiveness. In this hierarchy, other designs or methods that do not include randomisation are perceived as producing lower forms of evidence. Although the RCT is considered by many as a useful research design to evaluate the effectiveness of clinical interventions, in particular drugs and surgery, it is considered by others as having a number of limitations. RCTs are believed not to reflect the reality of clinical situations, in that participants are carefully selected in an attempt to control confounding variables and to have a sample who can complete the study. Thus, exclusion criteria are set, and these are often used to exclude the very frail, those who cannot speak the country's language and those with multiple conditions. The findings from these 'sanitised' samples are therefore not readily generalisable to all types of patient who seek help from health professionals.

Large-scale, multi-site RCTs are often required to establish the superiority of one treatment over another. RCTs are not, however, appropriate for all types of intervention. Archie Cochrane himself was sceptical about encouraging 'widespread RCTs in the care sector' because the objectives are more difficult to define and the RCT technique was less developed in that sector (Cochrane, 1972).

According to Clemence (1998), the interactive nature of much therapy and rehabilitation is not easily measured by RCTs. Even if the treatment is the same, the input of therapists would depend on their individual interactions with their clients. Some of the behavioural and therapeutic interventions used by nurses are complex and take place over a period of time. They are not as clearly defined as some medical interventions such as drugs or surgery. Advocates of evidence-based practice acknowledge that RCTs are not appropriate for all types of interventions (Sackett et al., 1996).

Booth (2010) rejects the notion of a hierarchy or ranking of evidence because each research design has its own strength and limitations in answering questions. Instead he believes that we need to consider which types of study are more appropriate for answering different types of question. For example, if we want to develop an evidence-base guideline on assessing patients' needs following a diagnosis of myocardial infarction (MI), it is more appropriate to use evidence from qualitative studies of patients' experience following an MI. On the other hand, if we want to know the effects of an intervention on quality of life of patients following an MI, an RCT (or evidence from a systematic review of RCTs) is more appropriate.

Evidence-based nursing

Evidence-based nursing has its roots in the evidence-based medicine movement. Most nursing authors have derived their definition or description of evidence-based nursing from Sackett et al.'s (1996) definition of evidence-based medicine. For example, The Royal College of Nursing (1996), while not using the term 'evidence-based nursing', describes evidence-based healthcare as being:

> rooted in best available scientific evidence and [taking] into account patients' views of effectiveness and clinical expertise in order to promote clinically effective services. This is essential in ensuring that health care practitioners do the things that work and are acceptable to patients and do not do the things which do not work.

What is different in this definition when compared with Sackett et al.'s (1996) is that patients' views of effectiveness are given prominence.

Most nurses and allied health professionals would probably say that this is what they have been doing all the time. Nursing, in particular, claims that evidence-based practice began with Florence Nightingale, who collected statistical data to inform policy in the British military hospitals during the Crimean War (Lang, 1999). Briggs (1972), in the Report of the Committee on Nursing in the UK, called for nursing to be research-based, and the phrase not only became one of the most quoted in nursing literature, but also influenced the development of nursing research in the UK in the decades that followed.

The nature of nursing knowledge

Nursing and medical interventions differ. Doctors deal mainly with the diagnosis and treatment of patients; their responses consist mainly of drugs and surgical interventions. The needs of people cared for by nurses are varied and complex, and require both technical and humanistic responses. Many nursing interventions are, in fact, interactions between nurses, patients and their families. Giving reassurance, allaying fears and anxiety, 'preparing' patients for surgery or counselling patients on how to stop smoking involve interactions in which the use of self is an important intervention. Of course, doctors, too, listen to and counsel their patients, but these are not the core focus of medical practice. Mulhall (1998) explains that 'nursing is not merely concerned with the body, but is also in an "intimate" and ongoing relationship with the person within the body. Thus, nursing becomes concerned with 'untidy' things such as emotions and feelings, which traditional natural and social sciences have difficulty accommodating.'

Much of what nurses do with patients is about the effects that their presence, personalities and themselves have on patients. As well as expecting their symptoms to be relieved or their disease to be cured, patients want to be treated with respect and dignity. They value confidence, trust, privacy and want their rights respected. Such patients' outcomes are difficult to assess and are rarely used as measures of the effectiveness of nursing care. Closs and Cheater (1999) point out that 'there is abundant evidence demonstrating wide discrepancies between patients' and professionals' judgements about what constitutes desirable or successful outcomes'.

Mulhall (1998) argues that because of the nature of nursing, nurses rely on many different ways of knowing and many different kinds of knowledge. To assess and respond to people's emotions, feelings or anxieties requires more than scales and questionnaires. It involves the use of self and all the senses that humans possess, and it happens in ways that are often beyond human consciousness. Assessing a patient or a situation often involves not just hearing and seeing, but also smelling and touching, as well as processing all this information while 'being there' with and for the patient. Professional expertise comprises intuition, personal and professional experience, tacit knowledge and external knowledge from research and other literature. Professionals often find it difficult to identify the sources of knowledge that led to particular decisions. This is because they build up their expertise from many different clinical situations as well as acquiring knowledge from a number of sources.

Nursing research is pluralistic in its use of methodologies. In particular, qualitative research seems to be popular with nurses. Although the debates about the value of RCTs and qualitative research have sometimes been polarised, there is abundant recognition that nurses are prepared to use the most appropriate methods to study nursing phenomena. The increase in the number of publications in nursing journals of studies using a combination of methods attests to the willingness of nurse researchers to be eclectic rather than dogmatic.

Medical treatments such as drugs, surgical interventions or the use of diagnostic and screening equipment can be to some extent studied by means of RCTs. The greater the number of confounding variables, the less easy it is to control or to account for them. With RCTs, the less involvement professionals and researchers have with an intervention, the more likely it is that the results will be attributed to the intervention itself rather than to other factors. Thus, there are fewer variables to control if the treatment consists of patients taking a particular drug. On the other hand, a nursing intervention such as 'giving information to patients prior to discharge' cannot be as neatly packaged as can tablets or injections. The number of confounding variables involved in the 'information-giving' session may be difficult to control or to account for, if an RCT is carried out.

RCTs, like other research approaches, have their strengths and limitations. What some have found objectionable is the pressure for practitioners to produce their evidence though RCTs and the downgrading of other forms of knowledge and evidence. Others see evidence-based practice, with its emphasis on RCTs, as an opportunity for nurses to use the experimental design to evaluate many of their practices. However, it is important, given the variety and complexity of nursing practice involving both technical and interactional activities, that researchers do not become entrenched in their preferred positions, refuse to listen to other viewpoints and impose their views on others.

Implementing evidence-based practice

In theory, evidence-based practice seems to be straightforward and simple. What could be more simple than asking a clinical question and looking for the evidence to justify one's decision? In practice, it is far from simple because it requires skills, knowledge, the right attitudes, a supportive environment, resources and, not least, the evidence itself. Evidence-based practice involves change – from the routine and traditional to new ways to practise based on evidence. Glasziou and Haynes (2005) warned that we should 'not just be concerned with clinical content but also the processes of changing care and systems of care'. Changing practice and mind sets are very difficult to achieve, as many studies on research utilisation have shown.

There are a number of change theories that practitioners can use in their attempt to change practice. These include diffusion of innovation (Rogers, 1983), the transtheoretical model of behaviour change (Prochaska and Di Clemente, 1983), health education theory (Green et al., 1980), social influence theory (Mittman et al., 1992), social ecology theory (Stokols, 1992) and the Promoting Action on Research Implementation in Health Services (PARIHs) framework (Kitson et al., 1998; Rycroft-Malone et al., 2002). Of these, Rogers' 'theory of diffusion of innovation' and the PARIHs framework are two that have been used to implement or investigate the integration of research into practice.

Funk et al. (1991) developed a Barriers to Research Utilisation Scale, based on Rogers' work, which consisted of four components (sub-scales): the characteristics of the adopter (for example, nurses' attitudes, knowledge, motivation, etc.), the characteristics of the organisation (support, resources, etc.), the characteristics of the innovation (types of and appropriateness of evidence) and the characteristics of the communication (access to research, user friendliness and so on).

The PARIHs framework consists of similar factors that facilitate or hinder change, but puts particular emphasis on the role of change agents or facilitators. As Kitson et al. (1998) explain:

> Successful implementation (SI) is represented as a function (f) of the nature and type of evidence (E) (including research, clinical experience, patient experience, and local information), the qualities of the context (C) of implementation (including culture, leadership and evaluation), and the way the process is facilitated (F) (internal and/or external person who enables implementation processes).

Nurses' use of research

Several studies have investigated nurses' use of research in their practice. Squires et al.'s (2011) review of 55 articles showed that, in 38 articles, nurses reported moderate to high research use, and that this level of reported use has remained unchanged since the 2000s. Squires et al. were doubtful of this optimistic picture of nurses' reported use of research. According to them, the self-reported method of measuring utilisation, the lack of rigour in the methodology of these studies and nurses' conceptualisation of what constitutes research use were three factors that could have led to an overestimation of research use. Squires et al. concluded that the unchanged self-reported system of research by nurses 'is troubling' given that over 40 years have elapsed since the first studies in this review were conducted and the increasing emphasis in the past 15 years is on evidence-based practice.

Wallin et al. (2012) carried out a longitudinal survey of the perceived use of research of a prospective cohort of 1,501 newly graduated Swedish nurses over a period of 5 years. These nurses reported that they made 'instrumental' use of research more frequently than 'conceptual' and 'persuasive' use. There was an upward trend in their use of research; by year five, their instrumental use of research had reached 54 per cent, from 34 per cent in year one and two.

In a study of US nurses' state of evidence-based practice, Melnyk and Fineout-Overholt (2012) concluded that 'although nurses believe in evidence-based care, barriers remain prevalent, including resistance from colleagues, nurse leaders and managers'. When asked about 'one thing that prevents them from implementing evidence-based practice', the results were time, organisational culture, lack of evidenced-based knowledge/skills, lack of access to information/evidence and leader/manager resistance (Melnyk and Fineout-Overholt, 2012).

These findings are similar to those reported in Kajermo et al.'s (2010) review of 63 studies, carried out by researchers worldwide, using the Barriers Scale. The review concluded that the main barriers reported by nurses were related to the setting (six out of the top 10 barriers) and the presentation of the research findings. Three factors that ranked eighth, ninth and 10th among the top 10 barriers in Kajermo et al.'s review were 'the nurse is unaware of the research', 'the nurse does not feel capable of evaluating the quality of the research' and 'the nurse is isolated from knowledgeable colleagues with whom to discuss research'.

Evidence-based practice is clearly a complex issue, involving a number of factors related to the setting where it is to be implemented, the evidence and the skills, knowledge and attitudes of nurses. The overall picture of evidence-based practice in nursing shows some signs of progress but not a wholesale embrace of the policy. The comments of Burns and Foley (2005) that evidence-based practice remains a relatively new concept in nursing, despite a recognition by nurses that research evidence has a crucial role in decision-making, seem to be an apt description of the current status of evidence-based nursing.

Table 21.1 Stakeholders' roles and responsibility in promoting evidence-based practice

Front-line nurses	Managers	Healthcare organisations	Educators	Researchers	Professional organisations (e.g. nurses associations)	Government
Critically reflect on their practice	Take a leadership role in evidence-based practice	Ensure that a written strategy and action plan is developed and accessible to all staff	Educate nurses to think critically and question what they (and others) do	Carry out research to meet the needs of practitioners and policy-makers	Develop strategies for promoting evidence-based practice in their professions	Recognise that nursing (including 'bedside nursing') requires evidence to underpin its practice
Ask the right questions	Assess the resource and support needs of staff	Provide resources and facilities for staff to access evidence	Help students to develop the skill of asking relevant evidence-based practice questions	Work collaboratively (as appropriate) to identify clinical practices for which there is little or no evidence	Provide opportunities for discussing/sharing evidence-based practice issues (e.g. conferences, workshops)	Recognise that nurses need to be educated to the same level as other health professionals
Search for the evidence	Create support structures for staff	Create a research culture within the entire organisation	Educate students to acquire evidence-based practice skills (e.g. searching, appraising, implementing, evaluating)	Translate research findings into accessible and user friendly information (e.g. avoid statistical details, academic language, etc.)	Develop and disseminate relevant material to enhance evidence-based practice	Develop and implement strategies for evidence-based healthcare
Appraise the evidence	Promote a culture to encourage staff to question practice	Create reward mechanisms to celebrate achievements	Educate students to resist the pressure to conform to traditional non-evidence-based practice	Carry out systematic reviews	Advocate the need for evidence-based practice and for nurses to acquire the skills, knowledge and opportunities to use research	Provide funding and other resources to make evidence-based practice a reality
Implement/evaluate change as appropriate	Assess the barriers and facilitators to evidence-based practice in their setting		Provide students with the skills to work as autonomous practitioners within multidisciplinary teams	Involve practitioners in research activities, as appropriate and feasible		
Seek opportunities to continue to develop professionally (participation in courses, conferences, etc.)	Facilitate staff to develop their evidence-based practice skills and knowledge		Put less emphasis on teaching undergraduate students how to do research and more on how to use research and implement change			
Take part in research projects where relevant and appropriate	Learn from experience of implementing evidence-based practice and celebrate success					

Evidence-based practice: whose responsibility?

The findings from Kajermo et al. (2010), Melnyk and Fineout-Overholt (2012) and Squires et al. (2011), as well as other similar studies, show how complex and challenging the implementation of evidence-based practice is. It is clear that a number of stakeholders have key roles and direct or indirect responsibility for promoting evidence-based practice. These include front-line nurses, managers, healthcare organisations, educators, researchers, professional organisations and governments. A brief outline of these roles (based on the literature) is given in Table 21.1. Underpinning each of these roles should be a genuine commitment to evidence-based practice from all stakeholders.

In this chapter, we have traced the emergence of evidence-based practice as a movement whose objective is to revolutionise the basis on which clinical and other decisions are made. Its aim is to ensure the cost-effectiveness of health services and reduce variations in healthcare and unnecessary interventions.

The nature of nursing and nursing knowledge does not seem to fit neatly into (what is perceived as) the medical model of evidence-based practice. Nursing research draws from a range of methodologies including, but not relying solely upon, the RCT.

While there are signs of interest in using research in their practice, nurses worldwide continue to identify a number of factors that act as barriers to their use of research in their practice. The responsibility for implementing evidence-based practice lies with a number of key stakeholders. When everyone fulfils their role, evidence-based practice will move from rhetoric to reality.

Summary

References

American Academy of Family Physicians (2013). Encouraging conversations between physicians and patients to improve care. Retrieved from http://www.aafp.org/about/initiatives/choosing-wisely.html?cmpid=van 533 (accessed 26 July 2013).

Booth A (2010) Using evidence in practice. *Health Information and Libraries Journal*, **27**, 1:84–8.

Briggs A (1972) *Report of the Committee on Nursing* (Briggs Report). Cmnd 5115 (London: HMSO).

Burns H K and Foley S M (2005) Building a foundation for an evidence-based approach to practice: teaching basic concepts to undergraduate freshman students. *Journal of Professional Nursing*, **21**, 6:351–7.

Centre for Reviews and Dissemination (2008) *Systematic Reviews* (York: CRD, York University).

Clemence M L (1998) Evidence-based physiotherapy: seeking the unattainable. *British Journal of Therapy and Rehabilitation*, **5**, 5:257–60.

Closs S J and Cheater F M (1999) Evidence for nursing practice: a clarification of the issues. *Journal of Advanced Nursing*, **30**, 1:10–17.

Cochrane A L (1972) *Effectiveness and Efficiency: Random Reflections on Health Services* (London: Nuffield Provincial Hospitals Trust).

Creedon S A, Slevin B, De Souza V et al. (2008) Hand hygiene compliance: exploring variations in practice between hospitals. *Nursing Times*, **104**, 49:32–5.

Department of Health (2013) Increasing research and innovation in health and social care. Retrieved from https://www.gov.uk/government/organisations/department-of-health (accessed 24 July 2013).

EBSCO (2013) CINAHL. Retrieved from: http://www.ebscohost.com/biomedical-libraries/cinahl-plus-with-full-text (accessed 15 January 2014).

Estabrooks C A, Wallin L and Milner M (2003) Measuring knowledge utilization in health care. *International Journal of Policy Analysis and Evaluation*, 1:3–36.

Evidence-Based Medicine Working Group (1992) Evidence based medicine: a new approach to teaching the practice of medicine. *Journal of the American Medical Association*, **268**, 17:2420–5.

Fraser A G and Dunstan F D (2010) On the impossibility of being an expert. *British Medical Journal*, **341**:1314–15.

Funk S G, Champagne M T, Wiese R A and Tornquist E M (1991) Barriers to using research findings in practice: the clinician's perspective. *Applied Nursing Research*, **4**, 2:90–5.

Gerrish K and Clayton J (1998) Improving clinical effectiveness through an evidence-based approach: meeting the challenge for nursing in the United Kingdom. *Nursing Administration Quarterly*, **22**, 4:55–65.

Glasziou P and Haynes B (2005) The paths from research to improved health outcomes. *Evidence-Based Medicine*, **10**:4–7.

Goode C J and Piedalue F (1999) Evidence-based clinical practice. *Journal of Nursing Administration*, **29**, 6:15–21.

Graverholt B, Riise T, Jaintvedt C, Husebo B S and Nortvedt M W (2013) Acute hospital admissions from nursing homes: predictors of unwarranted variation. *Scandinavian Journal of Public Health*, **41**, 4:359–65.

Green L, Kreuter M and Deeds S et al. (1980) *Health Education Planning: A Diagnostic Approach* (Palo Alto, CA: Mayfield Press).

Harris R, Probst H, Beardmore C et al. (2011) Radiotherapy skin care: a survey of practice in the UK. *Radiotherapy*, **18**, 1:21–7.

Ingersoll G L (2000) Evidence-based nursing: what it is and what it isn't. *Nursing Outlook*, **48**, 4:151–2.

Kajermo K N, Boström A-M, Thompson D S et al. (2010) The BARRIERS scale – the barriers to research utilization scale: a systematic review. *Implementation Science*, **5**:32.

Kitson A, Harvey G and McCormack B (1998) Enabling the implementation of evidence based practice: a conceptual framework. *Quality in Health Care*, **7**:149–58.

Lang N M (1999) Discipline-based approaches to evidence-based practice: a view from nursing. *Journal on Quality Improvement*, **25**, 10:539–44.

Lavery B A (1995) Skin care during radiotherapy: a survey of UK practice. *Clinical Oncology*, **7**, 3:184–7.

McMaster University Evidence-Based Medicine Group (1996) Evidence based medicine: the new paradigm [online]. Retrieved from http://www.hiru.mcmaster.ca/ebm (accessed 18 November 2005).

Melnyk B M and Fineout-Overholt E (2012). The state of evidence-based practice in US nurses. *Journal of Nursing Administration*, **42**, 9:410–17.

Millar B (1998) Failing the acid test. *Health Service Journal*, 26 March: 24–7.

Mittman B S, Tonesk X and Jacobson P D (1992) Implementing clinical practice guidelines: social influence strategies and practitioner behavior change. *Quality Review Bulletin*, **18**:413–22.

Mulhall A (1998) Nursing, research, and the evidence. *Evidence-Based Nursing*, **1**, 1:4–6.

New K, Bogossian F, East C and Davies MV (2010). Practice variation in the transfer of premature infants from incubators to open cots in Australian and New Zealand neonatal nurseries: results of an electronic survey. *International Journal of Nursing Studies*, **47**, 6: 678–87.

NHS Confederation (2013) Key statistics on the NHS. Retrieved from http://www.nhsconfed.org/priorities/political-engagement/Pages/NHS-statistics.aspx#funding (accessed 24 July 2013).

Pang T, Sadana R, Hanney S, Bhutta Z, Huder A and Simon J (2003) Knowledge for better health – a conceptual framework and foundation for health research systems. *Bulletin of the World Health Organization*, **81**:815–20.

Parahoo K (2011) Review: ways of assessing the economic value or impact of research: is it a step too far for nursing research? *Journal of Research in Nursing*, **16**, 2:167–8.

Prochaska J O and DiClemente C C (1983) Stages and processes of self-change of smoking: toward an integrative model of change. *Journal of Consultative Clinical Psychology*, **51**:390–5.

Research Councils UK (2003) Excellence with impact. Retrieved from http://www.rcuk.ac.uk/kei/ktportal/pages/home.aspx (accessed 26 July 2013).

Rogers E (1983) *Diffusion of Innovations* (New York: Free Press/Macmillan).

Royal College of Nursing (1996) *The RCN Clinical Effectiveness Initiative: A Strategic Framework* (London: Royal College of Nursing).

Rycroft-Malone J, Kitson A, Harvey G et al. (2002) Ingredients for change: revisiting a conceptual framework. *Quality and Safety in Health Care*, **11**:174–80.

Sackett D L, Rosenberg W M C, Muir Gray J A, Haynes R B and Richardson W S (1996) Evidence based medicine: what it is and what it isn't. *British Medical Journal*, **312**:71–2.

Squires J E, Hutchinson A M, Bostrom A-M, O'Rourke H M, Cobban S J and Estabrooks C A (2011) To what extent do nurses use research in clinical practice? A systematic review. *Implementation Science*, **6**:21.

Stokols D (1992) Establishing and maintaining health environments: toward a social ecology of health promotion. *American Psychology*, **47**:6–22.

Wallin L, Gustavsson P, Ehrenberg A and Rudman A (2012) A modest start, but a steady rise in research use: a longitudinal study of nurses during the first five years in professional life. *Implementation Science*, **7**: 19.

Wellcome Trust (2013) Global health: making a difference around the world. London: Wellcome Trust.

Glossary

abstract A brief summary usually found at the beginning of an article. It states briefly the aim of the study, the design – including the method(s), sample(s) and sampling – and the main relevant findings.

accidental sample A sample of convenience in which only those units which are available have a chance of being selected.

action research Action research involves using research in order to plan, implement and evaluate change in practice.

alternate-form test The alternate-form reliability test (also known as equivalence) is carried out by asking questions in different forms and comparing the data.

anonymity In research, the term is used to describe circumstances when respondents remain unknown to the researcher. This happens mainly when questionnaires are filled and posted by respondents without revealing their names.

attrition The loss of participants to a study due to mortality or to withdrawal for other reasons such as refusals, being too ill to continue or having moved away.

audit trail The process used by qualitative researchers to track and record their crucial decisions and actions that could have influenced the collection of the data and the interpretation of the findings.

axial coding In grounded theory, the term refers to the search for relationships between codes and themes to start to make sense of what is happening in the data. During this coding phase, researchers explore the contexts, causal and intervening conditions and consequences of social processes.

baseline The time or point (normally at the start of a study) at which measurements are taken so that they can be compared with other measurements taken subsequently.

bias Factors, other than those investigated, that may influence a study's findings.

bracketing The suspension of the researcher's preconceptions, prejudices and beliefs so that they do not interfere with or influence her description and interpretation of the respondent's experience.

case study Case studies focus on specific populations (usually small) and events that are bounded by time and well defined. In-depth information can be collected by using a variety of methods.

central tendency Refers to 'average' or 'typical' scores, not extreme ones. The statistical measures of central tendency are the mode, median and mean.

clinical effectiveness The most efficient and cost-effective way to assess, organise, deliver and evaluate care and treatment in order to achieve optimum benefit for clients.

cluster random sample A cluster or multistage random sample involves sampling the clusters before drawing samples from the selected clusters.

cluster randomisation The random allocation of clusters (for example, hospitals or schools) instead of individuals to the control or experimental groups.

coding The process of breaking up the data into segments to make sense of them.

comparative studies The purpose of a comparative study is to compare policies, practices, events and people.

conceptual/theoretical framework The use of concepts and/or theories to underpin a study.

confidentiality Refers to the assurance given by researchers that data collected from participants will not be revealed to others who are not connected with the study.

confirmability A strategy in qualitative research to ensure that participants recognise the findings as reflecting their responses.

confounders Variables that can work with or against the independent variable to produce an outcome in an experiment. It is sometimes difficult to separate the effects of each of these variables on the outcome.

constant comparison The process of comparing and contrasting responses from the same participant and between participants in the same study. It is also about comparing the emerging concepts or theories with similar ones in other situations or disciplines.

construct validity Refers to the extent to which the questionnaire or scale reflects the construct that is being assessed or measured.

constructivism A qualitative approach based on the belief that meanings are constructed through the interaction of researchers and participants.

content validity The degree to which the questions or items in a questionnaire or observation schedule can adequately study or measure the phenomenon being researched.

control To account for the effect of unwanted variables, researchers introduce control into their experiments by making sure that another group (the control group), similar in all respects (except for the intervention) to the experimental group, takes part in the experiment. Control is also exercised by the objective allocation of subjects to groups.

core category In grounded theory, this term refers to the overarching social process that captures the essence of what is happening in the way participants attempt to resolve what they are undertaking.

correlation The statistical association between two or more variables.

covert observation A form of participant observation in which researchers do not divulge that they are making observations for research purposes and 'participants' are not aware they are being observed as part of a research study. Covert observation has serious ethical implications.

credibility The extent to which the findings of a study reflect the experience and perceptions of those who provided the data. The findings must also be credible to those who subsequently read the report.

criterion-related, concurrent and predictive validity A questionnaire's criterion-related validity can be assessed by comparing the data collected with data from other sources. When other such data are currently available, the concurrent validity of the questionnaire can thus be assessed. Predictive validity refers to data that may be available in the future and may confirm the validity of the data from the present questionnaire.

culture The process that binds members of a group together, sets the rules for how they should behave, defines their roles within the group and distinguishes them from others outside the group.

data The information collected by researchers during the course of a study.

database A register of published materials, mostly in terms of articles, books, reports and audiovisual material.

deduction The process of knowledge acquisition by the formulation of a theory or hypothesis and the collection of data thereafter in order to support or reject it.

Delphi technique A form of survey that consists of gathering the views of experts, normally individually, on a particular issue. It involves a number of rounds during which feedback is provided to the respondents to allow them to reconsider their initial opinion, if necessary, for the purpose of reaching a consensus.

descriptive and correlational studies In descriptive studies, researchers describe phenomena about which little is normally known. From the data collected, patterns or trends may emerge and possible links between variables can be observed, but the emphasis is on the description of phenomena. In correlational studies, the primary aim is to examine or explore relationships between variables.

descriptive statistics This type of statistics answers descriptive questions and does so by such measures as frequency, central tendency and dispersion.

determinism The belief that phenomena have causes and effects and that experiments can find the answer to them.

discourse analysis An approach based on the analysis of discourse (verbal, non-verbal and written communication). The purpose of this type of analysis is to uncover the values, meanings and intentions in interactions between people.

dispersion Measures of dispersion such as standard deviation, variance, range and quartiles are used to describe how scores vary.

dissemination The communication of research findings in a range of formats including published papers, conference presentations, reports and seminars.

eidetic reduction The process of reducing experiences to what is absolutely necessary to describe the phenomenon. By this process, the 'essence' of a phenomenon is revealed.

emergence The process of allowing ideas, concepts or theories to come out of data collected from participants. Reliance on emergence is the fundamental principle that underpins the grounded theory method.

emic An ethnographic term to describe the insiders' (group members) perspectives.

ethics The moral principles providing the framework for conducting research studies.

ethnography A research approach developed by anthropologists who go and live among the people they study. Ethnographers study human behaviour as it is influenced or mediated by the culture in which it takes place.

etic An ethnographic term to describe the outsiders' (mainly researchers) perspectives.

evaluative studies An evaluative study is normally carried out when a researcher wants to find out if, how and to what extent the objectives of particular activities, policies or practices have been or are being met.

evidence-based practice Practice based on the most valid and reliable research findings, the judgement and experience of practitioners and the views of clients.

explanatory trials An experimental design that is used to study the efficacy of interventions, in ideal circumstances, in order to gain a scientific understanding of interventions and their effects.

face validity Face validity is one form of content validity. It involves giving the questionnaire to anyone, not necessarily an expert on the subject, who can 'on the face of it' assess whether the questions or items reflect the phenomenon being studied.

factorial design A design (either a survey or a trial) in which the effect of one or more independent variables can be tested in the same study.

feminist research Research carried out by women for women and on topics of relevance to women.

fittingness The degree to which the findings of qualitative studies 'fit' the reality of those who wish to use them.

focus groups A research method in which groups of participants take part in interviews or conversations with one or more researchers in order to provide data.

focused group interview This can be described as interactions between one or more researchers and more than one respondent for the purpose of collecting data on a specific topic.

frequency This involves describing scores in absolute numbers, percentages and proportion.

generalisability The extent to which the findings from a study can be applied to similar populations and settings elsewhere.

grounded theory This term was coined by Glaser and Strauss (1967) to mean an inductive approach to research whereby hypotheses and theories emerge out of, or are 'grounded' in, data.

Heiddegerian phenomenology The philosophy of Martin Heiddeger which explains that the key to understanding how we experience phenomena is to understand our own existence in the world. By 'being with' each other, participants and researchers bring their own subjective interpretations into the encounter, and together they co-create knowledge.

hermeneutics The science of the interpretation of texts. In an interview situation, the dialogues between participants and researchers, when transcribed, become contemporary texts that can be interpreted in the same way that scholars interpret classical texts.

Husserlian phenomenology The philosophy of Edmund Husserl to underpin the 'scientific study of consciousness'. Husserlian phenomenology has three key features: intentionality, phenomenological reduction and eidetic reduction.

hypothesis A statement that normally specifies the relationship between variables.

hypothetico-deductive An approach whereby hypotheses and theories are put to the test by the deductive process (see *deduction* above) during the course of research, especially experiments.

induction This means that after a large number of observations have been made, it is possible to draw conclusions or theorise about particular phenomena.

inferential statistics Inferential statistics describe correlational or casual links between variables.

informed consent The process of agreeing to take part in a study based on access to all relevant and easily digestible information about what participation means, in particular in terms of harms and benefits.

intentionality The act of consciously experiencing a phenomenon.

internal and external validity of experiments Internal validity is the extent to which changes, if any, in the dependent variable can be said to have been caused by the independent variable alone. External validity is the extent to which the findings of an experiment can be applied or generalised to other similar populations or settings.

interpretivism The belief that people continuously make sense of the world around them, and different people may have different interpretations of the same phenomena. Interpretivism is a blanket term for a collection of approaches broadly called 'qualitative' that share an opposition to the notion of logical positivists (see *positivism* below) that humans should be studied as objects or particles.

interval scale In this, the numbers allocated to variables signify the order or hierarchy of the variables and indicate the precise distance between them.

intervention/manipulation The term 'intervention' is used in an experiment to describe the independent variable whose effect the researcher is trying to assess or measure. Examples of interventions include medications, information programmes and therapies. By giving different medications (or the same medication in varying amounts) to different groups, the researcher is in fact manipulating the intervention, hence the term 'manipulation'.

intra- and inter-observer reliability Intra-observer reliability is the consistency with which the same observer records the same behaviours in the same way on different occasions. Inter-observer reliability is the consistency with which two or more observers record the same behaviours in the same way on different occasions.

intuition A form of knowing and behaving not apparently based on rational reasoning.

key informants In ethnographic studies, a term to describe the main person or persons who can provide insights into the group's behaviour and can help the researcher to gain access to others, events or activities.

longitudinal and cross-sectional studies A longitudinal study is one in which data are collected at intervals in order to capture any change that may take place over time. The same sample (cohort) is usually 'followed up' over a period of time. In cross-sectional studies, data are collected from different groups of people who are at different stages in their experience of the same phenomenon.

matched pairs Matched-pairs allocation takes place when researchers try to pair a subject in the experiment with another in the control group in terms of characteristics such as age, gender, illness condition and so on. Researchers usually enter a subject into one of the two groups and allocate someone else with similar characteristics to the other group.

mean The arithmetical average of a set of values.

median The midpoint value when the scores are arranged in ascending order.

meta-analysis A form of research on research. In its pure form, it involves the statistical analysis of research findings of similar studes in order to arrive at one final finding.

mixed method The use of different methods to answer research questions in the same study.

mode The most frequent value.

molar and molecular These are observation units or categories. Molar units are broad and sometimes abstract. Molecular units are more detailed and precise.

nominal group technique A structured meeting (led by a researcher or facilitator) designed to seek the views of a group of participants on a particular topic and to seek a consensus or agreement by asking them to rank or rate their responses.

nominal scale In a nominal scale, the numbers allocated to variables have no value and are only used to label them.

non-respondents All those included in a survey who do not return the questionnaire or do not answer some questions on the questionnaire.

normal distribution In a normal distribution of scores, most of the scores cluster around the mean; the extreme scores are few and are (more or less) equally distributed above or below the mean.

null hypothesis The hypothesis that is tested in experimental research. It is stated in a format suggesting that no correlation (or link) exists between two or more variables. Data are collected in order to reject or confirm the hypothesis.

nursing research All research that pertains to the organisation, delivery, uses and outcomes of nursing care. It therefore includes research on clients, nurses, resources and nursing practice.

objectivity This term is used in research approaches in which researchers remain detached from respondents by not letting their subjective views influence the data they collect and analyse.

observer's effect 'Observer's effect', 'reactivity' and 'Hawthorne effect' are terms used to describe changes in the participants' 'usual' or 'normal' behaviour as a reaction to being observed for research purposes.

open coding In this coding stage, the researcher carries out line-by-line and sentence-by-sentence analysis, and many codes, their properties and dimensions are constructed.

operational definition The process of communicating precisely the meaning of concepts and the ways in which they can be observed and recorded.

ordinal scale In an ordinal scale, the numbers allocated to variables signify the order or hierarchy of these variables, but cannot specify the exact difference between them.

paradigm A research paradigm can be described as the beliefs and values that particular research communities share about the types of phenomena that can or cannot be researched and the methodologies to be adopted.

Pearson product moment correlation coefficient A statistical test to measure the association between interval-ratio variables.

phenomenological reduction The process of 'bracketing' or 'suspending' previous knowledge of the experience in order to reveal what the phenomenon really means for us, not how we are expected to experience it.

phenomenology A philosophical theory about the way humans experience consciousness. The phenomenological approach focuses on individuals' interpretations of their lived experiences and the ways in which they express them.

placebo A substance of no pharmacological or therapeutic property that resembles, in all its physical characteristics, the intervention used in the experimental group. Placebos are used in experiments to overcome the possible suggestive effect of new interventions.

population The units (people, events, objects or institutions) from which data are collected.

positivism A movement in the social sciences that evolved in the eighteenth century as a critique of the supernatural and metaphysical interpretations of phenomena. It is based on the belief that the methods of the natural sciences can be used to study human behaviour as well. It is the belief that only what can be observed by the human senses can be called facts. Logical positivism is one branch of positivism that makes use of mathematics in the interpretation of research findings.

postmodernism An intellectual movement (from towards the end of the 1950s) that rejects the notion of 'truth' and 'reality' as objective, and rationalism as the only way to think. Postmodernists believe that knowledge is co-created (by participants and researchers).

primary and secondary sources Original publications are primary sources, while publications that report, quote from or comment on original works are known as secondary sources.

probability and non-probability samples With probability samples, every unit in the sample frame has a more than zero chance (known in advance) of being selected. Non-probability samples are made up of units whose chances of selection are not known.

prospective, retrospective and historical studies A prospective study is one in which the researcher investigates a current phenomenon by seeking data that are to be collected in the future. A retrospective study relies on information from the past in order to understand a current problem. Both prospective and retrospective studies have a 'foot' in the present. A historical study does not need to have a link with the present. It seeks to understand phenomena embedded in the past.

purposive or judgemental sample This involves making a judgement or relying on the judgement of others in selecting a sample. Researchers use their knowledge of potential participants to recruit them. The purpose of this type of sampling is to obtain as many perspectives of the phenomenon as possible.

qualitative interview A broad term to denote a family of interviews with varying degrees of flexibility for the purpose of studying phenomena from the perspective of the respondents.

qualitative research A research approach that aims to explore phenomena from people's perspectives through the use of inductive, interactive and flexible methods.

quantitative research A research approach that relies on the measurement of phenomena. The tools used in quantitative research are predetermined, structured and standardised.

quasi-experiment Such an experiment does not meet all three components of a true experiment, but it must have an intervention. A quasi-experiment may or may not have a control group – and if it does, it does not have randomisation.

quota sample When different groups of people take part in a study, the researcher allocates the number in each group beforehand and then uses non-probability sampling methods to select the units.

random sampling A probability sampling technique to select representative samples from target populations.

randomisation The process of allocating subjects to experimental and control groups by an objective method.

randomised controlled trial These are true experiments that are normally carried out in clinical practice.

range The lowest and highest value. It is sometimes expressed as the difference between these two values.

ratio scale An interval scale with an absolute zero. The numbers on a ratio scale tell us not only the amount by which they differ but also by how many times.

reductionism This means reducing complex phenomena to simple units that can be observed or recorded.

reflexivity The continuous process of reflection by researchers on how their own values, perceptions, behaviour or presence and those of the respondents can affect the data they collect.

replication This refers to the process of repeating the same study in the same or similar settings using the same method(s) with the same or equivalent sample(s).

research The study of phenomena by a rigorous and systematic collection and analysis of data. It is a private enterprise made public for the purpose of exposing it to the scrutiny of others, to allow for replication, verification or falsification, where possible.

research awareness This term has three main components: the adoption of a questioning stance to one's practice, a knowledge of existing research and the ability to use it.

research-based practice A term to denote the use of research to inform and justify one's practice.

research design A plan of how, when and where data are to be collected and analysed.

research questions Research involves asking questions. The term 'research question' is used mainly to describe the broad question that is set at the start of a study. Some researchers may prefer to state aims, objectives or hypotheses instead.

response rate The proportion of people who actually complete questionnaires or take part in interviews from those who were asked to take part in a study. It is usually expressed in percentage terms.

rigour The decisions and actions taken by researchers to ensure that their studies are carried out thoroughly and carefully in order to be of the highest quality.

sample and population A proportion or subset of the population is known as a sample. A population can be defined as the total number of units (such as individuals, organisations, events or artefacts) from which data can potentially be collected.

sample frame A list of all the units of the target population from which random samples are normally drawn.

semi-quartile, lower quartile and upper quartile The semi-quartile ranges are scores that fall below and above the median. The lower quartile is the midpoint between the lowest value and the median. The upper quartile is the midpoint between the highest value and the median.

semi-structured interview In this type of interview, respondents are all asked the questions from a predetermined list, but there is flexibility in the phrasing and sequence of the questions.

simple random sample Each unit in the sample frame has an equal chance of selection.

single-blind and double-blind trials A single-blind trial is when either the subjects or researchers are unaware which group is control or experimental. A design in which both subjects and researchers are unaware of which intervention each group is receiving is called a double-blind trial.

snowball sample In this type of sampling, the first respondent refers someone they know to the study, who in turn refers someone they know until the researcher has an adequate sample.

social processes The interactive processes that human beings use in their daily activities such as making decisions, seeking information, taking control of situations or recovering from illness. These processes are dynamic and take place in a social context.

split-half test This test (of reliability) involves dividing or splitting the instrument (normally a scale) into two equal halves and finding out if their scores are similar.

standard deviation An average deviation of the scores from the mean.

stratified random sample A stratified random sample is drawn by separating the units in the sample frame into strata (layers), according to the variables the researcher believes are important for inclusion in the sample, before drawing simple random samples from each stratum.

structured interview In this type of interview, researchers ask all the questions as they are formulated on an interview schedule. They have some flexibility to rephrase the question but cannot alter the content or sequence of the questions.

structured observation A structured observation is one in which aspects of the phenomenon to be observed are decided in advance (predetermined), a schedule or checklist is constructed (structured) and the same information is required of all observations (standardised).

survey A a research design that aims to obtain descriptive and correlational data usually from large populations, and usually by questionnaires interviews and to a lesser extent by observations.

systematic random sample A systematic random sample is drawn by choosing units on a list at intervals decided by the researcher in advance. Every unit on the list has an equal chance of selection.

systematic review This is one form of literature review in which all the available research studies on a particular topic are identified, analysed and synthesised.

target population The target or study population is the population that meets the criteria for inclusion that have been stipulated by the researcher.

test–retest Test–retest involves administering the questionnaire to the same respondents on two or more occasions and comparing their responses for the purpose of assessing the reliability of the questionnaire.

theoretical sampling A grounded theory technique to explore new avenues and test the emerging theory. It means that researchers can interview or observe 'new' participants (or carry out more interviews with the same participants) in order to follow the leads to where the emerging theory is taking them.

theory In its basic form, a theory is an explanation of how and why a phenomenon occurs. Scientific theories are more precise in that they specify relationships between variables.

theory-generating research The aim of this type of theory is to generate hypotheses and/or theories. Researchers identify themes, patterns or relationships from the data collected.

theory-testing research The aim of this type of research is to test particular hypotheses and/or theories. Researchers set hypotheses (often derived from theories) and collect data to confirm, modify or reject them.

thick description A process in ethnographic research of describing, in relevant details, events, activities or behaviour in order to make readers 'feel' as if they were there.

time and event sampling These types of sampling are used mostly in studies that use observation. In time sampling, the sampling unit is time instead of people. Researchers may decide to sample the first 15 minutes of every hour of the day instead of observing the whole day. When 'events' are the focus of a study, the events become the units from which a sample is drawn.

transferability A qualitative term similar to 'generalisability' to denote the applicability of the findings to other similar situations.

triangulation The use of more than one method to answer exactly the same research question.

true experiment In research terms, a true experiment is characterised by three components: intervention (manipulation), control and randomisation.

validity and reliability Validity refers to the degree or extent to which a questionnaire, interview or observation schedule and other methods of data collection study or measure the phenomenon under investigation. Reliability refers to the consistency of a particular method in measuring or observing the same phenomena.

variables, dependent and independent Anything that varies can be called a variable. Variables can be dependent or independent. In the statement 'lack of exercise causes constipation', the independent variable is 'lack of exercise' and the dependent variable is 'constipation'. It is the relationship between variables, and not the variables themselves, that determines whether they are dependent or independent. In the statement 'the degree of constipation determines one's level of well-being', constipation is the independent variable.

variables, extraneous and confounding Extraneous variables are those which researchers are aware of at the start of the study but do not seek to study. They need to be controlled so that they do not interfere with the experiment. Confounding variables are extraneous variables that researchers fail to or cannot control but that may work in the same or opposite direction to the independent variable. The two terms are sometimes used interchangeably.

volunteer sample A sample of convenience over which the researcher has little control but is instead dependent on the sample volunteering to take part.

within-subject and between-subject designs When the same group of subjects receive the usual intervention and the experimental intervention alternately, the design is described as within-subject or crossover. A between-subject (or parallel groups) design is one in which different subjects constitute the control and experimental groups.

Index